CAROTID ARTERY STENTING: CURRENT PRACTICE AND TECHNIQUES

CAROTID ARTERY STENTING: CURRENT PRACTICE AND TECHNIQUES

Editors

NADIM AL-MUBARAK, M.D.
Director
Interventional Cardiology
Fairview General Hospital
Cleveland Clinic Health System
Cleveland, Ohio

GARY S. ROUBIN, M.D., Ph.D.
Director
Endovascular Services
Lenox Hill Heart and Vascular Institute
New York, New York

SRIRAM S. IYER, M.D.
Clinical Associate Professor of Medicine
New York University School of Medicine
New York, New York

JIRI J. VITEK, M.D., Ph.D.
Department of Radiology
Lenox Hill Heart and Vascular Institute
New York, New York

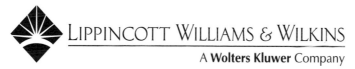

LIPPINCOTT WILLIAMS & WILKINS
A **Wolters Kluwer** Company

Philadelphia • Baltimore • New York • London
Buenos Aires • Hong Kong • Sydney • Tokyo

Acquisition Editor: Ruth W. Weinberg
Developmental Editor: Joanne Bersin
Production Editor: Emily Lerman
Manufacturing Manager: Benjamin Rivera
Cover Designer: David Levy
Compositor: Maryland Composition, Inc.
Printer: Quebecor World-Kingsport

© 2004 by LIPPINCOTT WILLIAMS & WILKINS
530 Walnut Street
Philadelphia, PA 19106 USA
LWW.com

Printed in the USA

Library of Congress Cataloging-in-Publication Data

Carotid artery stenting : current practice and techniques / editors, Nadim Al-Mubarak ... [et al].
   p. ; cm.
   Includes index.
   ISBN 0-7817-4385-0
1. Carotid artery—Surgery. 2. Stents (Surgery) I. Al-Mubarak, Nadim.
   [DNLM: 1. Carotid Stenosis. 2. Carotid Artery Diseases—therapy. 3. Embolization, Therapeutic—methods. WL 355 C2928 2004]
   RD598.6.C37 2004
   617.4′13—dc22

                                    2004007839

Care has been taken to confirm the accuracy of the information presented and to describe generally accepted practices. However, the author, editors, and publisher are not responsible for errors or omissions or for any consequences from application of the information in this book and make no warranty, expressed or implied, with respect to the currency, completeness, or accuracy of the contents of the publication. Application of this information in a particular situation remains the professional responsibility of the practitioner.

The authors, editors, and publisher have exerted every effort to ensure that drug selection and dosage set forth in this text are in accordance with current recommendations and practice at the time of publication. However, in view of ongoing research, changes in government regulations, and the constant flow of information relating to drug therapy and drug reactions, the reader is urged to check the package insert for each drug for any change in indications and dosage and for added warnings and precautions. This is particularly important when the recommended agent is a new or infrequently employed drug.

Some drugs and medical devices presented in this publication have Food and Drug Administration (FDA) clearance for limited use in restricted research settings. It is the responsibility of the health care provider to ascertain the FDA status of each drug or device planned for use in their clinical practice.

10 9 8 7 6 5 4 3 2 1

CONTENTS

Section III: FUTURE DIRECTIONS 291

CONTRIBUTING AUTHORS

Nadim Al-Mubarak, M.D.
Director, Interventional Cardiology
Fairview General Hospital
Cleveland Clinic Health System
Cleveland, Ohio

Mark C. Bates, M.D., F.A.C.C., F.S.C.A
Clinical Professor, Medicine and Surgery
Robert C. Byrd Health Sciences Center
Charleston, West Virginia

José Biller, M.D., F.A.H.A., F.A.C.P.
Professor of Neurology and Neurological
    Surgery
Department of Neurology
Loyola University
Maywood, Illinois

Christina M. Brennan, M.D.
Manager, Department of Endovascular
    Research
Lenox Hill Hospital
New York, New York

**Trevor J. Cleveland, M.B.B.S., F.R.C.S.,
F.R.C.R.**
Sheffield Vascular Institute
Northern General Hospital
Sheffield, United Kingdom

Antonio Colombo, M.D.
Chief Cardiac Catheterization Laboratory
    and Interventional Cardiology
Universita Vita-Salute San Raffaele
Milan, Italy

Edward B. Diethrich, M.D.
Medical Director, Arizona Heart Institute
    and Arizona Heart Hospital
Phoenix, Arizona

**Peter A. Gaines, M.B.B.S., F.R.C.S,
F.R.C.R.**
Freeman Hospital
Newcastle, United Kingdom

Randall T. Higashida, M.D.
Clinical Professor of Radiology and
    Neurological Surgery
Chief, Division of Interventional
    Neurovascular Radiology
University of California at
San Francisco Medical Center
San Francisco, CA

Isabelle Henry
ILRMDT
Nancy, France

**Michel Henry, M.D., F.A.C.A.,
    F.A.H.A., F.A.S.A.**
Interventional Cardiologist
Nancy, France

Robert W. Hobson II, M.D.
Professor of Surgery
Program Director in Vascular Surgery
UMDNJ-New Jersey Medical School
Newark, New Jersey

George Howard, Dr.PH
Professor and Chairman, Department of
    Biostatistics
University of Alabama at Birmingham
Birmingham, Alabama

Virginia J. Howard, M.S.P.H.
Assistant Professor, Department of
    Epidemiology
University of Alabama at Birmingham
Birmingham, Alabama

Michèle Hugel
ILRMDT
Nancy, France

Sriram S. Iyer, M.D.
Director, Endovascular Medicine
The Lenox Hill Heart and Vascular
    Institute
New York, NY

Pallavi Kumar, M.S.
Research Coordinator, Department of
  Endovascular Research
Lenox Hill Hospital
New York, New York

Brajesh K. Lal, M.D.
Assistant Professor of Surgery
Division of Vascular Surgery
UMDNJ-New Jersey Medical School
Newark, New Jersey

Francesco Liistro, M.D.
Consultant Cardiologist
Emodinamica
San Raffaele Hospital
Milan, Italy

Alfredo M. Lopez-Yuñez, M.D.
Department of Neurology
Indiana University School of Medicine
Indianapolis, Indiana

**Sumaira Macdonald, M.B.Ch.B.(Comm),
  M.R.C.P., F.R.C.R.**
Freeman Hospital
Consultant Vascular Radiologist
Newcastle, United Kingdom

Klaus Mathias, M.D.
Department of Radiology
Academic Teaching Hospital;
Department of Radiology
Klinikum Dortmund
Dortmund, Germany

Philip M. Meyers, M.D.
Assistant Professor, Departments of
  Radiology and Neurological Surgery
Columbia University
New York, New York

J. P. Mohr, M.D.
Sciarra Professor of Neurology
New York Presbyterian Hospital
New York, New York

Takao Ohki, M.D., Ph.D.
Associate Professor, Department of Surgery
Albert Einstein College of Medicine
Bronx, New York

Juan Carlos Parodi, M.D.
Professor of Surgery and Radiology
Washington University
St. Louis, Missouri

Antonios Polydorou
ILRMDT
Nancy, France

Kasja Rabe
Cardiovascular Center Frankfurt,
  Sanht Katharinen
Frankfurt, Germany

Gary S. Roubin, M.D., Ph.D.
Chief, Endovascular Services,
St. John's Hospital,
Jackson, WY
USA

H. Christian Schumacher, M.D.
Clinical Fellow, Doris and Stanley
  Tananbaum
Stroke Center Neurological Institute
Department of Neurology
College of Physicians and Surgeons
Columbia University

Fayaz Shawl, M.D., F.A.C.P., F.A.C.C.
Clinical Professor of Medicine
  (Cardiology)
George Washington University School of
  Medicine
Tacoma Park, Maryland

Brent J. Shelton, Ph.D.
UAB School of Public Health
Birmingham Alabama

Horst Sievert, M.D.
Chief, Department of Cardiology and
    Vascular Medicine
Santa Katharinen Hospital
Frankfurt, Germany

Goran Stankovic, M.D.
Assistant Professor, Institute for
    Cardiovascular Diseases
Medical Faculty of Belgrade
Belgrade, SCG

Jiri J. Vitek, M.D., Ph.D.
Director Interventional Neuroradiology
The Lenox Hill Heart and Vascular
    Institute
New York, NY

Mark H. Wholey, M.D.
Clinical Professor of Radiology
School of Medicine
University of Pittsburgh
Pittsburgh, Pennsylvania

Michael H. Wholey, M.D., M.B.A.
Associate Professor, Departments of
    Radiology and Cardiology
University of Texas Health Science Center
San Antonio, Texas

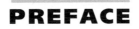

PREFACE

Carotid artery stenting (CAS) is attracting an ever-greater number of vascular specialists from the various disciplines of cardiology, radiology, surgery and neurology. This interest has recently been boosted by the introduction of Anti-Embolization devices and accumulating evidence that support the safety and efficacy of these strategies in minimizing the risk of embolization during the procedure. Particularly important are the recent reports of two randomized trials (CAVATAS and SAPHIRE) that demonstrated favorable outcomes of stenting as compared to the traditional treatment: carotid endarterectomy. Growing evidence also supports the late efficacy of CAS in preventing stroke resulting from obstructive extracranial carotid artery disease. It is now evident that CAS has a legitimate indication in the high-surgical-risk patients. The Food and Drug Administration is expected to approve the first stent and protection device for treatment of this disorder this year.

Outcomes of CAS are highly dependent on the operator's skills and performance. No single vascular specialty is well equipped with the depth of skills and knowledge necessary for the safe execution of this procedure. A significant gap exists between the limited number of experienced carotid stent operators and the increasing interest in this treatment. This book is intended to be a comprehensive, multidisciplinary resource for the growing number of vascular specialists interested in learning the carotid stenting techniques. Special emphasis is made on the clinical role of this treatment, essential angiographic anatomy, appropriate patient selection, periprocedural care, and a step-by-step technical description of the procedure and the various anti-embolization strategies.

We are greatly appreciative to the pioneers of this field for their valuable contributions to this book.

Nadim Al-Mubarak
Gary S. Roubin
Sriram S. Iyer
Jiri J. Vitek

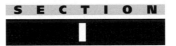

SECTION
I

CLINICAL RESULTS AND INDICATIONS

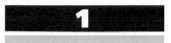

OBSTRUCTIVE CAROTID ARTERY DISEASE AND EVIDENCE-BASED BENEFITS OF REVASCULARIZATION

ALFREDO M. LOPEZ-YUÑEZ
JOSÉ BILLER

Approximately 10% to 20% of cases of cerebral infarction are secondary to carotid atherosclerosis (1). Carotid atherosclerosis develops in areas of low vessel-wall shear stress, most commonly the carotid bulb. In addition to the degree of carotid artery stenosis, plaque structure has been postulated as a critical factor in defining stroke risk. Complicated plaques characterized by cellular proliferation, tissue factor activation, oxidized low-density lipoprotein (LDL), ulceration, hemorrhage, and thrombosis may increase the risk of stroke in surgical and nonsurgical patients (2). Stabilization of the plaque with statins and modification of other risk factors may decrease the perioperative and long-term stroke risk. We discuss these new data in our first section.

The association between carotid artery stenosis and transient ischemic attack and stroke was first described by Fisher and Fisher et al. (3,4), who suggested surgical plaque removal as a potential therapy. Despite early proposal of revascularization of the carotid artery to prevent stroke, the benefit of carotid endarterectomy (CEA) was demonstrated only decades later, after a careful analysis of the natural history of carotid artery occlusive disease and the completion of large multicenter, randomized trials. These trials have unequivocally established the benefit of CEA proportional to the degree of carotid stenosis in symptomatic patients. The role of CEA in symptomatic patients with severe stenosis (70% to 99%) and moderate stenosis (50% to 69%) defined by contrast angiography is widely accepted. CEA in asymptomatic patients with high-grade stenosis has generated more controversy because of a perceived unacceptably high surgical risk in the community and a modest annual absolute risk reduction of ipsilateral stroke (5,6). In this review, we discuss revascularization in these two groups of patients in our first section. We also include a review of the current thinking on revascularization of symptomatic patients with recent internal carotid artery (ICA) occlusion. Despite the well-known negative results of the extracranial–intracranial bypass trial, there is renewed interest in revisiting the value of this procedure in a specific subset of patients with symptomatic ICA occlusion and high rates of recurrent ischemic stroke. Positron emission tomography with determination of oxygen extraction fraction identifies a high-risk group of patients who will be studied in the Carotid Occlusion Stroke Study (COSS). Finally, we summarize the current recommendations regarding CEA in diverse clinical scenarios.

STABLIZATION OF THE ATHEROSCLEROTIC CAROTID PLAQUE

Myocardial infarction (MI) and stroke are the leading cause of morbidity and death in the United States—for the most part, as a consequence of atherosclerosis. The earliest lesion of atherosclerosis is the fatty streak, which is an infiltration of monocyte-derived macrophages and T-lymphocytes in the arterial wall. Fatty streaks occur early in life, involving the aorta in the first decade of life and the coronary and extracranial carotid arteries in the second decade. The fatty streak starts as an infiltration of LDL cholesterol in the arterial wall, followed by its oxidation. The process continues when macrophages secrete chemokines and mitogens that induce smooth muscle cell proliferation. This may lead to plaque growth and eventual narrowing of the vessel lumen.

In the carotid bifurcation, atherosclerosis is most severe in the posterior wall of the carotid bulb, where there is low shear stress and greater turbulence. Disturbed laminar flow in the carotid bulb may lead to high adhesion molecule expression, activation of prescription factors, low expression of antioxidant enzymes, and high expression of endothelin, among other changes. Most MIs have been associated with thrombosis in plaques with high inflammatory cell content and large necrotic lipid cores, so-called unstable plaques. This mechanism has not been established as clearly in the carotid artery, although recent evidence suggests that occlusion of the extracranial carotid artery bifurcation has a similar pathophysiology (7,8).

Reversal from unstable to stable plaque has been demonstrated in coronary arteries and, more recently, in carotid arteries. Many strategies to stabilize the plaque have been focused on treatment of hypercholesterolemia, improvement of endothelial dysfunction by using statins, modifying the renin-angiotensin system, or lowering homocysteine levels. Clinically, there are extensive data supporting the use of statins to lower LDL cholesterol, increasing high-density lipoprotein (HDL) cholesterol slightly, and, overall, improving endothelial dysfunction independently of cholesterol effects. Ramipril, an angiotensin-converting enzyme inhibitor with a long half-life, demonstrated a reduction in MI, stroke, and other vascular events, independently of its effects on blood pressure (9). Vitamin supplementation with folate, vitamin B_6, and vitamin B_{12} may decrease levels of homocysteine, but its impact in reducing carotid artery atherosclerosis or recurrent ischemic stroke remains to be determined.

Current evidence from several large randomized trials has demonstrated that the risk of ipsilateral transient ischemic attack or stroke is proportional to the degree of the arterial stenosis. However, based on the data presented above, there is growing interest in investigating the relationship between the carotid plaque characteristics and the risk of embolization. Ultrasound data have shown a fair correlation between the plaque content of fibrin, elastin, calcium, hemorrhage, or lipids using B mode technology (10). Furthermore, the risk of embolization in previously asymptomatic patients has been found to be higher in those patients with hypoechoic plaques compared to hyperechoic plaques. Sabetai et al. found that when the gray scale median (GSM) of the plaque on B mode ultrasound was lower in those patients who became symptomatic with amaurosis fugax, transient ischemic attack (TIA), or stroke (GSM range of 7.4–14.9) compared to those patients who remained asymptomatic (GSM range of 26.2–34.7) (11).

Using magnetic resonance (MR) technology, stabilization and even regression of atherosclerotic plaques have been demonstrated in coronary artery lesions and, more recently, in the aortic arch and the carotids. When asymptomatic patients received simvastatin, serial black blood magnetic resonance imaging (MRI) measurements of the aorta and carotid artery showed stabilization of the lumen area, vessel wall thickness, and vessel wall area at 6 months and actual improvement of these measurements at 12 months. Several authors have shown the application of this stabilization concept in patients undergoing CEA (12,13). Consecutive patients with symptomatic carotid stenosis were treated with either pravastatin 40 mg per day versus no lipid-lowering agents 3 months prior to scheduled CEA. Detailed immunocytochemical and histological analysis of the removed carotid plaques showed stabilization of the atherosclerotic process. Plaques from the group treated with pravastatin showed less lipid content of the plaque area, less oxidized LDL immunoreactivity, fewer macrophages, fewer T-lymphocytes, less matrix metalloproteinase to immunoreactivity, greater tissue inhibitor of metalloproteinase immunoreactivity, and less apoptosis as measured by TdT-mediated dUTP-Biotin nick end labeling (TUNEL) staining, whereas there was a higher collagen content. All of these measures were statistically significant. These provocative results raise the possibility of preoperative or preprocedural medical interventions to stabilize the carotid atherosclerotic plaque, although their impact in decreasing perioperative vascular complications remains to be determined.

APPROACH TO THE PATIENT WITH CAROTID ARTERY OCCLUSIVE DISEASE

The first and most important approach to the patient with carotid atherosclerosis is to initiate strategies to modify vascular risk factors and to stabilize and prevent the progression of carotid atherosclerotic plaque. Hypertension, diabetes, cigarette smoking, elevated cholesterol, elevated homocysteine, obesity, excessive alcohol use, and sedentary lifestyle have been associated with carotid atherosclerosis and ischemic stroke. Table 1-1 summarizes the current recommendations for vascular risk factor modification.

The second approach is the initiation of antithrombotic therapy. Strong evidence supports the use of antiplatelet therapy for secondary stroke prevention (14–17). All available antiplatelet agents have demonstrated benefit in reducing recurrent stroke rates. The choice between aspirin, clopidogrel, ticlopidine, or the combination aspirin and modified release dipyridamole will depend on the patient's risk factor profile, side effects, and cost. Warfarin is not superior to aspirin in reducing recurrence of noncardioembolic ischemic events and

TABLE 1-1. APPROACH TO THE PATIENT WITH CAROTID ATHEROSCLEROSIS: RISK FACTOR MODIFICATION

Risk Factor	Aim	Intervention
Arterial hypertension	SBP < 140 mm Hg and DBP < 90 mm Hg	Tailored antihypertensive therapy, low sodium diet
	BP < 130/85 in diabetics	Exercise
Diabetes mellitus	Fasting blood glucose levels < 126 mg/dL	Diet, oral hypoglycemic agents, insulin
Cigarette smoking	Smoking cessation	Smoking cessation programs, nicotine replacement, bupropion
Elevated cholesterol and elevated LDL	LDL < 100 mg/dL	Diet low in saturated fat, weight reduction, HMG CoA reductase inhibitors (statins), niacin, fibrates
Excessive alcohol	Stop alcohol or moderate use (1 to 2 drinks/d)	Cessation programs
Sedentary lifestyle	Exercise regularly	Exercise 30–60 min 3 times/week
Elevated homocysteine	Plasma level < 15 μmol/L (may vary in different laboratories)	Folic acid, pyridoxine, vitamin B_{12}

SBP, systolic blood pressure; DBP, diastolic blood pressure; BP, blood pressure; LDL, low-density lipoprotein; HMG CoA, hepatic hydroxymethyl glutaryl coenzyme A.

probably should not be used routinely in this population owing to its potential hemorrhagic complications (18). A possible exception is the presence of intraluminal thrombus in the ICA. These patients are managed preferably with anticoagulation for few weeks, followed by CEA (19,20).

The third approach is the removal of the atherosclerotic plaque through surgery or an endovascular procedure (carotid artery stenting; CAS). The next section reviews the role of CEA in symptomatic and asymptomatic patients, including some areas of ongoing controversy. The technique and role of CAS are discussed elsewhere in this textbook. To date, there is no evidence that the endovascular approach is more effective than CEA, and early trials have shown either worse or, at best, similar outcomes when compared to CEA (Table 1-2) (21–24). Two preliminary studies comparing stenting and CEA were abandoned prematurely because of a high rate of serious morbidity associated with the endovascular procedure (21,24). However, these two trials had serious limitations. In the study by Naylor et al. (24), an interventional radiologist with little experience in carotid angioplasty was compared to a skilled surgeon. Not surprisingly, the complications were more commonly seen among those who were treated with angioplasty/stenting. The details of the second study (21) have not been published.

The study by Brooks et al. showed that surgery and angioplasty were approximately equal in terms of safety, and angioplasty was slightly more costly than CEA (22). The Carotid and Vertebral Artery Transluminal Angioplasty Study (CAVATAS) was a multicenter international trial that compared angioplasty (most patients did not have stenting) and CEA (23). Outcome measures were similar in both groups. Recurrent carotid stenosis was more common in patients having angioplasty, although these changes were asymptomatic. These data are helpful but not definite. Additional data comparing the safety and efficacy of endovascular treatment and carotid surgery are needed. The Carotid Revascularization

TABLE 1-2. TRIALS COMPARING CAROTID ENDARTERECTOMY VERSUS STENTING

Trial	Inclusion	Outcomes	Stent vs. CEA
Naylor et al. (24) n = 7 stent n = 10 CEA	Symptomatic >70% ICA stenosis	Death, total strokes at 30 d	70% vs. 0% ($p < 0.003$)
Alberts (21)[a] n = 107 stent n = 112 CEA	Symptomatic 60%–90% ICA stenosis	Ipsilateral stroke, procedure-related death, vascular death	12.1% vs. 4.5% ($p = 0.022$)
CAVATAS (23) n = 251 stent n = 253 CEA	Symptomatic and asymptomatic	Stroke or death within 30 d	10% vs. 10% (NS)
Brooks et al. (22) n = 53 stent n = 51 CEA	Symptomatic >70% ICA stenosis		2% vs. 1.9% (NS)

[a]Presented as abstract. Periprocedural stent complications 5% for sites with >10 procedures versus 11% for sites with <10 procedures.
CEA, carotid endarterectomy; ICA, internal carotid artery; CAVATAS, Carotid Vertebral Artery Transluminal Angioplasty Study; NS, not significant.

With Carotid Endarterectomy or Stent Trial (CREST) will include symptomatic patients (TIA or stroke) with more than 50% stenosis by angiography or more than 70% stenosis by ultrasound. This study should, it is hoped, provide more reliable evidence about the best revascularization option (25).

REVASCULARIZATION OF CAROTID STENOSIS

Technical Aspects

This section does not intend to provide an exhaustive description of the surgical technique of CEA, but rather intends to illustrate basic points of the procedure in order to understand the potential complications at every stage.

According to Loftus (26), there are several cardinal principles of carotid reconstruction: complete knowledge of the patient's vascular anatomy, complete vascular control at all times, anatomic knowledge to prevent harm to adjacent structures, and assurance of a widely patent vessel free of technical errors.

The first plane of dissection includes skin, subcutaneous tissue, and the platysma, after which the anterior edge of the sternocleidomastoid muscle is identified. In cases of high dissection, the greater auricular nerve may be observed (Fig. 1-1A). Dissection then proceeds

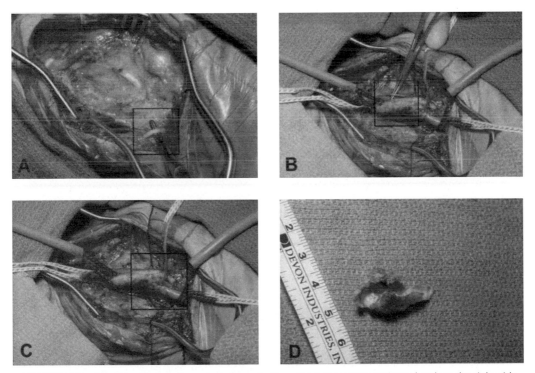

FIGURE 1-1. Carotid endarterectomy technique. **A:** Superficial dissection: patient's head on the right side of the figure, left carotid intervention. Detail: greater auricular nerve. **B:** Deeper plane: The jugular vein has been retracted, the facial vein ligated. Exposure of common carotid artery. Detail: ansa hypoglossi. **C:** Detail: The bifurcation of the common carotid artery has been exposed; the internal carotid artery lays in the lower part of the picture (initially runs lateral to the external carotid artery). **D:** Removed atherosclerotic plaque. Photographs courtesy of Mitesh Shah, MD, Section of Neurological Surgery, Indiana University School of Medicine, Indianapolis, Indiana. (See also color section following page 164 of this text.)

on the sternocleidomastoid muscle until the jugular vein is identified. The jugular vein is retracted back, constituting the key landmark (Fig. 1-1B). The next step in the procedure is dissection of the carotid complex (Fig. 1-1C). Dissection of the ICA is completed clearly beyond the distal extent of the plaque before cross clamping is performed. This is crucial to prevent embolism at a time of cross clamping. The plane between the lateral carotid wall and the medial jugular border is then followed to identify the hypoglossal nerve to prevent injury (Fig. 1-1B). A clamp is then placed on the ICA lying underneath the vessel, at which moment the decision to shunt is made based on the ancillary testing results: electroencephalogram (EEG), transcranial Doppler (TCD), or stump pressure. Intraluminal shunt is indicated when EEG changes occur, the middle cerebral artery velocity decreases on TCD, or loss of somatosensory-evoked potentials occurs. With or without shunt, the arteriotomy incision is made in the midline of the vessel, and the plaque is dissected from the arterial wall. Following gross removal (Fig. 1-1D), a careful search is made for remaining fragments adhering to the arterial wall, and all loose fragments are removed. The clamps are then removed first from the external carotid artery (ECA), then from the common carotid artery, and finally, 10 seconds later, from the ICA in order to flush all debris and remaining microbubbles into the external carotid arteries. Careful inspection for leaks is conducted and hand-held Doppler ultrasound is commonly used to assure patency of all vessels.

EVIDENCE OF BENEFITS

Symptomatic Patients

The degree of arterial stenosis is the most important predictor of cerebral infarction among symptomatic patients with extracranial ICA occlusive disease. (27). The severity of carotid stenosis is directly related to stroke risk. Surgical removal of the atherosclerotic plaque reduces the risk of retinal and cerebral embolism and improves cerebral blood flow, particularly in patients with critical stenosis.

Three major prospective studies have provided compelling evidence for the benefit of CEA in reducing recurrent stroke in high-risk symptomatic patients (27–29). The North American Symptomatic Carotid Endarterectomy Trial (NASCET) demonstrated the effectiveness of CEA in preventing stroke among 659 patients who had TIAs or minor strokes with high-grade (70% to 99%) carotid stenosis. Stenosis was measured uniformly by contrast angiography using the formula: [1 − minimum residual lumen/normal distal cervical ICA diameter] × 100 = percentage of stenosis. The absolute risk reductions in favor of surgery were 17% for ipsilateral stroke, 15% for all strokes, 16.5% for all strokes and death, 10.6% for major ipsilateral stroke, 9.4% for all major strokes, and 10.1% for major stroke and death. Ipsilateral perioperative stroke risk increased with the degree of carotid artery stenosis. CEA was performed by experienced surgeons with an overall perioperative stroke and death rates less than 6%. The same authors published in 1998 the results of 2,226 patients with 50% to 69% symptomatic carotid stenosis randomized to CEA versus medical therapy (NASCET-2) (30). A modest benefit in favor of surgery over medical therapy alone was observed, especially among nondiabetic men with hemispheric, ischemic cerebrovascular events. In those patients with less than 50% stenosis, CEA added no benefit over medical therapy in preventing stroke.

The benefits of CEA in symptomatic patients have been confirmed by two additional randomized trials. The European Carotid Surgery Trial (ECST) compared CEA to best medical therapy among 1,152 patients with carotid circulation TIA or nondisabling ischemic stroke (28). The ECST method of measuring angiographic stenosis was different than the method used in NASCET. Among all patients with 70% to 99% stenosis (n = 778), those who underwent surgery had significantly fewer strokes or deaths, whereas patients with less then 70% stenosis (n = 374) had no benefit from surgery. Similarly, the Veterans Administration Cooperative Study, which was terminated early because of the publication of the results of NASCET and ECST, showed that patients with a history of carotid TIA or nondisabling ischemic stroke and angiographic ICA stenosis more than 50% (n = 189) had fewer ipsilateral TIAs and strokes when treated with CEA and aspirin versus those who received aspirin only (29).

Based on these data, a multidisciplinary group published guidelines for the management of symptomatic patients (31). The community experience with CEA in symptomatic patients has not always been comparable to the results of randomized trials. Therefore, quality assurance by monitoring perioperative complications is mandatory for any team performing CEA, and this information should be part of the decision-making process for patients and clinicians.

Asymptomatic Patients

Asymptomatic carotid atherosclerosis is relatively common in the general population, but high-grade asymptomatic stenosis (more than 70% occlusion) is rare. The risk of ipsilateral cerebral infarction in asymptomatic patients is lower than in symptomatic patients with TIA or nondisabling stroke. Asymptomatic carotid artery stenosis of less than 75% carries an annual stroke risk of 1.3%, whereas stenosis more than 75% carries an annual combined TIA/stroke risk of 10.5% (32).

Several randomized trials on the efficacy of CEA in patients with asymptomatic carotid artery have been published. The first three showed no benefit of the procedure over medical therapy. The Carotid Artery Surgery Asymptomatic Narrowing Operation Versus Aspirin Trial (CASANOVA) studied CEA in asymptomatic patients with ICA stenosis between 50% and 90% versus medical therapy with aspirin and dipyridamole (33). No difference in outcomes was seen. Interestingly, patients with 90% to 99% ICA stenosis were excluded from the study. The Mayo Asymptomatic Carotid Endarterectomy Trial was terminated early because of higher rates of MI and TIA in the surgical group (34). Patients in the surgical group did not receive aspirin, probably explaining those results. The Veterans Affairs Asymptomatic Carotid Endarterectomy Trial randomized 444 patients with angiographically proven 50% to 99% stenosis to CEA versus medical therapy. Even though there was a trend favoring the surgical group in reducing ipsilateral hemispheric TIA, transient monocular blindness, and stroke as endpoints, there was no significant difference in the composite outcome of all strokes and death (35).

The Asymptomatic Carotid Atherosclerosis Study (ACAS) examined the combined use of CEA, aspirin therapy, and vascular risk factor modification in asymptomatic patients with more than 60% stenosis. The degree of stenosis was calculated by contrast angiography (using a method similar to that used in NASCET), by Doppler ultrasound, or by a combination of Doppler ultrasound and oculopneumoplethysmography. Patients randomized to surgery based on noninvasive testing received postrandomization presurgical angiography. Surgery was not performed in those patients with less than 60% stenosis, distal arteriovenous malformation, intracranial aneurysm, or intracranial ipsilateral distal carotid stenosis greater than the proximal stenosis. These patients were included in the intention-to-treat analysis. The primary endpoints were ipsilateral stroke, any perioperative stroke, or death. This study was stopped after a median follow-up of 2.7 years because of an absolute difference in these endpoints of 5.9% in favor of surgery. This translates into an annual absolute risk reduction of 1.2% based on a 5-year projection using the Kaplan-Meier estimation. After 5 years, 5.1% of patients in the surgical group versus 11% of patients in the medical group would have reached an endpoint, representing an aggregate relative risk reduction of 53% in the surgical group. The perioperative stroke and death rates in this study were at a low 2.3%, including a 1.2% angiography stroke complication rate.

The highly selective nature of patients in these surgical trials has led to questions about generalizing these results. For example, ACAS randomized 1,662 patients from 42,000 screened patients. Patients with multiple concomitant medical problems or life expectancy of less than 5 years are unlikely to benefit from CEA (36). Patients with asymptomatic progressive carotid artery stenosis or severe asymptomatic carotid stenosis with contralateral carotid occlusion represent a challenging clinical scenario (37,38).

Post hoc analysis has shown no obvious benefit from operating on the asymptomatic carotid artery stenosis in patients with severe asymptomatic carotid artery stenosis and symptomatic contralateral artery stenosis. Furthermore, therapeutic decisions should not be based on ultrasound data, as velocities may increase spuriously when the contralateral vessel is occluded or affected with high-grade stenosis (39).

The management of asymptomatic carotid artery stenosis in patients undergoing coronary artery surgery remains controversial (40). Perioperative stroke risk in patients undergoing coronary bypass grafting is approximately 2.2% irrespective of presence of carotid stenosis, and many mechanisms other than carotid artery atherosclerosis may be responsible for perioperative stroke after cardiac revascularization procedures (41).

For all these reasons, and despite the results from numerous randomized clinical studies, several authors consider that there is as yet insufficient evidence to recommend CEA in asymptomatic patients (5,42). It is estimated that approximately 19 patients need to undergo CEA to prevent one stroke or one death over a 5-year period. In addition, the radiologic/surgical risk should be less than 3% (31). Based on these caveats, along with a low stroke risk in asymptomatic patients, some experts consider it acceptable to delay CEA in asymptomatic patients until there is more than 80% stenosis.

Two ongoing trials in Europe may provide additional and useful information for the care of the asymptomatic patients (43,44). When considering management options in a patient with asymptomatic carotid stenosis, it is important to remember that surgery is not urgent or mandatory and that a detailed discussion of the risk/benefit ratio, along with modification of vascular risk factors, are necessary steps prior to surgery.

COST-EFFECTIVENESS OF CAROTID ENDARTERECTOMY IN ASYMPTOMATIC PATIENTS

CEA is expensive, with an estimated cost ranging from $8,000 to $15,000 per procedure (45). Since the publication of the ACAS results, there has been a significant increase in the number of CEAs performed in the community (46). The potential public health impact of operating on patients with asymptomatic stenosis has been questioned (5). Hanke (47) estimated the cost of 1.24 million Australian dollars if all Australians with asymptomatic stenosis greater than 60% were operated, resulting in prevention of 88 strokes. Conversely, Cronenwett et al. (48) found that CEA was effective in patients over 75 years of age with 60% or greater asymptomatic stenosis using assumptions from the ACAS study. Given the low frequency of asymptomatic carotid artery atherosclerosis in the population, mass screening is not likely to be as effective and may lead to complications from angiography or surgery (49).

More selective screening in patients with atherosclerotic risk factors, cervical bruits (50), and peripheral vascular or coronary artery disease would be more cost-effective, as it may detect clinically significant stenosis in 10% to 30% of patients with these characteristics (51).

Another factor to consider in the cost-effectiveness analysis is that at least 45% of the strokes in patients with asymptomatic carotid artery stenosis of 60% to 99% are either due to lacunar or cardiac embolic mechanisms. Analysis of stroke risk according to cause is therefore necessary to avoid overestimation of the potential benefit of CEA among asymptomatic patients (52).

COMPLICATIONS ASSOCIATED WITH CAROTID ENDARTERECTOMY

Stroke

Perioperative vascular complications, particularly stroke, are the most feared complications associated with CEA. Furthermore, the benefits of CEA over medical therapy are strictly dependent on low perioperative morbidity and mortality surgical risks. Surgery is beneficial only when the surgical risk is kept at a low rate: less than 3% among asymptomatic patients and less than 6.7% among symptomatic patients (31).

Etiology of perioperative ischemic stroke following CEA is multifactorial; ischemic stroke may occur as a consequence of atheromatous plaque thromboembolism, technical error, or clamp ischemia. Hemorrhagic stroke may occur as a result of the hyperperfusion syndrome (53). Plaque thromboembolism may occur at the time of surgery when plaque material dislodges and embolizes to intracranial vessels, particularly in cases of complicated atherosclerotic plaques. It may also occur at a later time, when platelet aggregates accumulate in the intimal surgical site, most commonly in patients with exaggerated platelet function. Incomplete endarterectomy with a residual intimal flap is the most common technical error leading to perioperative stroke (54). This residual flap partially obstructs the ICA lumen and becomes a nidus for further thrombus formation and potential embolism. Approximately 15% of patients undergoing CEA are intolerant of the temporary clamp time that is required for the procedure (35,55). This may occur in asymptomatic patients or among patients with TIAs and insufficient collateral intracranial circulation, or in patients with recent stroke in whom there is periinfarction tissue at risk. This ischemic mechanism usually leads to watershed infarctions. Techniques such as EEG monitoring (56), determination of back pressure, TCD (57), or somatosensory-evoked responses (58) may detect ongoing cerebral ischemia and may alert the surgeon to the need to place a shunt to prevent cerebral infarction in these patients.

Intracerebral hemorrhage is a rare complication of CEA. It may occur as part of the hyperperfusion syndrome in patients with poor cerebral autoregulation (typically those with critical ICA stenosis) and uncontrolled hypertension. Rapid reestablishment of cerebral flow in chronically ischemic brain regions may lead to hyperperfusion. Affected patients may present with headaches, confusion, and, occasionally, intracerebral hemorrhage. Careful blood pressure control is the best preventive and therapeutic measure in these high-risk patients (59). Alternatively, hemorrhages may occur in patients with recent, large infarctions associated with disruption of the blood–brain barrier.

Several groups have analyzed ways to increase safety and efficacy of CEA. A coordinated educational program for physicians in Iowa resulted in fewer perioperative complications

(60). Peer-reviewed monitoring of CEA complications also produced similar results (61). Other important factors in determining CEA efficacy are the number of operations performed at a specific institution and the skills of its surgeons (62,63). Selection of patients undergoing CEA can also improve efficacy of the operation. Careful risk-benefit analysis is recommended when considering CEA among patients over 75 years of age, patients with distal intracranial atherosclerotic disease (tandem arterial stenosis), and patients with contralateral ICA occlusion. However, Alamowitch et al. (64), analyzing NASCET, found no increase in perioperative stroke in older patients, and patients with intracranial stenosis distal to high-grade extracranial stenosis still benefit from CEA (65). Contralateral ICA stenosis increases the perioperative risk following CEA (66).

Other Complications

The large prospective studies on CEA have shown wound complication rates ranging from 3% to 5% (67). Most of these hematomas are small and without clinical significance. Rarely, hematomas enlarge to such extent that surgical evacuation is warranted in order to prevent obstruction of the upper airway. Aside form local compression, no other interventions are recommended to prevent hematoma formation. A trial of protamine sulfate to reverse heparin effect was terminated prematurely because of a 6.3% rate of thrombosis in the active arm, despite a significant reduction in the wound drainage volumes in the same group (68). Wound infections following CEA are very rare (69). A case of cerebral abscess of a previous hematoma following CEA has been reported (70). Routine perioperative antibiotic use is not indicated.

Cranial nerve injuries are the most common complications associated with CEA. Rates of cranial nerve injury vary greatly depending on the type of study and diagnostic methodology. Large prospective studies showed cranial nerve injury rates of 2.2% in ACAS (71), 5% in the VA cooperative study (29), and 7.6% in NASCET (27). Retrospective series showed rates ranging from 3% to 19% and decreasing in follow-up to 0% to 5% (72,73), whereas a large prospective series showed initial cranial nerve injury rates of 12.5% with only 0.3% being permanent (74). These transient deficits are consistent with neurapraxia rather than neurotmesis in most cases. Table 1-3 shows the most common cranial nerve injuries and their clinical significance.

Medical complications may also occur following CEA, although they are rare. Pneumonia, pulmonary embolism, respiratory distress, urinary retention, urinary tract infection, renal insufficiency, neovascular glaucoma, and cardiovascular complications have been described. Hemodynamic instability is more common following CEA than with other peripheral vascular surgeries. Myocardial ischemia is the most serious cause of these complications. Severe coronary artery disease (more than 70% stenosis in one or more vessels) has been found in 32% of vascular surgery patients (75). The main causes of perioperative mortality in CEA patients are MI and cardiac arrhythmias with rates ranging from 1.5% to 5% (27,76).

Timing of Carotid Endarterectomy

Many physicians have been reluctant to recommend CEA within a few weeks following ischemic stroke because of safety concerns. However, the perioperative risk varies widely depending on the severity of neurologic impairments, extent of neuroimaging ischemic lesions, and concomitant disease (77). Patients with minimal neurological impairments and small or no lesions on neuroimaging may be treated similarly to patients with TIA with

TABLE 1-3. CRANIAL NERVE INJURIES

Cranial Nerve	Mechanism of Injury	Clinical Presentation
Marginal mandibular branch of facial nerve	High exposure of carotid bifurcation	Weakness of depressor labii inferioris muscle
Hypoglossal nerve and ansa hypoglossi	Facial vein separation, bifurcation traction	Tongue deviation, dysphagia, dysarthria
Vagus nerve, branches (most commonly superior laryngeal nerve)	Posterolateral to carotid artery	Hoarseness, dysphagia
Greater auricular nerve	High carotid bifurcations (C2–3)	Hypoesthesia of the earlobe and angle of the jaw
Spinal accessory nerve	Aggressive sternomastoid retraction	Drooping of the shoulder, ipsilateral shoulder pain
Glossopharyngeal nerve and nerve of Hering	Traction of tissue between ICA/ECA	Dysphagia, hypotension, and bradycardia

ICA, internal carotid artery; ECA, external carotid artery.

minimal surgical delay. Recent reports suggest that carefully selected patients can have CEA safely within days of a stroke (78,79). Delaying surgery for more than 6 weeks is no longer recommended.

REVASCULARIZATION OF SYMPTOMATIC INTERNAL CAROTID OCCLUSION

The neurological consequences of internal carotid occlusion are diverse, ranging from no symptoms to a major cerebral infarction possibly leading to death (80). Approximately 10% to 15% of patients presenting with carotid territory stroke or TIA are found to have carotid occlusion. However, prevention of recurrent stroke in this group of patients constitutes a difficult challenge. The most important factor in predicting the effects of internal carotid occlusion is the status of the collateral circulation via pial arteries, circle of Willis, or from ECA branches. Inadequate collaterals may lead to poor hemispheric perfusion and increased stroke risk, particularly when the metabolic and oxygen demands increase. Several neuro-imaging techniques have been used to identify patients with internal carotid occlusion and high risk of ipsilateral stroke, including single photon emission computed tomography (SPECT), TCD, enhanced computed tomography (CT) and MRI (81,82), and positron-emission tomography (PET) determination of oxygen extraction fraction (OEF). This latter technique has demonstrated the best predictive value. Grubb et al. (83) found that patients with ICA occlusion and high OEF determined by PET had a 26% rate of strokes and TIAs at 2 years compared to approximately 5% risk in patients with normal OEF. These strokes occurred despite best medical therapy with antiplatelets or anticoagulants. These findings have been confirmed by other groups (84,85).

These data have kindled interest in the extracranial-intracranial (EC-IC) bypass surgery for symptomatic patients with recent ICA occlusion. As it is well known, the international trial of EC-IC bypass performed in 1985 failed to demonstrate the efficacy of this type of surgery despite excellent operative results and a high degree of bypass patency (86). This

TABLE 1-4. RECOMMENDATIONS FOR SYMPTOMATIC PATIENTS WITH CAROTID TERRITORY ISCHEMIA

Degree of Stenosis	CEA	Other Options
70–99%	Definite benefit	Antiplatelet therapy Angioplasty/stenting (ongoing evaluation)
50–69%	Potential benefit (especially men with hemispheric ischemia, nondiabetics)	Antiplatelet therapy
<50%	No benefit	Antiplatelet therapy

CEA, carotid endarterectomy.

well-designed and well-executed trial was, however, criticized, especially for the lack of a reliable way to screen patients with a high risk of ipsilateral stroke. The recently funded Carotid Occlusion Surgery Study (COSS) will test the usefulness of EC-IC bypass in preventing ischemic stroke among patients who have symptomatic carotid occlusion and an increased OEF determined by PET.

SUMMARY OF RECOMMENDATIONS

Table 1-4 summarizes the recommendations for symptomatic patients. CEA may be considered for asymptomatic patients with a 60% to 99% ICA stenosis as long as the procedure-related risk for stroke and death is less than 3%. Because the margin of error was narrow in the ACAS study, the authors prefer to recommend the procedure in selected asymptomatic patients when the ICA stenosis is 80% to 99%. Further studies may help clarify the usefulness of CEA in asymptomatic patients.

REFERENCES

1. Sacco RL, Ellenberg JA, Mohr JP, et al. Infarcts of undetermined cause: the NINCDS Stroke Data Bank. *Ann Neurol* 1989;25:382-390.
2. Garcia JH, Khang-Loon H. Carotid atherosclerosis. Definition, pathogenesis, and clinical significance. *Neuroimaging Clin N Am* 1996;6:801–810.
3. Fisher CM. Occlusion of the internal carotid artery. *Arch Neurol Psychiatr* 1951;65:346–377.
4. Fisher CM, Gore I, Okabe N, et al. Atherosclerosis of the carotid and vertebral arteries—extracranial and intracranial. *J Neuropathol Exp Neurol* 1965;24:455–476.
5. Chaturvedi S. Is carotid endarterectomy appropriate for asymptomatic stenosis? No. *Arch Neurol* 1999; 56:879–881.
6. Chaturvedi S. Public health impact of carotid endarterectomy. *Neuroepidemiology* 1999;18:15–21.
7. Carr S, Farb A, Pearce WH, et al. Atherosclerotic plaque rupture in symptomatic carotid artery stenosis. *J Vasc Surg* 1996;23:755–765.
8. Hatsukami TS, Ferguson MS, Beach KW, et al. Carotid plaque morphology and clinical events. *Stroke* 1997;28:95–100.
9. Heart Outcomes Prevention Evaluation (HOPE) Study Investigators. Vitamin E supplementation and cardiovascular events in high-risk patients. *N Engl J Med* 2000;342:154–160.
10. Rakebrandt F, Crawford DC, Havard D, et al. Relationship between ultrasound texture classification images and histology of atherosclerotic plaque. *Ultrasound Med Biol* 2000;26:1393–1402.

11. Sabetai MM, Tegos TJ, Nicolaides AN, et al. Hemispheric symptoms and carotid plaque echomorphology. *J Vasc Surg* 2000;31(Pt 1):39–49.
12. Crisby M, Nordin-Fredriksson G, Shah PK, et al. Pravastatin treatment increases collagen content and decreases lipid content, inflammation, metalloproteinases, and cell death in human carotid plaques: implications for plaque stabilization. *Circulation* 2001;103:926–933.
13. Corti R, Fayad ZA, Fuster V, et al. Effects of lipid-lowering by simvastatin on human atherosclerotic lesions: a longitudinal study by high-resolution, noninvasive magnetic resonance imaging. *Circulation* 2001;104:249–252.
14. Collaborative overview of randomized trials of antiplatelet therapy—I. Prevention of death, myocardial infarction, and stroke by prolonged antiplatelet therapy in various categories of patients. Antiplatelet Trialists' Collaboration. *Br Med J* 1994;308:81.
15. Hass WK, Easton JD, Adams HP. A randomized trial comparing ticlopidine hydrochloride with aspirin for the prevention of stroke in high-risk patients. *N Engl J Med* 1989;321:501–506.
16. Diener H, Cunha L, Forbes C. European Stroke Prevention Study. 2. Dipyridamole and acetylsalicylic acid in the secondary prevention of stroke. *J Neurol Sci.* 1996;143:1–13.
17. CAPRIE Steering Committee. A randomised, blinded, trial of clopidogrel versus aspirin in patients at risk of ischaemic events (CAPRIE). *Lancet* 1996;348:1329–1339.
18. Mohr JP, Thompson JL, Lazar B, et al. A comparison of warfarin and aspirin for the prevention of recurrent ischemic stroke. *N Engl J Med.* 2001;345:1444–1451.
19. Biller J, Adams HP, Boarini D. Intraluminal clot of the carotid artery. *Surg Neurol* 1986;25:467–477.
20. Buchan A, Gates P, Pelz D, Barnett HJM. Intraluminal thrombus in the cerebral circulation: implications for surgical management. *Stroke* 1988;19:681–698.
21. Alberts MJ. Results of a multicenter prospective randomized trial of carotid stenting vs. carotid endarterectomy. *Stroke* 2001;32:325(abst).
22. Brooks WH, McClure RR, Jones MR, et al. Carotid angioplasty and stenting versus carotid endarterectomy: randomized trial in a community hospital. *J Am Coll Cardiol* 2001;38:1589–1595.
23. Endovascular versus surgical treatment in patients with carotid stenosis in the Carotid and Vertebral Artery Transluminal Angioplasty Study (CAVATAS): a randomized trial. *Lancet* 2001;357:1729–1737.
24. Naylor AR, Bolia A, Abbott RJ, et al. Randomized study of carotid angioplasty and stenting versus carotid endarterectomy: a stopped trial. *J Vasc Surg* 1998;28:326–334.
25. Roubin GS, Hobson RW 2nd, White R, et al. CREST and CARESS to evaluate carotid stenting: time to get to work! *J Endovas Ther* 2001;8:107–110.
26. Loftus CM. Carotid endarterectomy: how the operation is done. *Clin Neurosurg* 1997;44:243–265.
27. Beneficial effect of carotid endarterectomy in symptomatic patients with high-grade carotid stenosis. North American Symptomatic Carotid Endarterectomy Trial (NASCET) Collaborators. *N Engl J Med* 1991;325:445–453.
28. MRC European Carotid Surgery Trial: interim results for symptomatic patients with severe (70-99%) or with mild (0-29%) carotid stenosis. European Carotid Surgery Trialists' Collaborative Group. *Lancet* 1991;337:1235–1243.
29. Mayberg MR, Wilson E, Yatsu F, et al. Carotid endarterectomy and prevention of cerebral ischemia in symptomatic carotid stenosis. *JAMA* 1991;266:3289–3294.
30. Barnett HJ, Taylor DW, Eliasziw M, et al. Benefit of carotid endarterectomy in patients with symptomatic moderate or severe stenosis. *N Engl J Med* 1998;339:1415–1425.
31. Biller J, Feinberg WM, Castaldo JE, et al. Guidelines for carotid endarterectomy: a statement for healthcare professionals from a special writing group of the Stroke Council, American Heart Association. *Stroke* 1998;29:554–562.
32. Norris JW, Zhu CA, Bornstein NM, et al. Vascular risks of asymptomatic carotid stenosis. *Stroke* 1991;22:1485–1490.
33. CASANOVA Study Group. Carotid surgery versus medical therapy in asymptomatic carotid stenosis. *Stroke* 1991;22:1229–1235.
34. Mayo Asymptomatic Carotid Endarterectomy Study Group. Results of a randomized controlled trial of carotid endarterectomy for asymptomatic carotid stenosis. *Mayo Clin Proc* 1992;67:513–518.
35. Hobson RW III, Weiss DG, Fields WS, et al. Efficacy of carotid endarterectomy for asymptomatic carotid stenosis. *N Engl J Med* 1993; 328:276–279.
36. Lepore MR Jr, Sternbergh WC 3rd, Salartash, K, et al. Influence of NASCET/ACAS trial eligibility on outcome after carotid endarterectomy. *J Vasc Surg* 2001;34:581–586.
37. Mukherjee D, Yadav JS. Effect of contralateral occlusion on long-term efficacy of endarterectomy in the Asymptomatic Carotid Atherosclerosis Study (ACAS). *Stroke* 2001;32:1443–1448.

38. Baker WH, Howard VJ, Howard G, et al. Effect of contralateral occlusion on long-term efficacy of endarterectomy in the asymptomatic carotid atherosclerosis study (ACAS). ACAS Investigators. *Stroke* 2000;Oct 31:2330–2334.

39. Henderson RD, Steinman DA, Eliaszi WM, et al. Effect of contralateral carotid artery stenosis on carotid ultrasound velocity measurements. *Stroke* 2000;31:2636–2640.

40. Char D, Cuadra S, Ricotta J, et al. Combined coronary artery bypass and carotid endarterectomy: long-term results. *Cardiovasc Surg* 2002;10:111–115.

41. Wijdicks EF, Jack CR. Coronary artery bypass-associated ischemic stroke. A clinical and neurological study. *J Neuroimaging* 1996;6:20–22.

42. Perry JR, Szalai JP, Norris JW. Consensus against both endarterectomy and routine screening for asymptomatic carotid artery stenosis. *Arch Neurol* 1997;54:25–28.

43. Halliday AW, Thomas D, Mansfield A. The Asymptomatic Carotid Surgery Trial (ACST): rationale and design. *Eur J Vasc Surg* 1994;8:703–710.

44. Nicolaides AN. Asymptomatic carotid stenosis and risk of stroke: identification of a high risk group (ACSRS): a natural history study. *Int Angiol* 1995;14:21–23.

45. Ballard JL, Deiparine MK, Bergan JJ, et al. Cost-effective evaluation and treatment for carotid disease. *Arch Surg* 1997;132:268–271.

46. Huber TS, Wheeler KG, Cuddeback JK, et al. Effect of the Asymptomatic Carotid Atherosclerosis Study on carotid endarterectomy in Florida. *Stroke* 1998;29:1099–1105.

47. Hanke J. Asymptomatic carotid stenosis: how should it be managed? *Med J Aust* 1995;163:197–200.

48. Cronenwett JL, Birkmeyer JE, Nackman GB. Cost effectiveness of carotid endarterectomy in asymptomatic patients. *J Vasc Surg* 1997;25:298–305.

49. Lee PT, Solomon NA, Heicenreich PA. Cost effectiveness of screening for carotid stenosis in asymptomatic persons. *Intern Med* 1997;126:337–342.

50. Obuchowski NA, Modic MT, Magdinec M, et al. Assessment of the efficacy of noninvasive screening for patients with asymptomatic neck bruits. *Stroke* 1997;28:1330–1339.

51. Derdeyn CP, Powers WJ. Cost effectiveness of screening for asymptomatic carotid artery disease. *Stroke* 1996;27:1944–1948.

52. Inzitari D, Eliasziw M, Gates P, et al. The causes and risk of stroke in patients with asymptomatic internal-carotid-artery stenosis. North American Symptomatic Carotid Endarterectomy Trial Collaborators. *N Engl J Med* 2000;342:1693–1700.

53. McKinsey JF, Desai TR, Bassiouny HS. Mechanisms of neurologic deficits and mortality with carotid endarterectomy. *Arch Surg* 1996;131:526–531.

54. Riles TS, Imparato AM, Jacobowitz GR. The cause of perioperative stroke after carotid endarterectomy. *J Vasc Surg* 1994;19:206.

55. Moore WS, Hall AD. Carotid artery back pressure: a test of cerebral tolerance to temporary carotid occlusion. *Arch Surg* 1969;99:702.

56. Sundt TM Jr, Sharbrough FW, Anderson E, et al. Cerebral blood flow measurements and electroencephalogram during carotid endarterectomy. *J Neurosurg* 1974;41:310–320.

57. Cao P, Giordano G, Zannetti S, et al. Transcranial Doppler monitoring during carotid endartectomy: is it appropriate for selecting patients in need of a shunt? *J Vasc Surg* 1997;26:973–979; discussion 979–980.

58. Horsch S, Knetidis K. Intraoperative use of sensory evoked potentials for brain monitoring during carotid surgery. *Neurosurg Clin North Am* 1996;7:693–696.

59. Mansoor GA, White WB, Grunnet M, et al. Intracerebral hemorrhage after carotid endarterectomy associated with ipsilateral fibrinoid necrosis: a consequence of the hyperperfusion syndrome? *J Vasc Surg* 1996;23:147–151.

60. Kresowik TF, Hemann RA, Grund SL, et al. Improving the outcomes of carotid endarterectomy: results of a statewide quality improvement project. *J Vasc Surg* 2000;31:918–926.

61. Olcott CI, Mitchell RS, Steinberg GK, et al. Institutional peer review can reduce the risk and cost of carotid endarterectomy. *Arch Surg* 2000;135:939–942.

62. O'Neill L, Lanska DJ, Hartz A. Surgeon characteristics associated with mortality and morbidity following carotid endarterectomy. *Neurology* 2000;55:773–781.

63. Pearce WH, Parker MA, Feinglass J, et al. The importance of surgeon volume and training in outcomes for vascular surgical procedures. *J Vasc Surg* 1999;29:768–776.

64. Alamowitch S, Eliasziw M, Algra A, et al. North American Symptomatic Carotid Endarterectomy Trial (NASCET) Group. Risk, causes, and prevention of ischaemic stroke in elderly patients with symptomatic internal-carotid-artery stenosis. *Lancet* 2001;357;1154–1160.

65. Kappelle LJ, Eliasziw M, Fox AJ, et al. Importance of intracranial atherosclerotic disease in patients with symptomatic stenosis of the internal carotid artery. The North American Symptomatic Carotid Endarterectomy Trial. *Stroke* 1999;30:282–286.
66. AbuRahma AF, Robinson P, Holt SM, et al. Perioperative and late stroke rates of carotid endarterectomy contralateral to carotid artery occlusion: results from randomized trial. *Stroke* 2000;31:1566–1571.
67. Young B, Moore WS, Robertson JT, et al. An analysis of perioperative surgical mortality and morbidity in the asymptomatic carotid atherosclerosis study. ACAS Investigators. Asymptomatic Carotid Atherosclerosis Study. *Stroke* 1996; 27:2216–2224 .
68. Fearn SJ, Parry AD, Picton A, et al. Should heparin be reversed after carotid endarterectomy? A randomised prospective trial. *Eur J Endovasc Surg* 1997;13:394–397.
69. Mora W, Hunter G, Malone J. Wound infection following carotid endarterectomy. *J Cardiovasc Surg* 1981;22:47–49.
70. Biller J, Baker WH, Quinn JP, et al. Intracranial hematoma with subsequent brain abscess after carotid endarterectomy. *Surg Neurol* 1985; 23:605–608.
71. Executive Committee for the Asymptomatic Carotid Atherosclerosis Study. Endarterectomy for asymptomatic carotid artery stenosis. *JAMA* 1995;273:1421–1428.
72. Hertzer NR, Feldman BJ, Bevin EG. A prospective study of the incidence of injury to the cranial nerves during carotid endarterectomy. *Surg Gynecol Obstetr* 1980;151:781–784.
73. Rogers W, Root HD. Cranial nerve injuries after carotid endarterectomy. *South Med J* 1988;81: 1006–1009.
74. Forsell C, Kitzing P, Bergqvist D. Cranial nerve injuries after carotid artery surgery. A prospective study of 663 operations. *Eur J Vasc Endovasc Surg* 1995;10:445–449.
75. Hertzer NR, Beven EG, Young JR, et al. Coronary artery disease in peripheral vascular patients. A classification of 1000 coronary angiograms and results of surgical management. *Ann Surg* 1984;199: 223–233.
76. Riles TS, Kopelman I, Imparato AM. Myocardial infarction following carotid endarterectomy: a review of 683 operations. *Surgery* 1979;85:249–252.
77. Pritz MB. Timing of carotid endarterectomy after stroke. *Stroke* 1997;28:2563–2567.
78. Parrino PE, Lovelock M, Shockey KS, et al. Early carotid endarterectomy after stroke. *Cardiovasc Surg* 2000;8:116–120.
79. Hoffmann M, Robbs J. Carotid endarterectomy after recent cerebral infarction. *Eur J Vasc Endovasc Surg* 1999;18:6–10.
80. Power WJ, Derdeyn CP, Fritsch SM, et al. Benign prognosis of never-symptomatic carotid occlusion. *Neurology* 2000;54:878–882.
81. Iwama T, Hashimoto N, Takagi Y, et al. Predictability of extracranial/intracranial bypass function: a retrospective study of patients with occlusive cerebrovascular disease. *Neurosurgery* 1997;40:53–59.
82. Yonas H. Predictability of extracranial/intracranial bypass function. A retrospective study of patients with occlusive cerebrovascular disease. *Neurosurgery* 1997;41:1447–1448.
83. Grubb RL Jr, Derdeyn CP, Fritsch SM, et al. Importance of hemodynamic factors in the prognosis of symptomatic carotid occlusion. *JAMA* 1998;280:1055–1060.
84. Klijn CJ, Kappelle LJ, Tulleken CA, et al. Symptomatic carotid artery occlusion. A reappraisal of hemodynamic factors. *Stroke* 1997;28:2084–2093.
85. Yamauchi H, Fukuyama H, Nagahama Y. Significance of increased oxygen extraction fraction in five-year prognosis of major cerebral occlusive diseases. *J Nucl Med* 1999;40:1992–1998.
86. The EC/IC Bypass Study Group. Failure of extracranial-intracranial arterial bypass to reduce the risk of ischemic stroke. Results of an international randomized trial. *N Engl J Med* 1985;313:1191–1200.

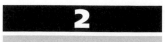

HISTORICAL BACKGROUND: 25 YEARS OF ENDOVASCULAR THERAPY FOR OBSTRUCTIVE CAROTID ARTERY DISEASE

KLAUS MATHIAS

Cerebrovascular disease is the third leading cause of death in Western countries, with an annual stroke rate of approximately 2.4% of the population. Moreover, it is the leading cause of adult disability. Carotid artery occlusive disease is responsible for about 25% of these strokes. The annual cost for treatment and lost productivity is estimated to be $30 billion in the United States. Large population-based studies indicate that the prevalence of carotid artery stenosis is about 0.5% in the sixth decade and increases to 10% in persons over 80 years of age. The majority of patients are asymptomatic.

Carotid endarterectomy (CEA) is currently accepted as the standard treatment for symptomatic carotid artery stenosis more than or equal to 50% (1). In the past two decades, endovascular techniques were developed and progressed to angioplasty and stent placement (2,3). This minimally invasive technique is gaining wider acceptance and is increasingly challenging the status of carotid surgery (4).

CAROTID REVASCULARIZATION

The first successful CEA was performed in 1953 by DeBakey (5), but the first written account detailing successful revascularization of the carotid artery was published in 1954 by Eastcott et al. (6). The number of CEAs increased steadily until the mid 1980s. Criticism appeared in the 1980s that the rates of perioperative strokes and deaths were unacceptably high and the indications often inappropriate. Between 1974 and 1985, approximately 1 million CEAs were performed worldwide with only anecdotal evidence of benefit. These unfavorable results stimulated critical neurologists and surgeons to start prospective, randomized clinical studies in Europe and the United States. Preliminary results of the European Carotid Surgery Trial (ECST) (7) and the North American Symptomatic Carotid Endarterectomy Trial (NASCET) (8) in 1991 showed a benefit of surgery compared to medical treatment alone in selected patients.

The ECST enrolled 3,024 patients stratified into 3 groups: 0% to 29%, 30% to 69%, and 70% to 99% carotid stenosis. The 3-year stroke or death risk in patients with a symptomatic stenosis of 80% or greater was reduced by CEA from 26.5% in the control group to 14.9% in the surgical group. The absolute risk reduction was 11.6% at 3 years. The rate of nonfatal stroke or death from surgery was 7% (7,9).

A total of 106 centers in the United States, Canada, Europe, and Australia participated in the NASCET trial. The 2,885 enrolled patients were divided into 2 groups according to the degree of stenosis. In 2,226 patients the diameter of stenosis was 30% to 60%, and in 659 patients it was 70% to 99% (8). High-risk patients were excluded from the trials (Table 2-1). The ipsilateral stroke incidence in the medical group was 26% and in the surgical group 9% within 2 years, yielding an absolute risk reduction of 17%. This means that in 100 patients, 17 strokes were prevented over a 2-year period. It was also shown that the benefit grows with the severity of stenosis. The risk reduction was twice as high in the patients with a degree of stenosis between 90% and 99% in comparison to those with a 70% to 79% stenosis. The long-term results emphasize the complexity of the treatment of carotid occlusive disease. At the 8-year follow-up, the risk of an ipsilateral disabling stroke was 6.7%, the risk of any ipsilateral stroke was 15.2%, the risk of any stroke was 29.4%, and the risk of any stroke and death was 46.6%. Despite the durability of CEA in preventing ipsilateral disabling stroke, the 8-year risk of stroke and death was nearly 50%. The complication rates for all 1,415 patients undergoing CEA (30% to 99% symptomatic stenosis) were recently reported (Table 2-2). The surgical risk was predictively increased in patients with irregular or ulcerated plaques, ipsilateral ischemic lesions on computed tomographic scans, hemispheric versus retinal transient ischemic attack as the qualifying event, and contralateral carotid occlusion.

Whereas there is proof of the benefit of CEA in preventing stroke in symptomatic patients under trial conditions, the evidence of risk reduction in patients with asymptomatic carotid artery stenosis is much less convincing. The only acceptable randomized controlled trial in patients with asymptomatic carotid stenosis comparing medical treatment and CEA is the Asymptomatic Carotid Atherosclerosis Study (ACAS), which enrolled 1,662 patients from 39 centers with a median follow-up of 2.7 years (10). The exclusion criteria were identical to NASCET. Patients in the medical group received 325 mg of aspirin daily. The ACAS trial calculated a 5-year risk for ipsilateral stroke or any perioperative stroke and death in patients with a carotid stenosis more than or equal to 60%, extrapolating the data of the 2.7-year follow-up. The patients undergoing surgery had an estimated risk of 5.1% versus 11% for patients who were medically treated. This is the equivalent of an absolute risk

TABLE 2-1. EXCLUSION CRITERIA FROM NASCET

Previous ipsilateral CEA
Severe intracranial lesion
Incomplete angiographic workup
Pulmonary failure
Renal failure
Hepatic failure
Uncontrolled diabetes mellitus
Hypertension
Unstable angina pectoris
Myocardial infarction within the preceding 6 mo
Contralateral CEA within the preceding 4 mo
Progressive neurological dysfunction
Major surgical procedure within the previous 30 d

NASCET, North American Symptomatic Carotid Endarterectomy Trial;
CEA, Carotid endarterectomy.

**TABLE 2-2. COMPLICATIONS OF
CAROTID SURGERY IN NASCET**

Complication	%
Perioperative death	—
Perioperative stroke	5.4
Stroke in contralateral occlusion	14.7
Perioperative wound complications	9.3
Perioperative cranial nerve damage	8.6
Medical complications	8.1
Myocardial infarction	—
Congestive heart failure	1.2
Hypotension	2.1

NASCET, North American Symptomatic Carotid
Endarterectomy Trial.

reduction of 5.9% (1.2% per year) or approximately one prevented stroke per year for every 85 patients operated on. When we count only the major strokes, the risk reduction decreases to 2.6%. A total of 170 patients with an asymptomatic carotid stenosis more than or equal to 60% must be surgically treated in order to prevent one disabling stroke. This result was obtained with a low 30-day morbidity and mortality of 2.3%. The stroke risk of female patients was not significantly reduced. Benefit and degree of stenosis did not correlate. One third of the neurological complications were due to angiography.

The Veterans Affairs Cooperative Study, with 444 recruited men with asymptomatic stenosis of 50% or more, could not demonstrate a statistically significant difference in the two groups during a follow-up of 47.9 months. The 30-day perioperative rate of permanent stroke or death was 4.7%, including a 0.4% stroke rate from diagnostic angiography. The ECST reported on the risk of stroke in 2,295 patients stratified into four groups: 0% to 29% stenosis, 1,270 patients; 30% to 60% stenosis, 843 patients; 70% to 99% stenosis, 127 patients; occlusion, 55 patients. The 3-year risk of ipsilateral stroke in patients with a 70% to 99 % stenosis was 5.7%, showing only a minor benefit of surgery in patients with a stenosis more than or equal to 80%.

The modest or missing benefit of CEA in asymptomatic patients, the low annual event rate in this group of patients, and the costs of surgery have stirred questions about the indications for CEA in asymptomatic carotid stenosis.

The risk of stroke or death due to CEA for symptomatic carotid stenosis was systematically reviewed by Rothwell et al. (1). The authors analyzed 51 studies performed between 1980 and 1996 and found an overall stroke and death rate of 5.64%. The results differed considerably when they were reported by neurologists (7.7%) or vascular surgeons (2.3%)(1). Wennberg et al. (11) assessed the perioperative mortality among 113,300 Medicare patients undergoing CEA in trial and nontrial hospitals for the years 1992 and 1993. The perioperative mortality rate was 1.4% at the trial hospitals versus 2.5% in the nontrial hospitals. Patients age 85 years and older were three times more likely to die from CEA than those younger than 70 years. From this observation, it can be concluded that trial results cannot be generalized, and everyday practice may show different, mostly worse, results (11).

CAROTID ARTERY ANGIOPLASTY AND STENTING

Percutaneous transluminal angioplasty (PTA) of the supraaortic arteries has been established in the last 25 years as an alternative procedure to surgical repair. After animal experiments in 1976 and 1977, the author and colleagues (2,3,12) treated the first carotid artery stenosis in a 32-year-old female patient suffering from fibromuscular dysplasia in 1979 and the first atherosclerotic stenosis in a symptomatic male patient in 1980. Balloon angioplasty had some limitations in atherosclerotic disease. In patients with morphologically presumably dangerous lesions, endovascular treatment seemed to be too risky to be offered to the patient as an alternative option to CEA. When we encountered an intimal flap after balloon angioplasty in 1989, we solved the problem with the placement of a self-expandable stent. The excellent result after stenting motivated us from 1989 onwards to place routinely self-expandable stents in the carotid artery. This addition to balloon angioplasty resulted in less residual stenosis, no plaque dissections, and no elastic recoil of the vessel wall. Using stents, complex carotid artery stenoses with ulceration and thrombus formation could be treated. With presently available devices, more than 95% of carotid artery stenoses can be treated successfully and with a very low risk by an endovascular approach (13).

Carotid artery disease has mainly an embolic and, in only about 5% of the patients, a hemodynamic pathophysiological background. Therefore, from the beginning of endovascular treatment of carotid artery stenosis, our major concern was the risk of embolization into the brain arteries with a consecutive stroke. To avoid this complication, we dilated the stenoses with undersized balloons with the intention to prevent plaque rupture and dissection. We accepted residual stenoses of 20% to 30%. Our attempts at cerebral protection with an umbrellalike filter in the 1980s failed because no manufacturer was interested in such a device. In 1984, Theron et al. (14) independently developed distal cerebral protection with balloons, which led to commercially available balloon protection devices. Also, the idea of blood filtering was revived, and different filter designs were developed with the aim of minimizing the risk of embolic cerebral damage. Today, more than half a dozen filters are available with profiles between 3.2 and 4 French and pore sizes between 80 and 150 μm. Kachel et al. (15) had the idea of proximal balloon protection in the 1990s, but it is through the work of Parodi that we have a ready product in the market. We changed our technique several times over the course of our experience: over-the-wire balloon dilatation, over-the-wire-stent angioplasty, coaxial technique with long sheaths and guiding catheters, routine use of cerebral protection, routine use of 0.014-inch guide wires, rapid exchange systems, and, presently, drug-eluting stents (16).

With the technical means of today, the success rate of CAS is in the range of 95% to 99%, with technical failure mainly due to an extremely elongated aortic arch. The complication rate is as least as low as in CEA, with a 30-day mortality rate of 0.5%; major strokes, 1%; and minor strokes, 1% to 3%. With arterial closure devices, the after-bleeding and groin hematomas are less than 1%. The long-term patency is astonishingly high in comparison to endovascular treatment in other regions of the arterial tree. Kaplan-Meier cumulative patency rates are about 90% after 5 years. The ipsilateral stroke rate within 5 years is less than 3%, which is in accordance with a risk reduction of about 90% (17).

The easy access to the lesion by endovascular techniques, the low complication rate, and the good primary and long-term results of the interventions have led to the wide and still increasing acceptance of the method. The patients favor CAS because it is less traumatic and shortens the hospital stay. The high-risk patients especially benefit from the gentle treatment of CAS.

REFERENCES

1. Rothwell PM, Slattery J, Warlow CP. A systematic review of the risks of stroke and death due to endarterectomy for symptomatic carotid stenosis. *Stroke* 1996;27:260–265.

2. Mathias K. Ein neuartiges Kathetersystem zur perkutanen transluminalen Angioplastie von Karotisstenosen. *Fortschr Med* 1977;95:1007–1011.

3. Mathias K, Mittermayer Ch, Ensinger H, et al. Perkutane Katheterdilatation von Karotisstenosen. *ROFO Fortschr Geb Röntgenstr Nuklearmed* 1980;133:258–261.

4. Zarin CK. Carotid endarterectomy: the gold standard. *J Endovasc Surg* 1966;3:10–15.

5. DeBakey ME. Carotid endarterectomy revisited. *J Endovasc Surg* 1996;3:4.

6. Eastcott HH, Pickering GW, Rob CG. Reconstruction of internal carotid artery in a patient with intermittent attacks of hemiplegia. *Lancet* 1954;267:994–996.

7. MRC European Carotid Surgery Trial: interim results for symptomatic patients with severe (70-99%) or mild (0-29%) carotid stenosis. European Carotid Surgery Trialists Collaborative Group. *Lancet* 1991;337:1235–1243.

8. Beneficial effect of carotid endarterectomy in symptomatic patients with high-grade carotid stenosis. North American Symptomatic Carotid Endarterectomy Trial Colloborators. *N Engl J Med* 1991;325: 445–453.

9. Randomised trial of endarterectomy for recently symptomatic carotid stenosis: final results of the MRC European Carotis Surgery Trial (ECST). *Lancet* 1998;351:1379–1387.

10. Endarterectomy for asymptomatic carotid artery stenosis. Executive Committee for the Asymptomatic Carotid Atherosclerosis Study. *JAMA* 1995;273:1421–1428.

11. Wennberg DE, Lucas FL, Birkmeyer JD, et al. Variation in carotid endarterectomy mortality in the Medicare population: trial hospitals, volume, and patient characteristics. *JAMA* 1998;279:1278–1281.

12. Mathias K. Perkutane transluminale Katheterbehandlung supraaortaler Arterienobstruktionen. *Angio* 1981;3:47–50.

13. Wholey MH, Wholey M, Bergeron P, et al. Current global status of carotid artery stent placement. *Cathet Cardiovasc Diagn* 1998;44:1–6.

14. Theron JG, Payelle GG, Coskun O, et al. Carotid artery stenosis: treatment with protected balloon angioplasty and stent placement. *Radiology* 1996;201:627–636.

15. Kachel R, Basche S, Heerklotz I, et al. Percutaneous transluminal angioplasty (PTA) of supra-aortic arteries especially the internal carotid artery. *Neuroradiology* 1991;33:191–194.

16. Jäger H, Mathias KD, Drescher R, et al. Zerebrale Protektion mit Ballonokklusion bei der Stentimplantation der A. carotis—erste Erfahrungen. *Fortschr Röntgenstr* 2001;173:139–146.

17. Mathias K, Jäger H, Hennigs S, et al. Endoluminal treatment of internal carotid artery stenosis. *World J Surg* 2001;25:328–336.

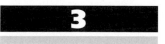

EVIDENCE-BASED EFFICACY IN PREVENTING STROKE

SUMAIRA MACDONALD
TREVOR J. CLEVELAND
PETER A. GAINES

The introduction of a novel procedure intended to be a less invasive alternative to an established surgical technique will gain acceptance only if it is as least as good as the surgery it is intended to replace. This mandates the accrual of sufficient evidence to effectively compare the alternative treatments. However, the evaluation of a new surgical technique or of a novel procedure that may replace it has not usually followed the protocols set for the introduction of a new drug, which is evaluated over a protracted timeline after extensive bench-top and animal work.

Carotid artery stenting (CAS) has recently emerged as an endovascular, and therefore potentially less invasive, alternative to carotid endarterectomy (CEA). Neither endarterectomy nor stenting underwent extensive bench-top or animal studies before introduction into use in humans, and although with time thousands of patients were treated by angioplasty or stenting and indeed millions by endarterectomy, they were largely treated outside of randomized trials.

In 1951, a patient with symptomatic thrombosis of the internal carotid artery (ICA) underwent surgical intervention with carotid-carotideal anastomosis (1). Following this, a patient with symptoms suggesting that a stroke was imminent underwent successful removal of a stenosed segment of the carotid artery (2). From that initial experience, endarterectomy evolved and was performed without convincing evidence to support the practice for nearly 40 years. Two randomized trials with poor outcomes were reported (3,4), yet despite this, and on the basis of anecdotal evidence, over 1 million endarterectomies were performed worldwide between 1974 and 1985 alone (5,6). Reflecting a paradigm shift in the way in which medicine was practiced, towards an evidence-based approach, endarterectomy was subsequently trialed in a randomized fashion. Three landmark trials reported outcomes in the 1990s and have been hugely influential, directing practice and justifying intervention in both symptomatic and, to a lesser extent, asymptomatic carotid stenosis (7–9). These were tightly controlled trials performed in centers of excellence by preselected high-volume surgeons who were allowed to participate only after proof of a low perioperative stroke and death rate. A number of patients were excluded on the grounds of anatomy or comorbidity. There were thus some limitations of these trials with respect to the fact that their outcomes could not necessarily be extrapolated to the general patient population or to the community hospital setting. On the basis of these trials, and despite some concerns about generalizability, CEA became the standard of care.

Following earlier innovations in peripheral and coronary percutaneous transluminal angioplasty, carotid angioplasty was first reported in 1980, albeit as a combined surgical and endovascular procedure. Proximal common carotid angioplasty was performed via carotid cutdown with concomitant bifurcation endarterectomy (10). Just over 20 years later, the first completed randomized trial comparing carotid angioplasty (with or without stenting) to CEA reported immediate and intermediate-term outcomes (conducted by investigators of the Carotid and Vertebral Artery Transluminal Angioplasty Study, or CAVATAS) (11). The relative speed with which this new procedure went from first report to first randomized trial reflects a number of things: (a) it had to compete with a reasonably well-evaluated gold standard; (b) the pioneering efforts of the interventionists involved were highly influential; and (c) the prevailing milieu of evidence-based practice was a significant factor.

This chapter focuses on the available evidence in support of the efficacy of carotid stenting in preventing future ipsilateral stroke. There is a body of evidence supporting the safety of stenting, a proportion of it level 1, but longer-term stroke prophylaxis is the parameter that is now of paramount importance in directing future recommendations.

CURRENT RECOMMENDATIONS FOR CAROTID STENTING

To date, recommendations with respect to carotid stenting have been based on the outcomes from the earliest randomized trials comparing endarterectomy and the endovascular approach. Two such trials were prematurely stopped (12,13), and the two completed trials were ongoing (11,14) when a number of the recommendations were made.

It is important to note that there has been substantial evolutionary change in the technique of percutaneous carotid intervention during the time frame of the reported randomized trials. The endovascular limb of the CAVATAS trial is hardly recognizable as current endovascular practice. Patients were primarily balloon angioplastied. Stents were used in only 26%, and procedures were performed without contemporary pharmacological support or cerebral protection. Modifications include a move towards primary stenting, the development of dedicated stents, lower profile balloons, coronary-type guide wires, the development of Anti-Embolization devices and closure devices for the femoral puncture site, and advances in the periprocedural antiplatelet regimen. Many of these changes are expected to further reduce the procedural adverse event rate, and this should be manifested in the outcomes of ongoing trials.

Current recommendations are given in Table 3-1.

The American Heart Association Science Advisory Councils' statements with respect to carotid stenting and angioplasty dating from 1998 (15) are as follows:

> "Despite several large studies...there is still debate about its relative efficacy and applicability compared with surgery, primarily because long-term patency after PTA (angioplasty) is limited by restenosis...."

The final statement of this document was:

> "The techniques of carotid angioplasty and carotid stenting are available, as are a limited degree of experience and a high level of interest. The existence of a technique, however, does not justify or mandate its use. We must remember a basic tenet of medicine: *primum non nocere*—first do no harm. At this point, with few exceptions, use of carotid stenting should be limited to well-designed, well-controlled randomized studies with careful, dispassionate oversight."

In the year 2000 (16), a Cochrane systematic review on percutaneous transluminal angioplasty and stenting for carotid artery stenosis concluded:

TABLE 3-1. CURRENT RECOMMENDATIONS FOR PRACTICE

Recommending Body	Year of Recommendation	Recommendation
American Heart Association (15)	1998	CAS should be limited to well-designed, well-controlled randomized studies with careful, dispassionate oversight
Cochrane systematic review (16)	2000	There is no evidence as yet to assess the relative effects of carotid PTA in people with carotid stenosis
Consensus of opinion leaders (17)	2001	CAS should not undergo widespread practice, which should await results of randomized trials. CAS is currently appropriate treatment for patients at high risk in experienced centers. CAS is not generally appropriate for patients at low risk
Intercollegiate Working Party for Stroke (18)	2002	CAS is an alternative to surgery but should only be carried out in centers with a proven low complication rate
European Stroke Initiative Committee (19)	2003	The use of CAS should be limited to well-designed, well-conducted randomized trials: 1. Carotid PTA may be performed for patients with contraindications to CEA or with stenosis at inaccessible sites (Level IV) 2. Carotid PTA/stenting may be indicated for patients with restenosis after initial CEA or stenosis following radiation (Level IV)

CAS, carotid artery stenting; PTA, percutaneous transluminal angioplasty; CEA, carotid endarterectomy.

"There is no evidence as yet to assess the relative effects of carotid percutaneous transluminal angioplasty in people with carotid stenosis."

CAVATAS (10) and the Lexington trial (13) were yet to report.

In 2001, in a document on the current status of carotid bifurcation angioplasty and stenting based on a consensus of opinion leaders (17), it was concluded:

"Carotid bifurcation angioplasty and stenting should not undergo widespread practice, which should await results of randomized trials. Carotid bifurcation angioplasty and stenting is currently appropriate treatment for patients at high risk in experienced centers. Carotid bifurcation angioplasty is not generally appropriate for patients at low risk."

There were divergent opinions regarding the proportions of patients presently acceptable for stenting, ranging from 5% to 100% with a mean of 44%.

In 2002, an Intercollegiate Working Party for Stroke (Royal College of Physicians, London, United Kingdom) produced guidelines on secondary stroke prevention as part of the National Clinical Guidelines for Stroke (18). It was stated that:

"Carotid angioplasty or stenting is an alternative to surgery but should only be carried out in centers with a proven low complication rate."

This was a grade A recommendation and reflects an early subtle change in emphasis. There was no stipulation that carotid stenting must be limited to trials or to patients deemed to be at high surgical risk.

The most recent documented recommendations date from 2003, from the *European Stroke Initiative Recommendations for Stroke Management-Update 2003* (19), and these recommendations are more restrictive than the UK Working Party guidelines (18). With respect to asymptomatic disease it was stated:

> "Carotid angioplasty, with or without stenting, is not routinely recommended for patients with asymptomatic carotid stenosis. It may be considered in the context of randomized clinical trials."

With respect to symptomatic disease, it was concluded that:

> "The use of carotid angioplasty and stenting should be limited to well-designed, well-conducted, randomized trials."

The specific recommendations were:

1. Carotid percutaneous transluminal angioplasty may be performed for patients with contraindications to endarterectomy or with stenosis at surgically inaccessible sites (level IV).
2. Carotid percutaneous transluminal angioplasty and stenting may be indicated for patients with restenosis after initial endarterectomy or stenosis following radiation (level IV).
3. Patients should receive a combination of clopidogrel and aspirin immediately before, during, and at least 1 month after stenting (level IV).

LEVEL-1 EVIDENCE SUPPORTING THE SAFETY OF CAROTID ANGIOPLASTY OR STENTING

The completed randomized trials include CAVATAS (11) and the Lexington trial set in a community hospital (14). Both trials reported fully in 2001.

CAVATAS was a multicenter clinical trial that randomized 504 patients with symptomatic carotid artery stenosis that the investigators "believed needed treatment" between endovascular and surgical treatments. In the endovascular limb, stents were used in 26% of cases. At 30 days, the rates of major outcome events within 30 days of first treatment did not differ significantly between endovascular and surgical treatment (6.4% versus 5.9%, respectively, for disabling stroke or death; 10% versus 9.9% for any stroke lasting more than 7 days, or death). Cranial neuropathy was reported after endarterectomy (8.7%) but not after endovascular treatment ($p < 0.0001$). Major groin or neck hematoma occurred less often after endovascular treatment than after surgery (1.2% versus 6.7%, $p < 0.0015$). The conclusions were that carotid surgery and angioplasty were equivalent in safety and efficacy, but that angioplasty had advantages with respect to nerve injury and cardiac complications (20). Detractors of this study would point out that the confidence intervals were wide and that the surgical event rate was higher than expected. The authors conceded that a clinically important difference in favor of either treatment could not be ruled out. With respect to the surgical event rate, it was concluded that the surgeons and anesthesiologists involved in CAVATAS were likely to have had similar skills and used similar techniques to those in the North American Symptomatic Carotid Endarterectomy Trial (NASCET); indeed, many CAVATAS centers had collaborated in the European Carotid Surgery Trial (ECST) and NASCET. The rate of non–stroke-related adverse events in CAVATAS and NASCET were very similar. The high morbidity rate in both limbs of the trial was attributed to the inclusion of patients at higher risk than average from treatment; case mix is known to be an important factor in surgical risk (21). The great strength of CAVATAS, apart from its randomized design, was the independent neurological review, common to NASCET and ECST but often lacking in many self-audited single-center experiences. The addition of a neurologist to the authorship of a paper evaluating outcomes following endarterectomy significantly increases the reported neurological event rate (22).

The Lexington trial randomized 104 patients with symptomatic carotid artery stenosis more than 70% (NASCET criteria) to carotid stenting versus endarterectomy. There was one death (from myocardial infarction) following endarterectomy and one transient ischemic attack (TIA) (following stenting). In the surgical limb, four surgical patients suffered peripheral neurological injury, and one had a neck hematoma requiring surgical intervention. Primary stenting was performed after routine predilatation without cerebral protection but with a dual antiplatelet regimen. The conclusions were that carotid stenting was equivalent to endarterectomy in reducing carotid stenosis without increased risk for major complications of death or stroke. Stenting was also considered to potentially challenge endarterectomy because of the shortened hospitalization and convalescence, if a reduction in costs could be achieved.

A systematic review published in 2000 and evaluating articles published between 1990 and 1999 concluded that the risk of stroke was significantly greater with angioplasty than with endarterectomy (7.1% versus 4%) (23). It is unfortunate that, as a systematic review, this comment may have considerable influence, as such reviews are expected to seek out the highest levels of evidence. However, this review was not prepared for the Cochrane Collaboration, and the studies included were nonrandomized, heterogeneous, sometimes single-center, and often self-audited. The reviewers did not assess the quality of the included studies, dual independent review was lacking, and there was no discussion of consistency, just a pooling and/or averaging of results. The patient populations treated by angioplasty and endarterectomy were different. Endovascular treatments were also heterogeneous. In short, this was a limited review that provided little clarification.

Some attention ought to be paid to the uncompleted trials. In a Cochrane review evaluating only level-1 evidence, stopped, unreported, and unpublished trials would necessarily all contribute to the final body of evidence.

The Wallstent trial (13) was stopped after only 219 patients out of the proposed 700 were recruited, and it aimed to compare carotid stenting and endarterectomy in patients with high-grade symptomatic carotid disease. The event rate in the stenting group was unacceptably high with an ipsilateral stroke, procedure-related death, or vascular death rate at 1 year of 12.1% versus 3.6% for endarterectomy ($p = 0.02$). Primary stenting was performed without Anti-Embolization, and the Wallstent was not a dedicated carotid device. Work from the Sheffield Vascular Institute demonstrated a significant reduction in the combined death or any neurological event rate when a dedicated stent was used in preference to a stent adapted from peripheral or coronary designs (8.9% versus 22.2%, $p = 0.05$) (10). Lastly, it is not clear whether the study was stopped owing to poor results or poor recruitment. The Leicester trial (12), which randomized patients with high-grade disease between surgery and stenting, was expected to recruit 300 patients but was stopped after only 17 had been treated because of an unacceptable complication rate in the stenting limb. Ten endarterectomies were performed without complication, but five of the seven patients undergoing stenting suffered a stroke. The structure of this study deserves special mention because the outcomes were so disparate compared with those of other centers. No prior imaging of the origin of the major vessels was undertaken to exclude disease that would ordinarily constitute a contraindication to an endovascular approach. Only a single antiplatelet agent was employed prior to carotid stenting, whereas major units were already recommending combining aspirin with clopidogrel or ticlopidine (24). The interventionist had performed only eight prior carotid procedures, most of these outside of an experienced unit, whereas the surgeons involved had considerable expertise. Predilatation was not routine, and it is observed from the data that of five of the cases in which there was failed initial passage of the stent, four suffered a stroke. A nondedicated Wallstent was used. It is clearly not possible to pass a 7F device (2.3 mm) through a 70% stenosis (best residual channel of 1.8 mm) without some uncontrolled plaque disruption. Anti-Embolization was not used.

Currently, a number of trials and registries are ongoing and hopefully will provide clinicians with further reliable data (Table 3-2). The Carotid Revascularization Endarterectomy Versus Stenting Trial (CREST), the International Carotid Stenting Study (ICSS or CAVATAS-II), Stent-protected Percutaneous Angioplasty of the Carotid Versus Endarterectomy (SPACE), and the Endarterectomy Versus Angioplasty in Patients with Severe Symptomatic Carotid Stenosis (EVA-3S) study are all multicenter randomized trials comparing carotid stenting and endarterectomy for symptomatic patients.

TABLE 3-2. ONGOING TRIALS AND REGISTRIES

Acronym	Title	Details
CREST	The Carotid Revascularization Endarterectomy Versus Stenting Trial	Multicenter RCT comparing CAS versus CEA in symptomatic high-grade carotid artery stenosis. Based in the U.S.
ICSS (CAVATAS II)	The International Carotid Stenting Study	Multicenter RCT comparing CAS versus CEA in symptomatic high-grade carotid artery stenosis. Based in the U.K.
SPACE	Stent-protected Percutaneous Angioplasty of the Carotid Versus Endarterectomy	Multicenter RCT comparing CAS versus CEA in symptomatic high-grade carotid artery stenosis. Based in Germany
EVA-S3	Endarterectomy versus angioplasty in patients with severe symptomatic carotid stenosis	Multicenter RCT comparing CAS versus CEA in symptomatic high-grade carotid artery stenosis. Based in France
SAPPHIRE[a]	Stenting and angioplasty with protection in patients at high risk for endarterectomy	RCT comparing CAS and CEA in patients at high surgical risk
CARESS	Carotid Revascularization with Endarterectomy or Stenting Systems	Registry to include patients excluded from CREST and to include some asymptomatic patients. Outcomes will be compared with registries of CEA undertaken at the study sites
SECURITY	Registry Study to Evaluate the NeuroShield Bare Wire Cerebral Protection System and X-Act Stent in Patients at High Risk for Carotid Endarterectomy	Registry of protected carotid stenting in surgically high-risk patients
ARCHER	ACCULINK for Revascularization of Carotids in High-Risk Patients	Registry of carotid stenting in surgically high-risk patients

[a]SAPPHIRE has now finished recruiting and 12-month outcomes have been presented.
RCT, randomized controlled trial; CAS, carotid artery stenting; PTA, percutaneous transluminal angioplasty; CEA, carotid endarterectomy.

The Stenting and Angioplasty with Protection in Patients at High Risk for Endarterectomy (SAPPHIRE) study was a randomized trial comparing carotid stenting and endarterectomy in those considered to be at high surgical risk. This has recently been completed and the 12-month results presented, showing a definitive advantage of stenting.

Carotid Revascularization with Endarterectomy or Stenting Systems (CARESS) is an observational study designed to include those patients excluded from CREST and include some asymptomatic patients. It is a registry, and the outcomes will be compared with those from a registry of endarterectomy undertaken at the study sites. The Registry Study to Evaluate the NeuroShield Bare Wire Anti-Embolization System and X-Act Stent in Patients at High Risk for Carotid Endarterectomy (SECURITY) and ACCULINK for Revascularization of Carotids in High-Risk Patients (ARCHER) are registries evaluating protected carotid stenting in surgically high-risk patients.

NON–LEVEL-1 EVIDENCE SUPPORTING THE SAFETY OF CAROTID ANGIOPLASTY OR STENTING

Large-series experience has gradually accrued within high-throughput centers, and the reported outcomes are favorable but do highlight the influence of both learning curve and the technological advances on the event rate. Many show a reduction in adverse event rates in more recently treated patients. Roubin et al. (25) performed a prospective evaluation in 528 patients, both symptomatic and asymptomatic. There was a 0.6% fatal stroke rate, a 1% non–stroke-death rate, a 1% major stroke rate, and a 4.8% minor stroke rate at 30 days. The overall 30-day stroke and death rate was 7.4%, but this improved from 7.1% for the first year (1994) to 3.1% for the fifth year (1999). Cremonesi et al. (26) evaluated 442 symptomatic and asymptomatic patients between 1999 and 2002. Cerebral protection was utilized for all cases. The all-stroke and death rate at 30 days was 1.1%. The Sheffield experience of 333 symptomatic patients was recently reported (27). At 30 days, the total major disabling stroke and all death rate was 3%. This outcome measure was chosen because it was thought to best reflect the net overall benefit of therapy according to a recent Cochrane systematic review on endarterectomy for symptomatic carotid stenosis (28). If the all stroke and death rate is considered, subset analysis shows a 7% event rate for angioplasty alone, 10% for stenting (largely adapted stent designs), and 5.2% for stenting (largely dedicated) with cerebral protection. Independent review was performed in these studies. A survey reporting outcomes of 12,392 carotid stent procedures worldwide (11,243 patients) demonstrated a combined all-stroke and procedure-related death rate of 4.75% (29). This was largely self-audited and comprised both symptomatic and asymptomatic patients, thus some caution must be exercised in the interpretation of this study. What is evident from the current available literature is that event rates from stenting may be comfortably below those recommended by the American Heart Association for endarterectomy (30).

EFFICACY AT PREVENTING FUTURE STROKE: LEVEL-1 EVIDENCE

At present, there are limited data on long-term outcomes following carotid stenting arising from randomized trials. Essentially, these data comprise the results of CAVATAS and the Lexington trial. There have been some concerns on the restenosis rate following carotid angioplasty or stenting. However, some important factors should be appreciated. First, the majority of patients treated within the endovascular limb of CAVATAS underwent angioplasty alone. Angioplasty may provide a less definitive lumen initially compared to stenting and may result in greater immediate recoil—this is not true restenosis as caused by neointimal hyperplasia or atheromatous disease progression. Secondly, there may be very different true restenosis rates following primary stenting compared to angioplasty due to the difference in mechanism of vascular wall injury. The pragmatic approach to restenosis is to consider the clinical relevance. Neointimal hyperplasia is not generally accepted to be an emboligenic surface, and the rationale for treatment in the carotid artery is for embolic risk and not, in the majority, for hypoperfusion. Asymptomatic restenosis is likely, therefore, to be of no clinical relevance.

At 1 year after treatment in CAVATAS, severe (70% to 99%) ipsilateral carotid stenosis was more usual after endovascular treatment than surgery (14% versus 4%, $p<0.001$), but symptomatic restenosis was low in both groups. Results from the survival analysis showed that both surgery and endovascular treatment were equally effective at preventing stroke

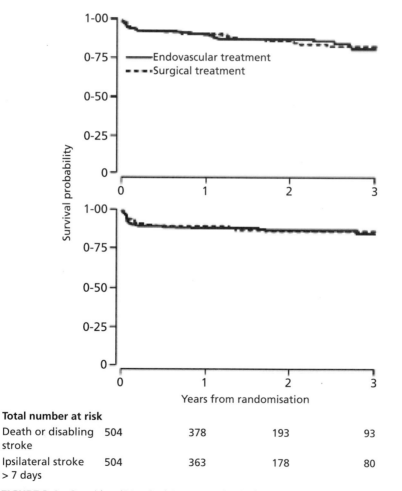

CAVATAS survival free of ipsilateral stroke:

Total number at risk			
Death or disabling stroke	504	378	193	93
Ipsilateral stroke > 7 days	504	363	178	80

FIGURE 3-1. Carotid and Vertebral Artery Transluminal Angioplasty Study (CAVA-TAS) survival free of ipsilateral stroke: death or disabling stroke in any vascular territory (*upper*) or ipsilateral stroke lasting more than 7 days (*lower*).

(Fig. 3-1). At the 3-year follow-up, the rate of death or disabling stroke (any territory) including treatment-related events was 14.3% in the endovascular group and 14.2% in the surgery patients. Survival analyses were done by Cox's proportional hazards regression, with adjustment for gender, age, and trial center. For any disabling stroke or death, the hazards ratio (endovascular treatment or surgery) was 1.03 (95% CI 0.64–1.64, $p = 0.09$). Secondary analyses were done for two other survival outcomes. For ipsilateral stroke lasting more than 7 days, the hazards ratio was 1.04 (0.63–1.70, $p = 0.9$). For disabling or fatal ipsilateral stroke, with other causes of treatment-related death excluded, the hazard ratio was 1.22 (0.63–2.36, $p = 0.4$).

NASECT reported a 15.8% 2-year any stroke or death rate and an 8% major stroke or death rate. The intermediate and longer-term outcomes from the surgical trials are given in Table 3-3, and the results following endovascular treatment are given in Table 3-4.

TABLE 3-3. INTERMEDIATE AND LONGER-TERM OUTCOMES FROM THE SURGICAL TRIALS

Trial	Follow-up Duration	Endpoint	Incidence	Restenosis	Asymptomatics Included?
NASCET (43) (70–99% stenosis subgroup)	5 yr	Disabling ipsilateral stroke	5.1%		No
		Ipsilateral stroke	13%		
		Any stroke	22.3%		
		Any stroke or death	31%		
	8 yr	Disabling ipsilateral stroke	6.7%		
		Ipsilateral stroke	15.2%		
		Any stroke	29.4%		
		Any stroke or death	46.6%		
ACAS (44)	Immediately postoperative			>60% on duplex at 95% PPV 4.1% (residual disease)	
	3–18 mo			7.6%	
	18–60 mo		5.9% reoperated (0.7% symptomatic)	1.9%	
ECST (45) (80–99% stenosis subgroup)	3 yr	Ipsilateral major stroke	2%		No
		Other major strokes	2.9%		
		Any major stroke/death	14.9%		

Figures exclude procedural events. The figures for NACSET are point estimates of the risks of each event. The aggregate incidence of residual/recurrent stenosis for all time intervals was 12.7% to 20.4% depending on whether the 90% or 95% PPV confidence interval was used.
NASCET, North American Symptomatic Carotid Endarterectomy Trial; ACAS, Asymptomatic Carotid Atherosclerosis Study; ECST, European Carotid Surgery Trial; PPV, positive predictive value.

TABLE 3-4. INTERMEDIATE AND LONGER-TERM OUTCOMES FROM CAROTID ANGIOPLASTY/STENTING TRIALS, REGISTRIES AND LARGER SERIES

Trial Series	Intervention	Duration of Follow-up	Endpoint	Rate of Outcome Event	Restenosis	Independent Review	Asymptomatic Patients Included
CAVATAS (11)	PTA/stent CEA	3 yr	Death/disabling stroke, any territory	14.3% 14.2%	(70–99%) 14% (70–99%) 4%	Yes	No
SAPPHIRE (31)	Protected stenting CEA	1 yr	MI/any stroke/death	11.9% 19.9%		Yes	Yes
Wholey et al. registry (29)	Stent	3 yr	All stroke/stroke-related death	1.7%	(>50%) 2.4%	No	Yes
Roubin et al. (25)	Stent	3 yr	Fatal and nonfatal stroke[a]	11% (symptomatic) 14% (asymptomatic)		Yes	Yes
McKevitt et al. (27)	PTA/stent	1 yr	All stroke Ipsilateral stroke	2.8% 0.8%	(>50%) 17.7% (>70%) 6.7% (100%) 2.9% (70–100%) 15.5%	Yes	No
Ahmadi et al. (35)	Stent	1 yr	All stroke Ipsilateral stroke	0.7% 0.3%	(>70%) 3%	Yes	Yes
Gray et al. (34)	Stent	2 yr	Ipsilateral stroke (including procedural) Ipsilateral stroke (major)	3.9% 1.3% 0%	(>50%) 4.8%	Yes	Yes
Cremonesi et al. (36)	PTA/stent	3 yr (6–36 mo)	All stroke Stroke mortality	6.7% 0%	(>50%) 5.04%	Yes	Yes
Becquemin et al. (37) (prospective cohort study)	Stent CEA	3 yr	Minor persistent stroke Major ipsilateral stroke Minor persistent stroke Major ipsilateral stroke	2.6% 1.8% 1.4% 0.5%	(>50%) 7.5% 1.4%	Yes	Yes

[a]Fatal and nonfatal stroke were chosen by Roubin et al. as the most appropriate outcome measure rather than stroke and all-cause mortality. This choice was made because selection criteria in trials of CEA often precluded life-threatening illnesses such as cancer, lung disease, and coronary ischemia, whereas these factors did not exclude patients from carotid stenting. Survival analysis in terms of all-cause mortality for carotid stenting may therefore reflect levels of comorbidity rather than efficacy of technique.

CAVATAS, Carotid and Vertebral Artery Transluminal Angioplasty Study; SAPPHIRE, Stenting and Angioplasty with Protection in Patients at High Risk for Endarterectomy; PTA, percutaneuous transluminal angioplasty; CEA, carotid endarterectomy; MI, myocardial infarction

The conclusion, therefore, is that the ability of carotid angioplasty or stenting to prevent stroke is the same as that of endarterectomy.

Provisional analysis of further follow-up data suggests that the benefit of carotid angioplasty or stenting persists for up to 8 years following treatment to a similar degree to that of endarterectomy.

Patients treated within the Lexington trial (14) have reported follow-up for 24 months to date. There were no strokes in either treatment limb within this period of follow-up and no evidence of asymptomatic focal cerebral ischemia on magnetic resonance imaging (MRI). The 24-month patency of the reconstructed artery was reported as "satisfactory" as determined by carotid ultrasound.

Twelve-month results have now been presented for the SAPPHIRE trial (31). In this population, deemed to be at high surgical risk, the 12-month major adverse event rate was 11.9% in patients randomized to stent plus a filter Anti-Embolization device compared with 19.9% in patients randomized to endarterectomy. Individual endpoints showed comparable or better results for stented patients versus surgically treated patients (death: 6.9% versus 12.6%, $p = 0.12$; stroke: 5.7% versus 7.3%, $p = 0.65$; myocardial infarction: 2.5% versus 7.9%, $p = 0.04$).

EFFICACY AT PREVENTING FUTURE STROKE: NON–LEVEL-1 EVIDENCE

There is a growing body of level-2 evidence providing data on the efficacy of stenting at preventing ipsilateral stroke in the intermediate term. There are some sizeable single-center series with independent review for 3 to 5 years.

In an updated review on the global carotid stent registry, Wholey et al. (29) reported 12,392 carotid stenting procedures in 11,243 patients. The patient population included patients with asymptomatic carotid stenoses. As a voluntary registry, this often included self-audited data. A total of 9,419 (85%) patients have been followed-up to date. The rates of restenosis, as assessed by duplex, greater than 50% were 2.7%, 2.6%, 2.4%, and 5.6% at 12, 36, and 48 months, respectively. It was accepted that there might have been errors in these determinations because of the inability to apply a Kaplan-Meier curve to each center. New ipsilateral neurological events (including TIAs, minor strokes, major strokes, and neurologic-related deaths) were reported for the 9,419 patients followed for the 4-year period. The rates for 12, 24, 36, and 48 months were 1.2%, 1.3%, 1.7%, and 4.5%, respectively.

Mathias and Jaeger (32) presented outcomes from 1,136 endovascular carotid procedures, reporting a sixth-month restenosis rate of 1.9% and a 5-year patency on duplex of 92%. Asymptomatic patients were treated and the series was independently reviewed.

Roubin et al. (25) followed 528 patients who had had carotid stents (604 arteries). Asymptomatic patients were included, and the outcomes were independently reviewed. Outside the 30-day procedural period, the incidence of late fatal and nonfatal stroke was 3.2%. The 3-year freedom from all fatal and nonfatal strokes was 88 ± 2% (mean ± standard error). Of those surviving the 30-day period, the 3-year freedom from all fatal and nonfatal strokes was 95 ± 2%. With respect to ipsilateral stroke after 30 days, the 3-year survival for fatal and nonfatal stroke was 99 ± 1%. A significant difference in outcomes was found in those over 80 years of age. The 3-year freedom from all fatal and nonfatal strokes including and excluding 30-day periprocedural period for less than 80 versus more than 80 years of age was 90 ± 2% versus 73 ± 4% ($p<0.0001$) and 95 ± 2% versus 91 ± 1% ($p<0.01$).

There were no differences in outcomes between men and women or between symptomatic and asymptomatic patients. Survival curves to 3 years in this series demonstrate an 11% rate of fatal and nonfatal stroke.

There is intermediate-term data from Wholey et al. at the Pittsburgh Vascular Institute (33). The purpose of their work was to compare the rates of neurological complications and restenosis for balloon-mounted and self-expanding stents. Of 496 patients, 247 (48%) received balloon-mounted stents and 273 (52%) self-expanding stents. Asymptomatic patients were included, and the series was independently reviewed. During a mean follow-up of 20.6 months (range up to 5.6 years), the 3-year freedom from all fatal and ipsilateral nonfatal strokes excluding the 30-day periprocedural period was 95% for balloon-mounted and 95.2% for self-expanding stents. Vessel patency (more than 50%) at 3 years was 92% in the population, 96.3% for balloon-mounted stents, and 83.7% for self-expanding stents ($p = 0.04$). One of the paper's conclusions was that vessel patency was excellent at 3 years, being slightly better in balloon-mounted stents, but that because of their vulnerability to compression, balloon-mounted stents would not replace self-expanding stents.

Of 333 procedures performed at the Sheffield Vascular Institute (27), 277 were eligible for 1-year follow-up. This series was homogeneous with respect to patients' symptoms (all were symptomatic) and lesion characteristics (all were atherosclerotic lesions more than or equal to 70% by NASCET criteria), but heterogeneous with respect to endovascular procedure. The series spanned developments in technique and included angioplasty alone, primary stenting with adapted and then with dedicated carotid stents, and latterly stenting with cerebral protection. Of those eligible for 1-year review, 29 were lost to follow-up; therefore, 248 procedures were reviewed. After the 30-day periprocedural time period, the all-stroke rate at 1 year was 2.8% (n = 7) and the ipsilateral all-stroke rate was 0.8% (n = 2). In addition, one patient had a suboptimal balloon dilatation and, on the repeat procedure, had a procedural nondisabling ipsilateral stroke. One-year duplex examination was available for 238 procedures. Forty-two patients (17.6%) had more than 50% restenosis or total occlusion, 6.7% (n = 16) had more than or equal to 70% restenosis or total occlusion, and 2.9% (n = 7) had a total occlusion. Twenty-one patients were documented as having a 50% to 79% stenosis. Therefore the 70% to 100% restenosis rate was 15.5% (n = 37) in this series.

Gray et al. (34) retrospectively reviewed 136 endarterectomies and 136 carotid stenting procedures at a tertiary-care community hospital. There was independent review of outcomes, and asymptomatic patients were included. Information on restenosis and late ipsilateral stroke for the stent group was available at the 2-year follow-up. At 6 months, Doppler velocities suggested significant restenosis (peak systolic velocity more than or equal to 2.5 m per second) in eight treated arteries. Subsequent angiography in these patients demonstrated restenosis (more than 50% diameter) in only four (3.1%), and in these cases, the peak systolic velocity was more than or equal to 3.4 m per second. Three of these patients had repeat percutaneous intervention, and one patient had endarterectomy with stent explantation; there were no clinical events arising from these secondary procedures. Between the 6- and 12-month evaluations, two additional stents had progression of neointimal hyperplasia on Doppler ultrasound. One of these patients presented with ipsilateral minor stroke and had repeat percutaneous intervention, and the remaining patient was asymptomatic. All 136 were followed to 6 months, 121 were followed to 12 months, and 78 to 24 months. The overall 2-year incidence of restenosis more than 50% was therefore 4.8%. This comprises 3.1% (to 6 months) plus an additional 1.7% (to 12 months) and no additional restenoses between 12 and 24 months. After the 30-day procedural period, there was one ipsilateral minor stroke, giving a total ipsilateral stroke rate of 0.8% at 12 months (1.3% at 24 months).

Ahmadi et al. (35) evaluated the intermediate-term morphological outcome in 303 patients undergoing carotid stenting. A total of 298 were successfully stented. Asymptomatic patients were included. Outcomes were independently reviewed. The procedural all-stroke and death rate was 3%. Over a median of 12 months (range 3–36), there was one contralateral stroke at 6 months and one ipsilateral stroke at 4 months. Duplex-documented recurrent stenosis more than or equal to 70% was identified in 9 (3%) of 298. Cumulative patency rates after 6, 12, and 36 months were 91%, 90%, and 90%, respectively.

Cremonesi et al. (36) evaluated the endovascular treatment of carotid atherosclerotic disease to include angioplasty and stenting in 110 patients. Asymptomatic patients were included, and the series was independently reviewed. The procedural all-stroke and death rate was 3.36%. Follow-up ranging from 6 to 36 months was available in all patients. All patients were reviewed at 6 months, and there were complete data to 12 months in 76 patients (63.86%). The combined minor and major neurological event and neurological death rate was 6.72% (8 patients). There were no neurological deaths. The overall in-stent restenosis rate (more than 50%) was 5.04%. There was one stent crush following a balloon-mounted stent placement (0.84%) and one stent migration (0.84%).

Becquemin et al. (37) carried out a prospective cohort study comparing carotid stenting and endarterectomy between 1995 and 2002. Asymptomatic patients were included in this series, and outcomes were independently reviewed. The procedural permanent-stroke and death rate was 2.6% in those stented and 1.1% in those operated upon (not statistically significant). The 3-year cumulative survival rate free from ipsilateral major neurological events was 95.2% in stent patients and 96.9% in the surgical group (significant). Restenosis was defined as a reduction of the carotid lumen more than 50% on duplex imaging and a velocity more than 120 cm per second. There was a 7.5% rate of restenosis in stented arteries versus 1.4% in the surgical group ($p = 0.001$).

With respect to stent deformation, this is a potential concern for balloon-mounted stents that have higher hoop strength and are generally less flexible than self-expanding stents. The updated world carotid stenting registry indicates a move towards the use of self-expanding Nitinol stents, which are not prone to this complication (29). Earlier experience indicates a 2.5% rate of deformation for the Palmaz stent over 6 months (38).

Care must be taken in the evaluation of carotid restenosis in a stented vessel. A study on the hemodynamic effects of ICA stenting using color-coded duplex sonography demonstrated a number of important findings (39). After stenting, the turbulent flow pattern in the stenotic segment of ICA recovers to laminar flow, and the reversed ophthalmic flow direction normalizes. Of the parameters applied to evaluate the effect of stenting, the ICA diameter, residual area, peak systolic velocity, diastolic velocity, and the ratio of systolic flow velocity in the ICA to that in the common carotid artery (CCA) were shown to be significantly altered. The mean and residual areas of the stenotic segment were significantly increased after stenting. The mean peak systolic flow velocity significantly decreased by 71% and the mean diastolic velocity by 77%. Both the systolic and diastolic velocities of the ipsilateral CCA significantly increased, whereas flow in the contralateral ICA decreased significantly. The change in vertebral artery flow was insignificant. These changes, particularly those involving the ICA to CCA velocity ratio, may be misinterpreted as restenosis on the basis of increased velocities. Those restenoses that are symptomatic are likely to be amenable to further endovascular intervention. The available data would suggest that restenosis might be reasonably common. However, just like the Asymptomatic Carotid Atherosclerosis Study (ACAS) trial, in which there was no correlation between late stroke and recurrent stenosis (40), following stenting, restenosis is infrequently symptomatic (41).

A recent study evaluated healing of the stented carotid artery on duplex (42). Three

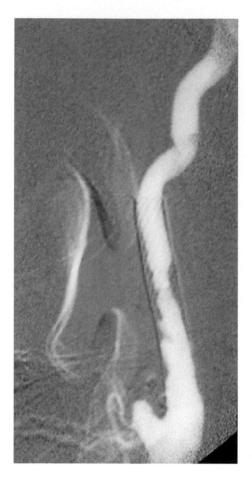

FIGURE 3-2. In-stent restenosis (neointimal hyperplasia).

phases of carotid stent incorporation were defined: an early unstable period soon after stent placement with an echolucent (thrombotic) layer that is seen to become negligible by 30 days, a moderately unstable phase with ingrowing neointima (1–12 months), and, lastly, a stable phase from the second year on. These data may indicate the need for different intensities of therapy and surveillance intervals. An example of carotid in-stent restenosis is given in Fig. 3-2.

SUMMARY

The emerging data on the efficacy of carotid stenting with respect to survival free of ipsilateral stroke is encouraging. Longer-term follow-up within CAVATAS shows equivalence between the treatment limbs, and SAPPHIRE suggests better outcomes in the stented population in the intermediate term. One- to 3-year results from high-throughput centers reporting results that are independently reviewed compare favorably with the results of endarterectomy within the high-grade stenosis subgroups of NASCET and ECST. Restenosis in excess of 50% luminal reduction ranges between 2.4% and 17.7% in the intermediate term, but these results reflect a heterogeneous population, comprising patients treated by angioplasty and those primarily stented. Restenosis does not necessarily herald the recurrence of symptoms.

The mechanisms of restenosis following carotid stenting are being investigated, and the time frame is now better understood. Caution must be taken regarding duplex assessment, which may be unreliable in delineating restenosis in a stented carotid bifurcation.

REFERENCES

1. Carrea R, Molins M, Murphy G. Surgical treatment of spontaneous thrombosis of the internal carotid artery in the neck. Carotid-carotideal anastomosis. Report of a case. *Acta Neurol Latinoamer* 1955;1: 17.
2. Eastcott HH, Pickering GW, Rob CG. Reconstruction of internal carotid artery in a patient with intermittent attacks of hemiplegia. *Lancet* 1954;267:994–996.
3. Fields WS, Maslenikov V, Meyer JS, et al. Joint study of extracranial arterial occlusion. V. Progress report of prognosis following surgery or nonsurgical treatment for transient cerebral ischemic attacks and cervical carotid artery lesions. *JAMA* 1970;211:1993–2003.
4. Shaw DA, Venables GS, Cartildge NEF, et al. Carotid endarterectomy in patients with transient cerebral ischemia. *J Neurol Sci* 1984;64:45–53.
5. Barnett HJ. Symptomatic carotid endarterectomy trials. *Stroke* 1990;21(Suppl 11):III2–III5.
6. Idem. Evaluating methods for prevention in stroke. *Ann R Coll Physicians Surg Can* 1991;24:33–42.
7. North American Symptomatic Carotid Endarterectomy Trial (NASCET) Steering Committee. North American Symptomatic Carotid Endarterectomy Trial: methods, patient characteristics, and progress. *Stroke* 1991;22:711–720.
8. Executive Committee for the Asymptomatic Carotid Atherosclerosis Study. Endarterectomy for asymptomatic carotid artery stenosis. *JAMA* 1995;275:1421–1428.
9. MRC European Carotid Surgery Trial: interim results for symptomatic patients with severe (70-99%) or with mild (0-29%) carotid stenosis. European Carotid Surgery Trialists' Collaborative Group. *Lancet* 1991;337:1235–1243.
10. Kerber CW, Cromwell LD, Loehden OL. Catheter dilatation of proximal stenosis during distal bifurcation endarterectomy. *AJNR Am J Neuroradiol* 1980;1:348–349.
11. Endovascular versus surgical treatment in patients with carotid stenosis in the Carotid and Vertebral Artery Transluminal Angioplasty Study (CAVATAS): a randomised trial. *Lancet* 2001;357:1729–1737.
12. Naylor AR, Bolia A, Abbott RJ, et al. Randomized study of carotid angioplasty and stenting versus carotid endarterectomy: a stopped trial. *J Vasc Surg* 1998;28:326–334.
13. Alberts MJ. Results of a multicenter prospective randomized trial of carotid artery stenting vs. carotid endarterectomy. *Stroke* 2001;32:325.
14. Brooks WH, McClure RR, Jones MR, et al. Carotid angioplasty and stenting versus carotid endarterectomy: randomized trial in a community hospital. *J Am Coll Cardiol* 2001;38:1589–1595.
15. Bettman MA, Katzen BT, Whisnant J, et al. AHA Science Advisory: carotid stenting and angioplasty. *Circulation* 1998;97:121–123.
16. Crawley F, Brown MM. Percutaneous transluminal angioplasty and stenting for carotid artery stenosis. *Cochrane Database Syst Rev* 2000:CD000515.
17. Veith FJ, Amor M, Ohki T, et al. Current status of carotid bifurcation angioplasty and stenting based on a consensus of opinion leaders. *J Vasc Surg* 2001;33:S111–S116.
18. Intercollegiate Working Party for Stroke. Section 11.3: Secondary prevention—update. In: *National Clinical Guidelines for Stroke*. London: Royal College of Physicians, 2002.
19. Hack W, Kaste M, Bogousslavsky J, et al. European Stroke Initiative Recommendations for Stroke Management—update 2003. *Cerebrovasc Dis* 2003;16:311–337.
20. Brown MM. Results of the carotid and vertebral artery transluminal angioplasty study. *Br J Surg* 1999; 86:710–711.
21. Sundt TM, Sandok BA, Whisnant JP. Carotid endarterectomy: complications and preoperative assessment of risk. *Mayo Clin Proc* 1975;50:301–306.
22. Rothwell P, Warlow C. Is self-audit reliable? *Lancet* 1995;346:1623.
23. Golledge J, Mitchell A, Greenhalgh RM. Systematic comparison of the early outcome of angioplasty and endarterectomy for symptomatic carotid artery disease. *Stroke* 2000;31:1439–1443.
24. Yadav JS, Roubin GS, Iyer S, et al. Elective stenting of the extracranial carotid arteries. *Circulation* 1996; 95:376–381.
25. Roubin G, Gishel N, Iyer SS, et al. Immediate and late clinical outcomes of carotid artery stenting

in patients with symptomatic and asymptomatic carotid artery stenosis. A 5-year prospective analysis. *Circulation* 2001;103:532.

26. Cremonesi A, Manetti R, Setacci F. Protected carotid stenting. Clinical advantages and complications of embolic protection devices in 442 consecutive patients. *Stroke* 2003;34:1936–1941.

27. McKevitt F, Macdonald S, Venables GS, et al. Complications following carotid angioplasty and carotid stenting in patients with symptomatic carotid artery disease. *Cerebrovasc Dis* 2004;17:28–34. (Epub 2003 Oct 03).

28. Cina CS, Clase CM, Haynes RB. Carotid endarterectomy for symptomatic carotid stenosis. *Cochrane Database Syst Rev* 2000:CD001081.

29. Wholey MH, Al-Mubarak N, Wholey MH. Updated review of the global carotid artery stent registry. *Catheter Cardiovasc Interv* 2003;60:259–266.

30. Moore WS, Barnett HJM, Beebe HG, et al. Guidelines for carotid endarterectomy. A multidisciplinary consensus statement from the Ad Hoc Committee, American Heart Association. *Stroke* 1995;26: 188–201.

31. Yadav J. SAPPHIRE 12-month results. Presented at: Transcatheter Cardiovascular Therapeutics (TCT); March 2003; Chicago, Illinois.

32. Mathias K, Jaeger M. How much cerebral embolization occurs during C.A.S? International Symposium on Endovascular Therapy; Miami 2001:73–75.

33. Wholey MH, Wholey MH, Tan WA, et al. Comparison of balloon-mounted and self-expanding stents in the carotid arteries: immediate and long-term results of more than 500 patients. *J Endovasc Ther* 2003;10:171–181.

34. Gray WA, White HJ, Barrett DM, et al. Carotid stenting and endarterectomy. A clinical and cost comparison of revascularization strategies. *Stroke* 2003;33:1063–1070.

35. Ahmadi R, Willfort A, Lang W, et al. Carotid artery stenting: effect of learning curve and intermediate-term morphological outcome. *J Endovasc Ther* 2001;8:539–546.

36. Cremonesi A, Castriota F, Manetti R, et al. Endovascular treatment of carotid atherosclerotic disease: early and late outcome in a non-selected population. *Ital Heart J* 2000;1:801–809.

37. Becquemin JP, Ben El Kadi H, Desgranges P, et al. Carotid stenting versus carotid surgery: a prospective cohort study. *J Endovasc Ther* 2003;10:687–694.

38. Wholey MH, Wholey M, Mathias K, et al. Global experience in cervical carotid artery stent placement. *Catheter Cardiovasc Interv* 2000;50:160–167.

39. Lu CJ, Kao HL, Sun Y, et al. The hemodynamic effects of internal carotid artery stenting: a study with color-coded duplex sonography. *Cerebrovasc Dis* 2003;15:264–269.

40. Moore WS, Kempczinski RF, Nelson JJ, et al. Recurrent carotid stenosis: results of the asymptomatic carotid atherosclerosis study. *Stroke* 1998;29:2018–2025.

41. Christiaans MH, Ernst JM, Suttorp MJ, et al. Restenosis after carotid angioplasty and stenting: a follow-up study with duplex ultrasonography. *Eur J Vasc Endovasc Surg* 2003;26:141–144.

42. Willfort-Ehringer A, Ahmadi R, Gschwandtner ME, et al. Healing of carotid stents: a prospective duplex ultrasound study. *J Endovasc Ther* 2003;10:636–642.

43. Barnett HJM, Taylor MA, Eliasziw M, et al. Benefit of carotid endarterectomy in patients with symptomatic moderate or severe stenosis. *N Engl J Med* 1998;339:1415–1425.

44. Moore WS, Kempczinski RF, Nelson JJ, et al. Recurrent carotid stenosis. Results of the Asymptomatic Carotid Atherosclerosis Study. *Stroke* 1998;29:2018–2025.

45. Randomised trial of endarterectomy for recently symptomatic carotid stenosis: final results of the MRC European Carotid Surgery Trial (ECST). *Lancet* 1998;351:1379–1387.

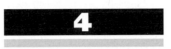

THE GLOBAL CAROTID ARTERY STENT REGISTRY

MICHAEL H. WHOLEY
NADIM AL-MUBARAK
MARK H. WHOLEY
THE INTERVENTIONALISTS AT THE PARTICIPATING
CAROTID STENT CENTERS

Stroke is the most common and disabling neurological disorder in the elderly population (1). In the United States, there are more than half a million strokes annually, accounting for more than 2 million stroke survivors with varying degrees of disability (1,2). After heart disease and cancer, cerebrovascular disease is the third leading cause of death, with 1.5 deaths per 1,000 people (2). Carotid artery occlusive disease is responsible for approximately 20% to 30% of strokes (3,4).

The traditional standard of care in treating cervical carotid artery stenosis has been carotid endarterectomy (CEA). The procedure was initially performed in the 1950s by such pioneers as Drs. Eascott, DeBakey, and Cooley (4). After the landmark studies of the North American Symptomatic Carotid Endarterectomy Trial (NASCET) and Asymptomatic Carotid Atherosclerosis Study (ACAS), CEA has been proven beneficial in reducing the stroke risks for symptomatic and asymptomatic patients with significant carotid artery stenoses (5–8).

However, in sets of patients, an alternative form of treatment has been the use of carotid artery stenting (CAS). CAS has been shown to be an effective and relatively safe means of treating cervical carotid artery disease (9–12). The purpose of this chapter is to provide a 5-year update of a world carotid registry that was started in 1997 and updated annually.

METHODS AND MATERIALS

In June 1997, 24 surveys were completed by major carotid interventional centers in Europe, South America, North America, and Asia (11). The data were then updated annually with most recent September 2002 addition. Twenty-eight additional centers were included for a total of 52 major carotid centers worldwide. This paper presents an overview of the recent results in carotid stenting (Table 4-1).

The survey asked a series of questions regarding the following:

- Number of procedures performed
- Technical success
- Types of stents used
- Complications including TIAs, minor and major strokes, and deaths
- Clinical follow-up
- Subset analyses of embolic protection devices

TABLE 4-1. ACTIVE PARTICPANTS IN CAROTID REGISTRY CENTER

Physicians	Location
Ansel	MidWest Cardiology, Columbus, OH
Bergeron	St. Joseph, Marseille, France
Calderon	San Juan de Dios Hospital, Costa Rica
Castroita/Cremonesi	Cotignola, Italy
Cates	Emory University, Atlanta, GA
Colombo	Centro Cuore Columbus, Milano, Italy
Criado	Union Memorial Hospital, Baltimore, MD
Escudero	Hospital Germans Trias, Barcelona, Spain
Gaines	Sheffield Vascular Institute, London, UK
Gomez	University of Alabama, Birmingham, AL
Gray	Swedish Hospital, Seattle, WA
Henry	Nancy, France
Higashida	University of California San Francisco, San Francisco, CA
Kracjer	St. Luke's Episcopal Hospital, Houston, TX
Laborde/Marco	Clinique Pasteur, Toulouse, France
Londero	Institut de Cardiologie Buenos Aires, Argentina
Mathias	Dortmund, Germany
Mesa	Unidad Cardiovascular Clinica, Medilin, Colombia
Mischell	Prairie Cardiovascular, Springfield, IL
Muhling	Dr. Muller Hospital, Munich, Germany
Musacchio	Interventional Neurorad, Sante Fe, Argentina
Myla	California Heart Association, Fountain Valley, CA
Parodi	Buenos Aires, Argentina
Ramee/White	Oschner Clinic, New Orleans, LA
Roubin/Iyer	Lenox Hill, New York, NY
Sakai	Kobe City General Hospital, Kobe, Japan
Schultz	Minneapolis, MN
Shofer	Center for Cardiology and Vascular Intervention, Hamburg, Germany
Sievert	Cardiology Center Bethien, Frankfurt, Germany
Smith	Duke University, Durham, NC
Tinoco	Itaperuna, Brazil
Van Den Berg	St. Antonius Hospital, Nieuwegein, Netherlands
Vaclav	Ostrava, Czech Republic
Vozzi	Hemodinamia Institute, Rosario, Argentina
Wholey	Pittsburgh Vascular Institute, Pittsburgh, PA
Wholey	University of Texas, San Antonio, TX

The National Institute of Health (NIH) classification of neurologic complication was employed in determination of endpoints (13). Percentage complication values used both denominators of total number of vessels treated (which the original 1997 study used) as well as patients enrolled in the study. Patients with bilateral diseased vessels were not counted twice.

A transient ischemic attack (TIA) was classified as any neurologic deficit that resolves within 24 hours and leaves no evidence of residual neurologic damage. In order to determine more about procedure-related TIAs, which are not frequently reported in surgical studies, a separate questionnaire was provided to centers.

A minor stroke was classified as a new neurological event that results in slight impairment of neurological function (speech, motor, or sensory skills) that either completely resolves within 7 days or causes an increase in the NIH stroke scale of less than four (13). A new neurological deficit that persisted after 7 days and increased the NIH stroke scale score by four or more was classified as major stroke (13). Deaths within 30 days after the procedure were recorded and further delineated into procedure-related and non–procedure-related. Non–procedure-related deaths included those from cardiopulmonary and other organ-based causes. The reason for the delineation was because in previous surveys only the procedure-related deaths were recorded.

Limitations exist in this study. Most of the data, volunteered by the 52 centers, have not been published or been subject to any peer-review process. The information is observational and retrospective.

RESULTS

Since the registry was started in 1997, there have been a total of 11,035 patients with 12,166 diseased carotid arteries who underwent CAS. There were 1,131 patients with diseased bilateral carotid arteries. A technical success of 98.8% was reported, with 12,030 carotid arteries being successfully stented. Technical success was defined as less than 30% residual stenosis covering a region no longer than the original lesion without any decreased or abnormal intracranial arterial anatomy.

The responding physicians stated that 55% of their patients had symptoms attributable to the carotid lesion. The range in symptomatic patients varied from 28% to 100%.

There were 11,910 carotid stents placed. The majority of the stents placed were the metallic self-expanding Boston Scientific Wallstent (Natick, MA), which was used in 4,600 (54%) cases and the newer carotid version in 1,831 (15.4%) (Fig. 4-1). The balloon expandable Palmaz stents were used in 2,037 (17%) of the cases. Self-expanding nitinol stents included the Cordis Johnson and Johnson SMART (Warren, NJ) with 1,401 (11.8%) and Precise 888 (7.5%). Other nitinol self-expanding stents included Guidant Acculink (Mountain View, CA), Endotex (Palo Alto, CA), Jomed Sito (Stockholm, Sweden), Boulton Expander (France), Medtronics (Santa Rosa, CA), Perclose X-Act (Mountain View, CA), and other companies. When the survey was started, the balloon-mounted stents had 54% (1110 out of 2037) of the market, reflecting the almost complete change away from balloon mounted, and hence, crushable stents in the cervical carotid area.

Complications that occurred during the carotid stent placement or within a 30-day period following placement were recorded (Fig. 4-2). Overall, there were 375 TIAs for a rate of 3.08%. Based on the total vessels treated, there were 264 minor strokes with a rate of occurrence of 2.17%. The total number of major strokes was 147 for a rate of 1.21%. There were 80 procedure-related deaths within a 30-day postprocedure period, resulting in a mortality rate of 0.66%. The combined minor and major strokes and procedure-related death rate was 4.04%. There were 95 (0.78%) non–procedure-related deaths within the 30-day period, resulting in a total stroke and death rate of 4.82%. Compared to the 5.70% rate found in the initial registry performed in June 1997, there has been a steady decrease in the complication rate (Fig. 4-3). Based upon the total number of patients, the current total stroke and death rate was 5.30%.

Subset Studies

Symptomatic Versus Asymptomatic Patient Population

A subset of questions was directed to determine the rate of complications based upon symptomatic versus asymptomatic patient populations. Thirty-two of the 52 centers responded,

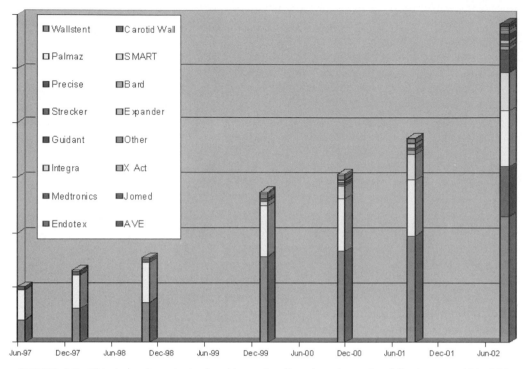

Wallstent	Carotid Wall
Palmaz	SMART
Precise	Bard
Strecker	Expander
Guidant	Other
Integra	X Act
Medtronics	Jomed
Endotex	AVE

Jun-97   Dec-97   Jun-98   Dec-98   Jun-99   Dec-99   Jun-00   Dec-00   Jun-01   Dec-01   Jun-02

FIGURE 4-1. Historical review: stents placed by center. (See also color section following page 164 of this text.)

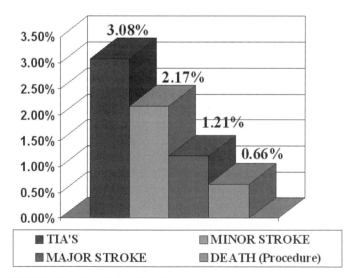

3.08%

2.17%

1.21%

0.66%

3.50%
3.00%
2.50%
2.00%
1.50%
1.00%
0.50%
0.00%

■ TIA'S   ■ MINOR STROKE
■ MAJOR STROKE   □ DEATH (Procedure)

FIGURE 4-2. Historical review of stent complications. (See also color section following page 164 of this text.)

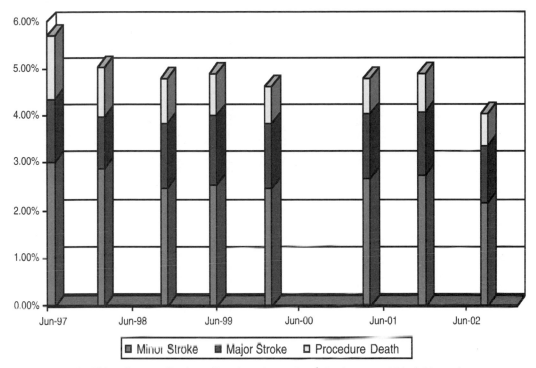

FIGURE 4-3. Thirty-day complications. (See also color section following page 164 of this text.)

representing 10,693 patients. This subset involved both Anti-Embolization protection and nonprotection patients. There was a combined minor and major stroke and procedure-related death rate of 5.04% involving 6,172 symptomatic patients and 2.96% involving 4,521 asymptomatic patients.

Anti-Embolization Protection

Thirty-three centers of the 52 have started to utilize embolic protection devices in CAS. These centers reported that embolic protection was used in approximately 4,005 (%) patients and no protection was used in the remaining 6,688 (%) of patients. Of the protected patients, the distal occlusion balloon system (GuardWire®, Medtronics, Perclose Division, Santa Rosa, CA) was used in 46% of the cases followed by 30% for the Angioguard filter (Cordis Johnson & Johnson, Miami Lakes, FL), 9% for the Microvena filter (White Bear, MN), and 8% for the Mednova filter (Mednova, Galway, Ireland).

Complications that occurred during the CAS or within a 30-day period following placement were recorded. The combined minor and major strokes and procedure-related death rate was 5.29% without Anti-Embolization protection compared to 2.27% with AntiEmbolization protection; this was statistically significant (Fig. 4-4). The protection versus no-protection subset was further divided into symptomatic and asymptomatic patients (Fig. 4-5). Symptomatic patients without Anti-Embolization protection (4,223 patients) had a stroke and procedure-related death rate of 6.07% compared to those symptomatic patients with Anti-Embolization protection (1,949 patients) who had a rate of 2.82%.

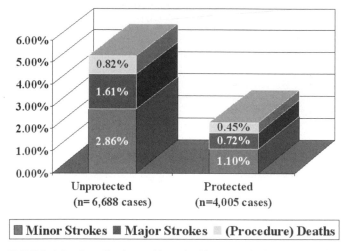

FIGURE 4-4. Complications with and without cerebral protection. (See also color section following page 164 of this text.)

Asymptomatic patients without Anti-Embolization protection (2,465 patients) had a stroke and procedure-related death rate of 3.97% compared to those asymptomatic patients with Anti-Embolization protection (2,056 patients) who had a rate of 1.75%. Both of these subsets were statistically significant. If non–procedure-related deaths were included, the rates of stroke and deaths were 6.69% for unprotected symptomatic patients versus 3.25% for protected symptomatic patients. The rates of stroke and deaths including both procedure and non–procedure-related deaths were 4.78% for unprotected asymptomatic patients versus 2.53% for protected asymptomatic patients.

A learning curve of 50 cases using Anti-Embolization protection was revealed by the study. Those centers that performed under 50 cases using embolic protection had a higher rate of minor and major strokes and procedure-related deaths (4.04%) compared to the rate of 3.60% for centers performing 50 to 100 cases and 2.85% for centers performing 200 to 500 cases. Those centers that have done more than 500 cases have a complication rate of 1.56%. Surprisingly, those centers performing between 100 and 200 embolic procedures had the best rate of 1.28%.

Clinical Follow-up

Follow-up ultrasound studies were performed at years 1 to 3 poststent placement at many of the institutions. Computed tomography (CT) scans and angiographic studies were done as needed clinically. At 12 months, the restenosis rate was approximately 2.70% cases with a residual stenosis greater than 50%. At years 2 and 3, the rates were 2.50% and 2.40%, respectively. Hence, at year 3, the overall restenosis rate was 7.60%. The rates of ipsilateral neurological events were also recorded. The rates of ipsilateral neurological events for years 1 through 3 were 1.20%, 1.30%, and 1.70%, respectively. Hence, the cumulative rate of ipsilateral neurological events at the end of year 3 was 4.2%.

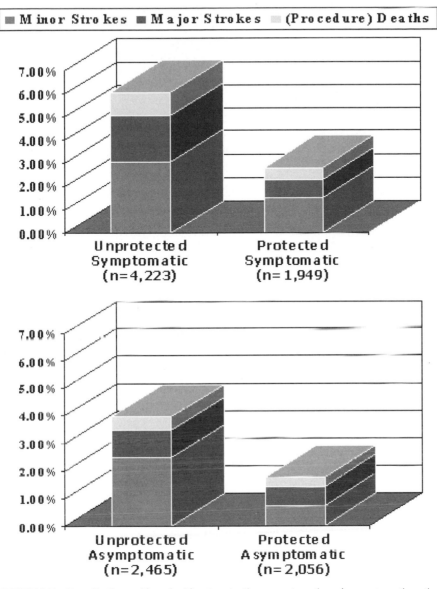

FIGURE 4-5. Complications with and without protection: symptomatic and asymptomatic patient populations. (See also color section following page 164 of this text.)

DISCUSSION

With the goal of effectively treating cervical atherosclerotic disease as a major cause of stroke, surgeons have refined CEAs over the past 40 years. However, CEA still has significant risks. The risks of perioperative stroke from CEA vary from 1.5% to 9% depending on the published series (14,15). The perioperative stroke and/or death rate is 7.5% in the European Carotid Surgery Trial (ECST), 5.8% in NASCET, and 2.3% in the ACAS (5–8,10,14,15).

Also, the NASCET perioperative stroke and/or death rate for contralateral occlusions was 14.3% (16). The risks for cranial nerve palsies occur in 7.6% to 27%, which are frequently not recorded as morbidity in surgical publications (10,15,17).

Hence, though it is relatively difficult to compare CAS with endarterectomy without a randomized study, some early comparisons can be made. There was a combined minor and major stroke and procedure-related death rate of 5.04% involving symptomatic patients and 2.96% involving asymptomatic patients. Hence, for symptomatic patients, the results appear equivocal with stenting compared to surgery. For asymptomatic patients, there was slight difference compared to the complication rates incurred in the ACAS (5–8). With the advent of Anti-Embolization protection devices, the combined rate of stroke and procedure-related death was decreased from 5.29% to 2.27%. In the subset, the stroke and procedure-related death rates for symptomatic patients with Anti-Embolization protection was 2.82% and for asymptomatic patients with cerebral protection was 1.75%. Hence, compared to NASCET and ACAS standards, carotid stenting with cerebral protection appears competitive for asymptomatic and especially for symptomatic patient groups.

The reported 1-year restenosis rate was 2.70% and cumulative 3-year rate was 7.60%. Vitek et al. (18) revealed a restenosis rate of 5% at 6 to 12 months postprocedure involving 350 vessels. Longer-term data from the Pittsburgh Vascular Institute (PVI) under Wholey et al. (22) revealed that vessel patency (more than or equal to 50% diameter obstruction) for 3 years was 96.3% for the balloon-mounted stents. One of the limitations of the study is the reliability of accurate follow-up by the different centers.

The risks of ipsilateral neurological sequelae remain impressive: in the study, we reported TIAs, stroke, and stroke-related deaths at a rate of 1.20% for 1 year and a cumulative 3.20% for 3 years. This is similar to the data from the PVI, which revealed a 3-year freedomfrom all fatal and ipsilateral nonfatal strokes without the inclusion of a 30-day periprocedural period of 95% (22).

CONCLUSION

Endovascular stent placement for carotid artery occlusive disease is evolving from its initial controversial position to that of a reasonable alternative of treating cervical carotid occlusive disease. The number of carotid stent procedures is increasing worldwide at a rate of 18% to 47% per year. The high technical success rate and advantages of endovascular treatment help to propel its growth. The complication rate at this early stage of development in cerebral protection is encouraging, especially for symptomatic patients. As technology improvements occur in stent, delivery, and thromboembolic protection designs, the complication rates should continue to decrease and approach rates below 2%. Still, the important test for CAS will be its long-term (1-, 3-, 5-year) patency as well as the results of randomized studies against the gold standard of CEA.

REFERENCES

1. Patient Outcomes Research Teams Study Groups. In: *Stroke clinical updates.* Englewood: National Stroke Association, 1994;9–12.
2. *Heart and stroke facts statistical supplement.* Dallas: American Heart Association, 1994:12.
3. Dorros G. Carotid arterial obliterative disease: should endovascular revascularization (stent supported angioplasty) today supplant carotid endarterectomy? *J Interv Cardiol* 1996;9:193–196.
4. DeBakey MH. Carotid endarterectomy revisited. *J Endovasc Surg* 1996;3:4.

5. North American Symptomatic Carotid Endarterectomy Trial Collaborators. Beneficial effect of carotid endarterectomy in symptomatic patients with high-grade carotid stenosis: *N Engl J Med* 1991;325: 445–453.

6. Asymptomatic Carotid Atherosclerosis Study Group. Endarterectomy for asymptomatic carotid artery stenosis. *JAMA* 1995;273:1421–1428.

7. Clinical advisory: carotid endarterectomy for patients with asymptomatic internal carotid artery stenosis. *J Neurol Sci* 1995;129:76–77.

8. Clinical advisory: carotid endarterectomy for patients with asymptomatic internal carotid artery stenosis. *Stroke* 1994;25:2523–2524.

9. Diethrich EB. Indications for carotid stenting: a preview of the potential derived from early clinical experience. *J Endovasc Surg* 1996;3:132–139.

10. Yadav JS, Roubin GS, King P, et al. Angioplasty and stenting for restenosis after carotid endarterectomy. *Stroke* 1996;27:2075-2079.

11. Wholey MH, Wholey M, Bergeron P, et al. Current global status of carotid artery stent placement. *Cathet Cardiovasc Diagn* 1998;44:1–6.

12. Wholey MH, Wholey M, Eles G, et al. Endovasacular stents for carotid occlusive disease. *J Endovasc Surg* 1997;4:326–338.

13. Brott T, Adams HP, Olinger CP, et al. Measurement of acute cerebral infarction: a clinical examination scale. *Stroke* 1989;20:864 870.

14. Zarins CK. Carotid endarterectomy: the gold standard. *J Endovasc Surg* 1996;3:10–15.

15. Lusby RJ, Wylie EJ. Complications of carotid endarterectomy. *Surg Clin North Am* 1983:63: 1293–1301.

16. Gasecki AP, Elliasziw M, Ferguson GG, et al. Long-term prognosis and effect of endarterectomy in patients with symptomatic severe carotid stenosis and contralateral carotid stenosis or occlusion: results from NASCET. *J Neurosurg* 1995;83:778–782.

17. Diethrich EB, Cerebrovascular disease therapy: the past, the present, and the future. *J Endovasc Surg* 1996;3:7–9.

18. Vitek J, Iyer S, Roubin G. Carotid stenting in 350 vessels: problems faced and solved. *J Invasive Cardiol* 1998;10:311–314.

19. Theron JG, Payelle GG, Coskun, O, et al. Carotid artery stenosis: treatment with protected balloon angioplasty and stent placement. *Radiology* 1996;201:627- 636.

20. Theron J, Courtheoux P, Alachkar F, et al. New triple coaxial catheter systems for carotid angioplasty with cerebral protection. *AJNR Am J Neuroradiol* 1990;11:869–874.

21. Theron J, Dorros G. A rationale for endovascular therapy with balloon occlusion during extracranial atherosclerotic carotid artery stenosis. *J Intervent Cardiol* 1996;9:209–213.

22. Wholey MH, Wholey M, Tan W, et al. Long term follow-up comparing balloon-mounted and self-expandable stents. *J Endovasc Ther* 2004 *(in press)*.

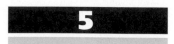

CURRENT INDICATIONS OF CAROTID ARTERY STENTING

NADIM AL-MUBARAK
GARY S. ROUBIN

Obstructive atherosclerotic carotid bifurcation disease is responsible for approximately 30% of stroke cases in the United States (1). Any successful treatment of this disease should demonstrate significant and durable reduction in the related risk for stroke without compromising the patient's safety. A favorable risk-benefit ratio of the treatment in the individual patient should satisfy three critical issues: (i) an acceptably low immediate risk for stroke or death, (ii) superiority to the natural course of the disease, if the patient were to continue conservative medical therapy only, and (iii) durable efficacy in preventing stroke. Randomized control trials have clearly documented the superiority of carotid endarterectomy (CEA) to medical therapy in reducing the risk of future stroke in a select group of patients with carotid stenosis, provided that a low perioperative rate of stroke and death is achieved (2–4). Based on these trials, the American Heart Association has set specific guidelines for the performance of CEA, which accordingly should be performed only if the combined perioperative stroke and death rates can be kept less than or equal to 6% in symptomatic and less than or equal to 3% in asymptomatic patients with severe carotid bifurcation stenosis (5).

Over the past decade, the utilization of carotid artery stenting (CAS) as a less-invasive alternative treatment to surgery has progressively increased (6–14). It is now evident that many experienced centers can perform carotid stenting with outcomes that compare favorably with those reported in the major CEA trials (6–14). Further, the results of a large randomized control trial of CAS versus CEA, which included a high-risk symptomatic population of patients with high-grade carotid artery stenoses, have recently been reported (9). In this trial, despite the suboptimal techniques and the deficiencies in the interventionists' experience compared with the participating experienced surgeons', both early and late outcomes were equivalent among the two treatment groups. These outcomes have recently been enhanced with improved patient selection, the availability of more suitable equipment for the procedure, and, most importantly, the introduction of "Anti-Embolization devices" that can capture embolic matter released during the intervention, preventing it from reaching the brain (10–14). The first reports of CAS with Anti-Embolization devices have clearly shown a significant reduction in the associated neurological embolic events. Importantly, a very low rate of major disabling stroke was achieved. Moreover, several investigators, reporting their late follow-up data, have clearly shown that CAS is effective in reducing the risk of late stroke and that its outcomes compare favorably to those reported for CEA (8,10).

CURRENT INDICATIONS

The current indications for CAS are determined predominantly by the operator's experience and results. As with CEA, poor outcomes from CAS may result from poor technical skills, limited experience, and inappropriate patient selection. Based on the current outcomes of the surgical treatment for obstructive carotid bifurcation disease, CAS should be applied only to lesions that have more than or equal to 50% diameter obstruction in the symptomatic and more than or equal to 70% diameter obstruction in the asymptomatic patients [as determined by the North American Symptomatic Carotid Endarterectomy Trial (NASCET) angiographic methodology] (2,3).

In principle, the indications for CAS can be divided into two main categories: the first includes patients at high risk for stroke from severe carotid stenoses in which CEA has been proven to be effective. Generally, there should be no contraindications to proceed with CAS in these patients *provided that* the procedure can be performed with acceptably low complication rates and in accordance with the American Heart Association (AHA) guidelines for CEA. In this category, CAS has the advantage of being a less-invasive treatment that does not require general anesthesia or skin incision and can safely be performed as an outpatient procedure (14). Combined carotid and coronary interventions can be performed during the same setting (15). Ultimately, the results of the ongoing randomized trials will be necessary to further define the role of CAS as a standard treatment in these patients (16).

The second category of indications for CAS includes patients with high-grade carotid artery obstructions in whom the surgical treatment has been shown to be technically challenging or impossible, requires extensive surgical incision, or is associated with high rates of complications, labeled the "high-risk surgical groups" (Table 5-1). Most of these groups have been excluded from the major CEA trials owing to a documented high surgical risk (2–4). Therefore, the benefits observed in the landmark trials of CEA cannot be extrapolated to this category of patients. CAS, as a less-invasive treatment, offers several advantages that make it a safer alternative treatment in these patients (17–22). The stenting procedure is performed in the nonsedated conscious patient, does not require surgical incision, and has a short recovery time. It must be emphasized that a prerequisite for the utilization of CAS in these patients is "the ability of the operator to execute a technically successful procedure with an acceptably low complication rate."

Most of the high-risk surgical patients are at low risk for stenting and therefore represent ideal indications for CAS (Table 5-1). The high surgical risk groups can be classified into

TABLE 5-1. SURGICAL HIGH-RISK GROUPS: OPTIMAL CANDIDATES FOR CAS

Anatomical high risks
  Proximal or ostial common carotid lesions
  Distal internal carotid artery lesion (≥3 cm above the bifurcation)
  High carotid bifurcation (at C-2 or higher)
  Obese short neck
  Patients with contralateral carotid artery occlusion
Medical high risks
  Coexisting severe coronary artery disease
  Severe cardiopulmonary disease contraindicating general
    anesthesia
  Severe renal failure contraindicating contrast medium use
Technical high risks
  Neck radiation/prior radial neck dissection
  Prior carotid endarterectomy

CAS, carotid artery stenting

(i) anatomically high surgical risk group, and includes patients with surgically difficult to access carotid artery lesions (such as proximal/ostial common carotid artery lesions and distal internal carotid artery lesions), (ii) medically high surgical risk group, and includes patients with severe medical comorbidities that significantly increase the perioperative risk for complications such as coexisting severe coronary artery disease or severe heart failure, and (iii) technically high surgical risk group, and includes patients in whom CEA is technically difficult or impossible, such as those with recurrent stenosis after CEA, patients with prior neck radiation and/or radical neck dissections, and those with fibromuscular dysplasia. In general, none of these conditions represents a technical challenge or increased risk for the endovascular treatment and, by consensus, they are currently acceptable indications for CAS (17–22).

ANATOMICALLY HIGH-RISH CAROTID ENDARTERECTOMY GROUP

These include patients with discrete proximal or ostial common carotid artery lesions; discrete distal internal carotid artery (ICA) lesions, lesions that involve high carotid bifurcations (C-2 and above), immobile neck (inability to extend the head due to cervical arthritis or other cervical disorders), and short obese neck (Figs. 5-1–5-3) (20). CEA is very difficult in these patients, and in most instances requires extensive surgical exposure of the carotid artery, adding a considerable risk to the surgery, which in these cases can be performed under only general anesthesia (20). In patients with high carotid bifurcation or stenosis that extends more than 3 cm distal into the ICA, extensive surgical dissection that frequently includes mobilization of the mandible may result in cranial nerve damage and potentially prolonged wound healing. It is also more difficult for the surgeon to track down the distal arm of the plaque and expose the artery for shunt placement. Similarly, lesions in the common carotid artery, particularly the ostial and very proximal lesions, require major surgical intervention

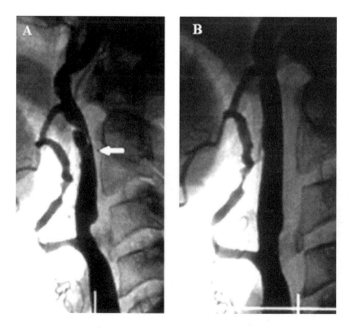

FIGURE 5-1. Carotid stenting of a severe stenosis within the distal internal carotid artery (ICA) at the level of C-2 (high ICA lesion): (**A**) prestenting and (**B**) poststenting.

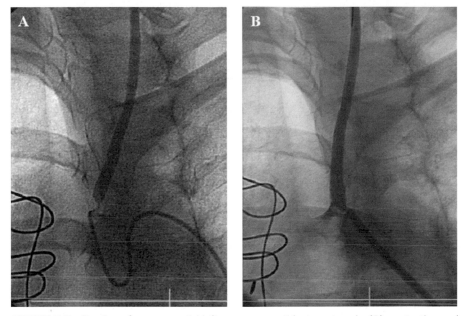

FIGURE 5-2. Stenting of a severe ostial left common carotid artery stenosis: (**A**) prestenting and (**B**) poststenting.

including bypassing the stenosis, mobilizing the clavicle, and entering the chest cavity. These patients are considered ideal candidates for CAS. Another anatomically high-risk group that can benefit from the endovascular treatment includes patients with severe carotid stenosis and occluded contralateral internal carotid artery. In these patients, CEA has been associated with a high risk for stroke and death (14% in NASCET). CAS in this patient subset is feasible, does not represent a technical challenge, and has been shown to be safe (20).

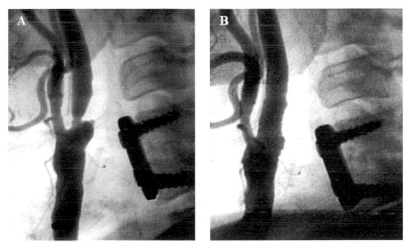

FIGURE 5-3. Stenting of severe internal carotid artery (ICA) lesion in a patient with an immobile neck following a spinal surgery: (**A**) prestenting and (**B**) poststenting.

MEDICALLY HIGH-RISK CAROTID ENDARTERECTOMY GROUP

The most important medical risk of complications during CEA is the presence of severe coronary artery disease (CAD), which frequently coexists with obstructive carotid artery disease as part of the systemic atherosclerotic process (23–26). It is estimated that more than 50% of patients undergoing CEA have significant CAD with prior angina, myocardial infarction, or ischemic electrocardiographic changes (23–26). Conversely, 10% to 20% of patients with symptomatic CAD have significant carotid artery stenosis of more than or equal to 70% diameter obstruction. Management of this patient group poses a major dilemma. The coexistence of severe obstructions in both systems substantially increases the risk of complications from one territory during the surgical revascularization of the other (26–32). General anesthesia, cardiopulmonary bypass, and associated hemodynamic instabilities during surgery pose a significant risk for hypotension and embolization of air or atherosclerotic matter. Staged and combined surgeries of both vascular territories in the same patient have been practiced at the expense of significant morbidity and mortality, mainly from myocardial infarction and stroke (28–32). CEA in patients with severe CAD has been associated with combined major event rates of 8.8% to 10% (including stroke, myocardial infarction, and death) (26–32). Likewise, coronary bypass surgery in the presence of severe carotid artery obstruction has been associated with 4% to 20% risk of perioperative stroke (26–32). Although simultaneous CEA and coronary artery bypass graft (CABG) have been advocated as the safest surgical approach, recent reports have shown that this resulted in combined stroke and death rates of 8% to 18% (28–32). Therefore, the current standards of surgical revascularization in these patients remain controversial, and the associated risks can at times be prohibitive.

As a less-invasive procedure, CAS has been explored as an alternative treatment in this high-risk group, either prior to CABG or in combination with percutaneous coronary intervention. Avoiding general anesthesia, hemodynamic instabilities, and the aortic bypass pump system required for surgery dramatically reduces the associated risk of comorbidities and improves the clinical outcomes (8,10,19). The feasibility and safety of simultaneous and staged CAS with coronary angioplasty or CABG have been demonstrated in multiple reports. Babatasi et al. (33) performed carotid balloon angioplasty with and without stenting in 10 patients with severe carotid artery disease prior to CABG for severe CAD and reported no mortalities and no neurological events. The authors have reported a series of 51 patients with severe coexistent carotid and CAD that were successfully treated by staged or combined coronary angioplasty and CAS (19). Two minor strokes with full recovery occurred in the hospital, and there were no major neurological events, myocardial infarctions, or deaths. A number of subsequent reports have documented favorable outcomes with low complications rates for CAS in this high surgical risk group (34–40). On a clinical note, staging the procedures in these patients is a clinical judgment that is undertaken on an individual basis. Generally, it is best to first treat the clinically unstable vascular territory. If both are stable, then the most severe obstruction should be approached first.

TECHNICALLY HIGH-RISK CAROTID ENDARTERECTOMY GROUP

Three groups of patients may represent a technical challenge during CEA. These include: (i) patients with recurrent stenosis after CEA, (ii) patients with radiation-induced obstructive carotid artery disease with or without radical neck dissection, termed "hostile neck," and (iii) those with fibromuscular dysplasia of the ICA (Figs. 5-4, 5-5). In these conditions, surgery can be very challenging, at times impossible, or may require extensive mobilization

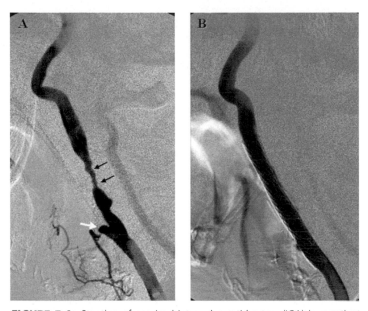

FIGURE 5-4. Stenting of proximal internal carotid artery (ICA) in a patient with severe radiation-induced obstructive carotid artery disease. **A:** preprocedural angiogram showing severe long lesion of the ICA distal to the carotid bifurcation. **B:** immediate results following successful stenting.

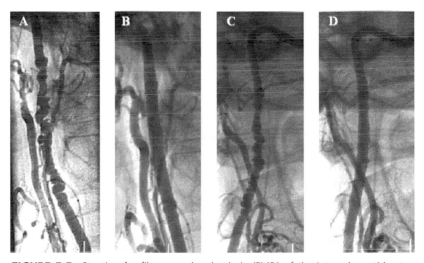

FIGURE 5-5. Stenting for fibromuscular dysplasia (FMD) of the internal carotid artery (ICA) in a woman who presented with an ipsilateral transient ischemic attack. **A** and **C:** Preprocedural angiography in two different projections with the typical "string of beads" appearance of FMD. **B** and **D:** Poststenting angiography: the carotid artery is now widely patent, and the lumenogram has been "smoothed" by the stent.

of the mandible or clavicle. It may also be very difficult for the surgeon to expose the artery for shunt placement or dissect through the very fibrotic arterial layers. The utilization of CAS in patients with prior CEA is addressed in the next chapter. In this section, we will address the rational in utilizing CAS in patients with prior neck radiation with radical neck dissection.

Radiation-induced Carotid Artery Disease

With improved survival of cancer patients, the long-term effects of radiation therapy have gained clinical significance. Radiation-induced carotid artery occlusive disease occurs 10 to 20 years following the radiation treatment and has been associated with increased incidence of stroke compared to a control group with no prior radiation (41–45). The disease typically involves the irradiated regions anywhere from the origin of the carotid artery to the cranial base, often rendering it inaccessible to the surgical treatment. The pathology is thought to be accelerated atherosclerosis or panarteritis. In the latter, intimal thickening and severe sclerosis of the arterial layers make it difficult or impossible to achieve adequate separation of the plaque from the media during CEA, often necessitating arterial bypass of the diseased segment (41–45). Many of these patients had undergone prior radical neck dissection with resultant extensive skin scarring and distorted neck anatomy. This, along with the radiation-induced cutaneous sclerosis, makes the external dissection and the carotid artery exposure extremely difficult during surgery. Subsequent wound closure and healing can be complicated and occasionally requires skin grafts. Further, frequently present tracheotomies increase the risk of wound infection (41–45).

The endovascular treatment in these patients bypasses these surgical challenges and offers several additional advantages that obviate the need for dissection through dense scar tissue, improving the procedural success and eliminating the risk of infection as well as cranial nerve palsies (Fig. 5-4). In addition to carotid bifurcation lesions, more distal or proximal lesions are accessible for the endovascular treatment. There is no need for general anesthesia, and therefore, tracheotomy does not interfere with the safety of the procedure (18,46).

The feasibility of percutaneous balloon dilatation for radiation-induced carotid artery disease has been previously reported (18,46). In an early report, Bergqvist et al. described successful balloon angioplasty in two patients who remained asymptomatic for 3 years (46). In another report, balloon dilatation of both carotid arteries was successfully performed in a patient with symptomatic radiation-induced stenosis (47). The patient remained asymptomatic during the 2-year follow-up. Stenting has dramatically improved the safety and efficacy of balloon angioplasty including the carotid arteries. The authors have reported a series of CAS in 14 patients (15 carotid arteries) with severe radiation-induced extracranial carotid artery stenoses (18).Technical success was achieved in all patients. Two patients also had combined stenting of severe vertebral artery lesions during the same setting. One patient had minor stroke after the procedure but completely recovered within 2 days. No other complications were encountered. Nine (64%) patients had 6-month follow-up imaging (angiography or duplex scanning) that showed no evidence of restenosis. At follow-up (18 ± 2 months), three patients had died from unrelated causes, but no neurological events occurred, and no repeat carotid artery interventions were required in the remaining patients. A number of subsequent reports supported these favorable outcomes of CAS (48–52).

Fibromuscular Dysplasia

Fibromuscular dysplasia (FMD) is an arteriopathy that affects medium-sized arteries in many locations (53). The ICA is involved in approximately three-fourths of the cases of

TABLE 5-2. CONTRAINDICATIONS FOR CAS

Severely tortuous and atheromatous aortic arch and arch vessels (Fig. 5-6)
Pedunculated thrombus at the lesion site or distal to it (angiographic filling defect: Fig. 5-7)
Heavy calcifications within and around the lesion (Fig. 5-7)
Severe tortuosities and angulations of the carotid arteries
Severe renal impairment precluding safe use of contrast agents
Recent stroke (within 3 wks prior to CAS)
Presence of contraindications to antiplatelet agents

CAS, carotid artery stenting.

brachiocephalic FMD, typically involving a long segment at C2-3 sparing the great vessel origins, carotid bifurcations, and bulbs. It is most often found in women between the ages of 30 and 50 years (53). Asymptomatic cases of FMD may be discovered incidentally, although transient ischemic attack, cerebral infarction, and subarachnoidal hemorrhage are common presentations. Angiographic finding of multifocal stenoses that alternate with areas of mural dilatations, called the "string of beads" appearance, may be observed to a variable degree depending on the histopathologic type (Fig. 5-5). The distal location and the long segments involved make this entity difficult or impossible to treat surgically. For the reasons detailed earlier, CAS in these patients clearly offers a suitable alternative treatment (Fig. 5-5).

CONTRAINDICATIONS OF CAROTID ARTERY STENTING

Conditions that place the patient at high risk for clinical neurological embolic events during the carotid intervention are contraindications for CAS (Table 5-2, Figs. 5-6, 5-7) (54).

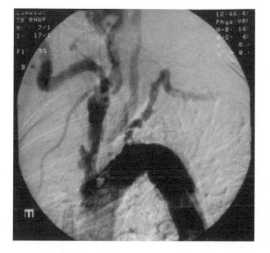

FIGURE 5-6. Carotid angiogram showing severe and diffuse atherosclerosis of the aortic arch and the aortic arch vasculature. In these patients, carotid artery stenting (CAS) is associated with increased risk of embolization and is therefore contraindicated.

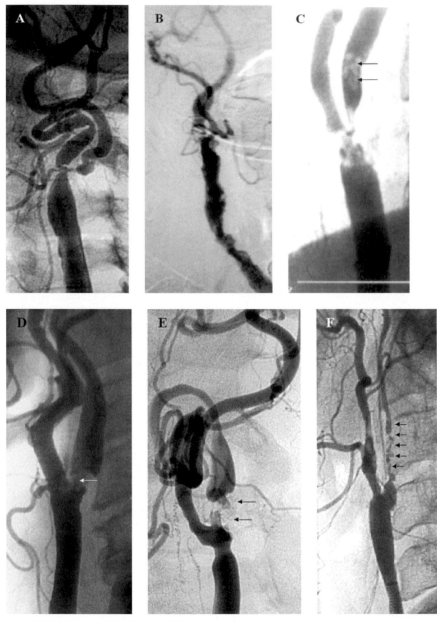

FIGURE 5-7. Anatomical contraindications for carotid artery stenting: (**A**) severely angulated internal carotid artery (ICA) origin with tortuous distal segments, (**B**) diffuse atherosclerosis of the ICA and common carotid artery (CCA), (**C**) pedunculated thrombus (*arrows*), (**D** and **E**) heavily calcified ICA lesions, and (**F**) subtotal occlusion of the ICA, called the "string sign."

Based on our learning-curve experience and considering the current carotid stent technology, we have identified a number of factors that are associated with either increased or decreased risk for procedural events (Table 5-3) (54). These unfavorable factors constitute less than 5% of the patients presenting for carotid stenting. It is extremely important for the interventionist to recognize the high-risk factors prior to the carotid stenting procedure and to

TABLE 5-3. CLINICAL AND ANATOMICAL VARIABLES AND THE RISK FOR EMBOLIC EVENTS DURING CAS

Patients at increased risk for embolic neurological complications
  Clinical factors
    1. Advanced age (<80 yr)
    2. Prior major disabling stroke
    3. Cerebral atrophy/dementia
    4. Unstable neurological symptoms (recent TIA or stroke)
  Anatomical factors
    1. Severely tortuous, calcified, and atherosclerotic aortic arch/arch vessels
    2. Severe tortuosities distal to the bifurcation
    3. Coexisting proximal common carotid artery lesions
    4. Total occlusion or long subtotal occlusions ("string sign lesions")
    5. Severe concentric calcification
    6. Angiographic evidence of a large thrombus
Patients at lower risk for embolic neurological complications
  Clinical factors
    1. Age ≤80 yr
    2. Less severe stenosis (within the guidelines)
  Anatomical factors
    1. Straight, noncalcified aortic arch vessels
    2. Nontortuous bifurcation
    3. Absence of kinks, loops, bend points at lesion site
    4. Short lesions
    5. Prior CEA

CAS, carotid artery stenting; TIA, transient ischemic attack; CEA, carotid endarterectomy.

establish a risk-benefit ratio for the individual patient. Higher-risk patients require much greater experience to achieve good outcomes and avoid complications. Therefore, during the initial experience of the operator, only cases with low procedural risk should be selected, and high-risk patients should be avoided. The low-risk patients, particularly those younger than 80 years, can be stented with a low rate of periprocedural events.

It should also be noted that several factors that increase the risk of CEA might also increase the risk for complications from the endovascular treatment. These factors include advanced age, a recent neurological event (particularly when a significant neurological deficit is present), and unstable neurological symptoms. At the beginning of the operator learning experience, there is a tendency to accept patients thought to be at high risk for CEA. This temptation should be avoided if the patient has one or more of the higher-risk descriptors listed in Table 5-2. The operator judgment is critical in order to ensure a low complication rate. It must be emphasized that unfavorable lesion characteristics may be apparent only following the initial angiography. The interventionist should be prepared to abandon the procedure at this point and consider an alternative treatment (CEA if suitable, or continuing medical therapy). It must also be emphasized that "failure to complete the procedure is acceptable but an avoidable complication is not."

Finally, the indications for CAS are evolving as the techniques, stents, and catheter technology advance. There is an ongoing need to improve the equipment suitable for carotid stenting and a need to enhance the safety of the procedure. Often, when a technical problem is encountered, it is attributed to the inadequacy of the devices currently available. As the technology improves, particularly with the application of the Anti-Embolization devices, the indications and contraindication may need to be revised.

REFERENCES

1. American Heart Association. *1999 heart and stroke statistical update.* Dallas: American Heart Association, 1999.
2. Beneficial effect of carotid endarterectomy in symptomatic patients with high-grade carotid stenosis. North American Symptomatic Carotid Endarterectomy Trial Collaborators. *N Engl J Med* 1991;325: 445–453.
3. Endarterectomy for asymptomatic carotid artery stenosis. Executive Committee for the Asymptomatic Carotid Atherosclerosis Study. *JAMA* 1995:1421–1428.
4. MRC European Carotid Surgery Trial: interim results for symptomatic patients with severe (70-99%) or with mild (0-29%) carotid stenosis. European Carotid Surgery Trialists' Collaborative Group. *Lancet* 1991;337:1235–1243.
5. Morey SS. AHA updates guidelines for carotid endarterectomy. *Am Fam Physician* 1998;58:1898, 1903–1904.
6. Yadav JS, Roubin GS, Iyer S, et al. Elective stenting of the extracranial carotid arteries. *Circulation* 1997;95:376–381.
7. Wholey MH, Al-Mubarak N, Wholey MH. Updated review of the global carotid artery stent registry. *Catheter Cardiovasc Interv* 2003;60:259–266.
8. Shawl F, Kadro W, Domanski MJ, et al. Safety and efficacy of elective carotid artery stenting in high-risk patients. *J Am Coll Cardiol* 2000;35:1721–1728.
9. Endovascular versus surgical treatment in patients with carotid stenosis in the Carotid and Vertebral Artery Transluminal Angioplasty Study (CAVATAS): a randomized trial. *Lancet* 2001;357:1729–1737.
10. Roubin GS, New G, Iyer SS, et al. Immediate and late clinical outcomes of carotid artery stenting in symptomatic and asymptomatic carotid stenosis: a 5-year prospective analysis. *Circulation* 2001:103: 532–537.
11. Parodi JC, La Mura R, Ferreira LM, et al. Initial evaluation of carotid angioplasty and stenting using three different cerebral protection devices. *J Vasc Surg* 2000;32:1127–1136.
12. Reimer B, Corvaja N, Moshiri S, et al. Cerebral protection with filter devices during carotid artery stenting. *Circulation* 2001:104;12–15.
13. Al-Mubarak N, Colombo A, Gaines PA, et al. Multicenter evaluation of carotid artery stenting with a filter protection system. *J Am Coll Cardiol* 2002;39:841–846.
14. Al-Mubarak N, Roubin GS, Vitek JJ, et al. Procedural safety and short-term efficacy of ambulatory carotid stenting. *Stroke* 2001;32:2305–2309.
15. New G, Roubin GS, Iyer SS, et al. Integrated minimally invasive approaches for the treatment of atherosclerotic vascular diseases: hybrid procedures. *Catheter Cardiovasc Interv* 2001;52:154–161.
16. Hobson RW 2nd. CREST (Carotid Revascularization Endarterectomy versus Stent Trial): background, design, and current status. *Semin Vasc Surg* 2000;13:139–143.
17. Shawl FA. Carotid stenting in patients with symptomatic coronary artery disease; a preferred approach. *J Invasive Cardiol* 1998;10:432–442.
18. Al-Mubarak N, Roubin GS, Gomez CR, et al. Carotid stenting for severe radiation-induced extacranial carotid artery occlusive disease. *J Endovasc Surg* 2000;7:36–40.
19. Al-Mubarak N, Roubin GS, Liu MW, et al. Early results of percutaneous intervention for severe coexisting carotid and coronary artery disease. *J Am Coll Cardiol* 1999;84:600–602.
20. Dangas G, Laird JR Jr, Mehran R, et al. Carotid artery stenting in patients with high-risk anatomy for carotid endarterectomy. *J Endovasc Ther* 2001;8:39–43.
21. Al-Mubarak N, Roubin GS, Vitek JJ, et al. Simultaneous bilateral carotid stenting for restenosis after endarterectomy. *Cathet Cardiovasc Diagn* 1998;45:11–15.
22. New G, Roubin GS, Iyer SS, et al. Safety, efficacy, and durability of carotid artery stenting for restenosis following carotid endarterectomy: a multicenter study. *J Endovasc Ther* 2000;7:345–352.
23. Mackey WC, O'Donnell TF, Callow AD. Cardiac risk in patients undergoing carotid endarterectomy: impact on perioperative and long-term mortality. *J Vasc Surg* 1990;11:226–234.

24. Craven TE, Ryu JE, Espeland MA. Evaluation of the association between carotid artery atherosclerosis and coronary artery stenosis. *Circulation* 1990;82:1230–1242.
25. Faggioli GL, Curl GR, Ricotta JJ. The role of carotid screening before coronary artery bypass. *J Vasc Surg* 1990;12:724–731.
26. Mackey WC, Khabbaz K, Bojar R, et al. Simultaneous carotid endarterectomy and coronary bypass: perioperative risk and long-term survival. *J Vasc Surg* 1996;24:58–64.
27. Takach TJ, Reul GJ, Cooley DA, et al. Is an integrated approach warranted for concomitant carotid and coronary artery disease? *Ann Thorac Surg* 1997;64:16–22.
28. Coyle KA, Gray BC, Smith RB 3rd, et al. Morbidity and mortality associated with carotid endarterectomy: effect of adjunctive coronary revascularization. *Ann Vasc Surg* 1995;9:21–27.
29. Hines GL, Scott WC, Schubach SL, et al. Prophylactic carotid endarterectomy in patients with high-grade carotid stenosis undergoing coronary bypass: does it decrease the incidence of perioperative stroke? *Ann Vasc Surg* 1998;12:23–27.
30. Herlitz J, Wognsen GB, Haglid M, et al. Risk indicators for cerebrovascular complications after coronary artery bypass grafting. *Thorac Cardiov Surg* 1998;46:20–24.
31. Akins WG, Moncure AC, Dagget WM, et al. Safety and efficacy of concomitant coronary artery operations. *Ann Thorac Surg* 1995;60:311–318.
32. Trachiotis GD, Pfister AJ. Management strategy for simultaneous carotid endarterectomy and coronary revascularization. *Ann Thorac Surg* 1997;64:1013–1018.
33. Babatasi G, Massetti M, Theron J, et al. Asymptomatic carotid stenosis in patients undergoing major cardiac surgery: can percutaneous carotid angioplasty be an alternative? *Eur J Cardiothorac Surg* 1997;11:547–553.
34. Matsuo T, Nishina T, Masumoto H, et al. Two successful cases of coronary artery bypass grafting followed by transluminal carotid angioplasty with stenting. *Kyobu Geka* 2001;54.1082–1086.
35. Cardaioli P, Giordan M, Isabella G. Percutaneous revascularization of coexisting severe carotid and coronary artery disease: a case report. *Ital Heart J* 2001;2:707–710.
36. Paniagua D, Howell M, Strickman N, et al. Outcomes following extracranial carotid artery stenting in high-risk patients. *J Invasive Cardiol* 2001;13:375–378.
37. Waigand J, Gross C. Carotid artery stent placement prior to coronary angioplasty or coronary bypass graft surgery. *Curr Interv Cardiol Rep* 2001;3:117–129.
38. Reifart N. Carotid percutaneous transluminal angioplasty in cardiological patients with increased surgical risk. *Z Kardiol* 2000;89(Suppl 8):27–31.
39. Yoon YS, Shim WH, Kim SM, et al. Carotid artery stenting in patients with symptomatic coronary artery disease. *Yonsei Med J* 2000;41:89–97.
40. Waigand J, Gross CM, Uhlich F, et al. Elective stenting of carotid artery stenosis in patients with severe coronary artery disease. *Eur Heart J* 1998;19:1365–1370.
41. Rockman CB, Riles TS, Fisher FS, et al. The surgical management of carotid artery stenosis in patients with previous neck radiation. *Am J Surg* 1996;172:191–195.
42. Atkinson JL, Sundt TM Jr, Dale AJ, et al. Radiation-associated atheromatous disease of the cervical carotid artery: report of seven cases and review of the literature. *Neurosurgery* 1989;24:171–178.
43. Melliere D, Becquemin JP, Berrahal D, et al. Management of radiation-induced occlusive arterial disease: a reassessment. *J Cardiovasc Surg* 1997;38:261–269.
44. Murros KE, Toole JF. The effect of radiation on carotid artery. A review article. *Arch Neurol* 1989;46:449–455.
45. Feeh RS, McGuirr WF, Bond MG, et al. A significant risk factor for carotid atherosclerosis. *Arch Otolaryngol Head Neck Surg* 1991;117:1135–1137.
46. Bergqvist D, Jonsson K, Nilsson M, et al. Treatment of arterial lesions after radiation therapy. *Surg Gynecol Obstet* 1987;165:116–120.
47. Ahuja A, Blatt GL, Guterman LR. Angioplasty for symptomatic radiation-induced extracranial carotid artery stenosis: case report. *Neurosurgery* 1995;36:399–403.
48. Houdart E, Mounayer C, Chapot R, et al. Carotid stenting for radiation-induced stenoses: a report of 7 cases. *Stroke* 2001;32:118–121.
49. Kitamura J, Kuroda S, Ushikoshi S, et al. Three cases of successful stenting for radiation-induced carotid arterial stenosis. *No Shinkei Geka* 2002;30:1097–1102.
50. Alric P, Branchereau P, Berthet JP, et al. Carotid artery stenting for stenosis following revascularization or cervical irradiation. *J Endovasc Ther* 2002;9:14–19.

51. Ohta H, Sakai N, Nagata I, et al. Bilateral carotid stenting for radiation-induced arterial stenosis. *No Shinkei Geka* 2001;29:559–563.
52. Hernandez-Vila E, Strickman NE, Skolkin M, et al. Carotid stenting for post-endarterectomy restenosis and radiation-induced occlusive disease. *Tex Heart Inst J* 2000;27:159–165.
53. Osborn AG. *Diagnostic cerebral angiography.* Philadelphia: Lippincott Williams & Wilkins, 1999.
54. Al-Mubarak N, Roubin GS, Iyer SS, et al. Techniques of carotid artery stenting: the state of the art. *Semin Vasc Surg* 2000;13:117–129.

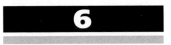

6

RECURRENT STENOSIS FOLLOWING CAROTID ENDARTERECTOMY

NADIM AL-MUBARAK
GARY S. ROUBIN

Restenosis following carotid endarterectomy (CEA) has been reported in up to 28% of patients with prior carotid surgery, although the more recent figure has averaged 13% (1–4). These figures have varied with the definition of restenosis, the follow-up duration, and the test used to detect carotid artery obstruction. In a meta-analysis of 29 studies that used noninvasive vascular testing, the average restenosis rate (defined as diameter obstruction of more than or equal to 50%) during the first year was 10% (4). Although the causative etiology remains controversial, the development of restenosis after CEA has been attributed to a number of factors, including trauma during the initial surgery and the presence of multiple risk factors for atherosclerosis (4,5). Clearly, the literature differentiates between an "early restenosis" (occurring within the first 24 months after CEA) that is pathologically attributed to myointimal hyperplasia and is usually located at the CEA site, and a "delayed restenosis" (occurring at or more than 24 months after CEA) that tends to occur distal or proximal to the prior CEA site and is presumed to be caused by progression of atherosclerosis (4,5). This dichotomy, however, is probably artifactual and represents two aspects of a continuum of progression. The literature is also ambiguous about the clinical relevance of restenosis after CEA as a risk for subsequent stroke. A recent multivariate analysis reported an increased risk of stroke in patients with recurrent carotid stenosis after CEA compared with medical therapy, although this analysis was limited by marked heterogeneity among the studies (3). In a recent long-term follow-up study, Ricotta and O'Brien-Irr (6) have suggested that these patients are at significantly increased risk for future ischemic events.

REPEAT SURGERY

Repeat surgery, until recently the only mode of revascularization available for restenosis following CEA, is more difficult than the initial surgery owing to the dense scarring within and around the arterial wall (7–11). External dissection through the surrounding scar tissue can be challenging and more traumatic, increasing the risk of cranial nerve damage and frequently requiring graft interposition. Intimal thickening and sclerosis of the arterial layers make it difficult to achieve adequate separation of the plaque from the media during CEA. Importantly, the combined rate of stroke and death associated with repeat CEA is approximately 11%, although improved outcomes have recently been reported (7–11). This is in part due to the advanced age and high prevalence of comorbidities such as hypertension, coronary artery disease, and myocardial infarction in these patients (7–11).

INDICATIONS FOR TREATMENT

Technical difficulty and high complication risks associated with repeat CEA, in addition to the fact that the majority of the patients with restenoses are asymptomatic, have led to some degree of controversy regarding the indication for carotid revascularization in these patients (11). The absence of controlled clinical trials that compare repeat CEA with medical therapy in this population further complicates this issue. Patients with restenosis after CEA have consistently been excluded from the major randomized carotid surgery trials because of a perceived increased risk for associated complications (12,13). Therefore, to justify revascularization in this setting, it is important to demonstrate that the treatment modality used has a low risk for complications and provides durable freedom from stroke. Nevertheless, a general consensus exists in the surgical community to treat those patients with high-grade symptomatic restenoses following CEA and asymptomatic patients with high risk for future stroke from severe restenosis, such as those undergoing coronary artery bypass surgery and patients with contralateral internal carotid artery occlusion (7–11).

ENDOVASCULAR TREATMENT

With the introduction of the endovascular techniques as an alternative to surgery for treatment of carotid artery stenosis, the application of this treatment in the high-risk surgical patients has increasingly gained popularity (14–23). This has been encouraged by the less-invasive nature of this treatment and the low risk for complications. Carotid artery stenting (CAS), by virtue of its percutaneous nature, does not require general anesthesia or skin incision, is safe in patients with severe coexisting coronary artery disease, and therefore is more suitable than surgery in treating patients with recurrent carotid stenosis after CEA. Recurrent stenosis following CEA poses no additional technical challenge for CAS (Fig. 6-1). The stenting technique used is identical to stenting *de novo* lesions, and its success rate is approximately 98% (14–23).

Prior to the vascular stenting era, the utilization of balloon angioplasty for treating carotid artery stenosis was limited owing to concerns about the risk of arterial wall dissection, acute closure, or embolic stroke during the intervention. The advent of intravascular stents and their subsequent successful application in the various vascular territories has led to a widespread utilization of stent-supported carotid angioplasty. Adjunctive stenting has the advantage of improving the immediate and late outcomes of endovascular revascularization. The risk of embolization may be reduced by trapping embolic material between the stent and the arterial wall. It is generally believed that recurrent stenoses following CEA, particularly those related to myointimal hyperplasia, are at low risk for embolic complications. Anecdotal observation from Lenox Hill using transcranial Doppler during CAS showed that stenting of these lesions is associated with a low microembolic load. Nevertheless, it remains our practice to use distal protection during CAS in these patients. On a technical note, we prefer predilation of the lesion using a compliant coronary balloon (standard size: 4 × 40 mm), which may reduce the risk of distal embolization of plaque material during the stent placement. Self-expanding stents are preferred mainly for their permanent radial expansion, preventing them from crimping under external pressure, as it has been our experience with balloon-expandable stents.

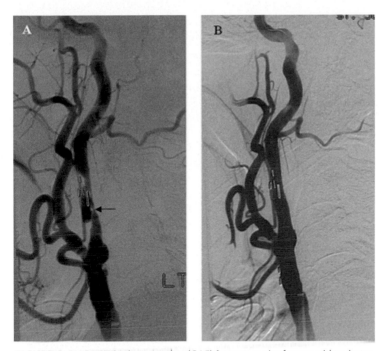

FIGURE 6-1. Carotid artery stenting (CAS) for restenosis after carotid endarterectomy (CEA). A 76-year-old man with history of CEA 11 years earlier was found to have a high-grade stenosis of the cervical left internal carotid artery at the prior CEA site (**A**; *arrows*) following a presentation with right sided weakness that completely resolved. Owing to the associated relatively high-located carotid bifurcation, the consultant surgeon deemed the patient to be at high risk for repeat CEA, which was potentially impossible to perform. CAS was successfully performed without complications (**B**).

Courtheoux et al. (14) reported successful balloon angioplasty in three patients for recurrent carotid artery stenosis without complications, but a fourth patient could not tolerate the balloon inflation and was managed surgically. Bergeron et al. (15) reported percutaneous angioplasty for restenosis after CEA in 15 patients. Stents were used to treat complications (dissection and acute closure) that occurred after balloon dilatation in two patients and residual stenosis in one patient.

More recent series of elective CAS in these patients have reported encouraging immediate outcomes and late freedom from stroke that compared favorably with the reported surgical results of low-risk surgical patients. Yadav et al. (16) reported the first series of elective CAS in 22 patients with recurrent stenosis after CEA (25 hemispheres). There was one procedural minor stroke, but no major stoke and no death. On late follow-up (mean of 8 months), no neurological events occurred. Among the eight patients who had 6-month angiographic follow-up, no restenosis (more than or equal to 50% diameter obstruction) was detected (16).

Two recent comparative studies of CAS versus surgery for recurrent stenosis after CEA have been published (17,18). Hobson et al. (17) examined outcomes of 16 consecutive CEAs and 17 consecutive CASs performed by the same operators. One (6%) minor stroke occurred in the CEA group, and no events occurred in the stented patients. However, the small patient number in this nonrandomized study has confounded the results. The authors also reported their experience with 1,065 repeat CEA with a combined 30-day stroke and death rate of 1.4%, cranial nerve palsies rate of 3.5%, and neck hematoma requiring surgical treatment occurred in 0.5% of the patients. In another nonrandomized comparative study (58 repeat CEA with 25 CAS) that included the interventionist's learning curve, Aburahma et al. (18) reported comparable 30-day outcomes in the two groups.

The largest experience of CAS for recurrent stenosis after CEA was reported in a mulicenter registry that included 14 centers from the United States (19). The registry included a total of 358 CAS procedures on 338 patients who developed recurrent stenosis after CEA at a mean of 5.5 months. The combined stroke and death rate at 30 days was 3.7%, including a minor stroke rate of 1.7%, major stroke rate of 0.8%, fatal stroke rate of 0.3%, and a nonneurological death rate of 0.9%. Although this study was limited by its retrospective design, it provided evidence for a significant freedom from stroke at 3 years and suggested that CAS is suitable and safe treatment for restenosis after CEA.

To further prospectively address the role of CAS in the treatment of recurrent stenosis following CEA, a number of high-risk registries evaluating CAS with distal protection in a variety of high-risk surgical subsets are currently underway. The most important of these is Carotid Revascularization with Endarterectomy or Stenting Systems (CARESS), a multicenter prospective study that includes a variety of high-risk surgical groups that are expected to be excluded from any randomized trial that compares CEA with CAS (24).

In summary, repeat surgery for restenosis following CEA can be technically challenging, and its attendant operative risk may preclude its benefits. In these patients, CAS is technically feasible and offers a less-invasive alternative to CEA. Current data support the safety of CAS in this patient population and the midterm effectiveness in preventing stroke. The application of Anti-Embolization devices is expected to further enhance the immediate outcomes of this treatment.

REFERENCES

1. Degroote RD, Lynch TG, Jamil Z, et al. Carotid stenosis: long-term noninvasive follow-up after carotid endarterectomy. *Stroke* 1987;18:1031–1036.
2. Kieny R, Seiller C, Petit H. Evolution of carotid restenosis after endarterectomy. *Cardiovasc Surg* 1994; 2:555–560.
3. Frericks H, Kievit J, van Baalen JM, et al. Carotid recurrent stenosis and risk of ipsilateral stroke: a systematic review of the literature. *Stroke* 1998;29:244–250.
4. Avaramovic JR, Fletcher JP. The incidence of recurrent carotid stenosis after carotid endarterectomy and its relationship to neurological events. *J Cardiovasc Surg* 1992;33:54–58.
5. Gelabert HA, El-Masssry S, Moore WS. Carotid endarterectomy with primary closure does not adversely affect the rate of recurrent stenosis. *Arch Surg* 1994;129:648–654.
6. Ricotta JJ, O'Brien-Irr MS. Conservative management of residual and recurrent lesions after carotid endarterectomy: long-term results. *J Vasc Surg* 1997;26:963–970, 970–972.
7. Das MB, Hertzer NR, Ratliff NB, et al. Recurrent carotid stenosis. A five-year series of 65 reoperations. *Ann Surg* 1985;202:28–35.
8. Lattimer CR, Burnand KG. Recurrent carotid stenosis after carotid endarterectomy. *Br J Surg* 1997; 84:1206–1219.
9. AbuRahma AF, Snodgrass KR, Robinson PA, et al. Safety and durability of redo carotid endarterectomy for recurrent carotid artery stenosis. *Am J Surg* 1994;168:175–178.
10. Sterpetti AV, Schultz RD, Feldhaus RJ, et al. Natural history of recurrent carotid artery disease. *Surg Gynecol Obstet* 1989;168:217–223.
11. Meyer FB, Piepgras DG, Fode NC. Surgical treatment of recurrent carotid artery stenosis. *J Neurosurg* 1994;80:781–787.
12. Beneficial effect of carotid endarterectomy in symptomatic patients with high-grade carotid stenosis. North American Symptomatic Carotid Endarterectomy Trial Collaborators. *N Engl J Med* 1991;325: 445–453.

13. Endarterectomy for asymptomatic carotid artery stenosis. Executive Committee for the Asymptomatic Carotid Atherosclerosis Study. *JAMA* 1995;273:1421–1428.
14. Courtheoux P, Theron J, Tournade A, et al. Percutaneous endoluminal angioplasty of post endarterectomy carotid stenoses. *Neuroradiology* 1987;29:186–189.
15. Bergeron P, Rudondy P, Benichou H, et al. Transluminal angioplasty for recurrent stenosis after carotid endarterectomy. Prognostic factors and indications. *Int Angiol* 1993;12:256–259.
16. Yadav JS, Roubin GS, King P, et al. Angioplasty and stenting for restenosis after carotid endarterectomy. Initial experience. *Stroke* 1996;27:2075–2079.
17. Hobson RW 2nd, Goldstein JE, Jamil Z, et al. Carotid restenosis: operative and endovascular management. *J Vasc Surg* 1999;29:228–235.
18. Abu Rahma AF, Bates MC, Stone PA, et al. Comparative study of operative treatment and percutaneous transluminal angioplasty/stenting for recurrent carotid disease. *J Vasc Surg* 2001;34:831–838.
19. New G, Roubin GS, Iyer SS, et al. Safety, efficacy, and durability of carotid artery stenting for restenosis following carotid endarterectomy: a multicenter study. *J Endovasc Ther* 2000;7:345–352.
20. Al-Mubarak N, Roubin GS, Vitek JJ, et al. Simultaneous bilateral carotid stenting for restenosis after endarterectomy. *Cathet Cardiovasc Diagn* 1998;45:11–15.
21. Lanzino G, Mericle RA, Lopes DK, et al. Percutaneous transluminal angioplasty and stent placement for recurrent carotid artery stenosis. *J Neurosurg* 1999;90:688–694.
22. Hernandez-Vila E, Strickman NE, Skolkin M, et al. Carotid stenting for post-endarterectomy restenosis and radiation-induced occlusive disease. *Tex Heart Inst J* 2000;27:159–165.
23. Shawl FA. Safety and efficacy of elective carotid artery stenting in high-risk patients. *J Am Coll Cardiol* 2000;35:1721–1728.
24. Roubin GS, Hobson RW 2nd, White R, et al. CREST and CARESS to evaluate carotid stenting: time to get to work! *J Endovasc Ther* 2001;8:107–110.

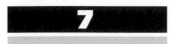

THE ROLE OF MULTISPECIALTY GROUPS IN CAROTID ARTERY STENTING

MICHAEL H. WHOLEY

The purpose of this chapter is to analyze the role of multispecialty groups in the growth and development of cervical carotid artery stenting (CAS). Despite its controversial beginning, CAS will continue to grow beyond its niche role for treatment of primarily high-risk surgical symptomatic patients and will envelop more asymptomatic patients. Part of the growth will come from the development of multispecialty groups involving interventional radiologists and neuroradiologists, interventional cardiologists, and endovascular-trained surgeons. This chapter addresses the need for multispecialty groups, the strategic planning that is required prior to forming such a group, and the process of how to start one.

THE NEED FOR MULTISPECIALTY GROUPS

In order to introduce the concept of multispecialty groups, it is necessary to jump to the conclusion that the current system needs improvement and agree to the following:

1. The old status quo was not beneficial for the various specialists and especially not for patients. There is a growing need for more patients with cervical carotid disease to receive treatment, be it endarterectomy or stent placement. Many of these patients not seen in the medical system would be better with stent placement. Though there are many excellent surgeons with low complication rates, carotid endarterectomy is not suitable to many patients. Hence, not only will the total number of patients to be intervened on increase, but also those patients receiving carotid stents will increase.
2. There must be a common goal to advance the field and understanding of CAS. Carotid stenting is a young field, having been pioneered by Drs. Mathias and Theron, and only recently receiving dedicated stents and Anti-Embolization devices. The best means to improve a field scientifically is to have a balanced input of ideas from the various specialists, each contributing their own expertise.
3. For effective and efficient use of available resources, peripheral vascular disease will have been treated by a team approach of radiology, surgery, and cardiology. In order to perform carotid stenting safely, an exhaustive supply of equipment is required, including a multitude of guidewires, diagnostic catheters, sheaths and guiding catheters, balloon catheters, stents, and Anti-Embolization devices. More daunting is the need for excellent imaging utilized in performing peripheral vascular imaging. The use of C-arms in the operating room as well as conventional cardiac imaging without adequate digital subtraction are steps backward in a field that is one of the most challenging. The nation's health care

system cannot afford to duplicate many of the imaging requirements needed for carotid imaging by various departments in the same hospital.

4. In order to achieve greater acceptance of CAS by the surgery community, greater representation by the surgical community will be required. One of the great roadblocks to the acceptance of carotid stenting by the medical community as well as by the government has been the general fear that CAS will replace carotid endarterectomy. Whether the surgery community should have such influence on the nation's medical policies is another debate, but, regardless, in order to achieve a better reception of carotid stenting, more surgeons will need to be involved. In comparison, the Food and Drug Administration (FDA) and Health Care Financing Administration (HCFA) accepted abdominal aortic stent grafts based only on historical data. There were no clinical trials. Likewise, small bowel transplants received acceptance. The question then comes, how do you train more surgeons without hurting the other specialties, primarily interventional radiology? This brings up the last assumption.

5. A team is required where all specialists share in the process. Whenever a team is created, in order to get full cooperation and maximum efficiency, it is necessary for all team members to share in risks and benefits. No one group should feel slighted or placed in a less than advantageous position. This includes establishing from the start an atmosphere where all parties have equal rights in the creation, management, and revenue sharing of CAS.

HISTORICAL REVIEW OF CAROTID ARTERY STENTING

CAS has grown significantly within the past decade. Early pioneers such as Kachel, Theron, and others performed percutaneous transluminal angioplasty of the carotid artery in the early 1980s using technology developed for peripheral angioplasty. Though limited in number, these procedures provided key insight into a potentially new field. Interventional techniques were developed and implemented almost entirely by interventional radiologists. As stents became commercially available in the early 1990s, carotid application began in 1994 and 1995 at several centers. The role of stents, as in other arterial applications, has been to hold back the arterial plaque, increase the treated diameter, and, thus, help prevent dissection and restenosis. Because cardiologists were familiar with stent placement and guiding catheters, it was a natural transition into the common and internal carotid artery. In 1997, from the world registry, approximately 24 centers performed the procedure worldwide. At this time, interventional cardiologists performed approximately one-half of the procedures. This has grown in the past 5 years to where almost 60% to 70% of carotid stents are placed by interventional cardiologists. Sharing the remaining portion of the market have been interventional radiologists and neuroradiologists as well as a growing number of surgeons including vascular, neurosurgery, and cardiothoracic surgeons.

STRATEGIC PLANNING FOR MULTISPECIALTY GROUPS

In order to decide whether forming a multispecialty group is right for you and your partners, it is important to form a brief strategic plan. Regardless, forming such a plan will be helpful for making many of the decisions needed in today's changing market in health care. Included in the strategic plan are the key steps.

MISSION STATEMENT

Determine what business you are in. Simply said, we are in the business of the diagnosis and treatment of cardiovascular disease regardless of our specialty.

ASSESS THE ENVIRONMENT

Know the background of the various specialists you may work with.

Positions of the Various Specialists

Who should be performing CAS? There are many strengths and weaknesses to each specialty (Table 7-1). Neuroradiologists are most skilled in intracranial applications with diagnostic and interventional procedures in the cerebral circulation, but lack some skills in clinical management and patient referrals. Interventional radiologists, likewise, have always regarded carotid diagnostic and intervention as their field, but also lack clinical management and patient referral skills. Vascular surgeons have had an over-50-year history treating cervical carotid disease but have only recently become involved in endovascular techniques. Cardiologists have tremendous control over patients and good catheter skills but are unfamiliar with neuroanatomy and neurologic rescue techniques. To understand each group's desires and goals, it is important to look carefully at their different backgrounds and situations.

Position of Interventional Radiologists

Interventional radiology, as we know it, is facing extinction. It has always had a tradition of pioneering most interventional procedures, including cardiac angiography. Long-standing turf battles including the "call to arms" by cardiologists performing peripheral vascular procedures have had devastating effects on the field. This year, less than half of the interventional fellowship positions were filled, and the near future does not look better. As interventional radiologists are forced into venous access and other nondescript fields, fewer are being trained in arterial intervention. The Society of Cardiovascular & Interventional Radiology (SCVIR) recently underwent a name change from SCVIR to The Society of Interventional Radiology (SIR), dropping the "Cardiovascular."

This decrease in training, culminated with the drop in fellows, will impact the interventional radiologist's role in standard arterial cases, but also in areas not as glamorous; embolization of arterial injuries in major trauma centers, pediatric intervention, and nonvascular intervention such as percutaneous biliary and nephrostomy procedures will all be severely affected. Some surgery colleagues think that all these areas could be taken over by other specialists, such as by cardiology to do embolization, gastroenterologists to do the biliary procedures, and so on. Unfortunately, this will not happen, at least in the short term, and the patients will suffer. It would take a long time to duplicate the skills and knowledge base. If you are not performing catheter manipulations 1 or 2 days a week, how can you replace a specialty that uses it every day?

Hence, interventional radiologists have been less than warmly receptive of the oncoming changes by cardiology and now vascular surgeons wishing to do all of their own diagnostic angiograms and the subsequent interventions.

Position of Vascular Surgeons

Vascular surgeons have maintained a dominant position in the management of peripheral vascular disease, including the carotids. Since the beginning of carotid endarterectomy by

TABLE 7-1. STRENGTHS AND WEAKNESSES OF VARIOUS SPECIALTIES PERFORMING CAROTID STENT PLACEMENT

Interventional Neuroradiology
   Greatest experience in neurologic anatomy
   Most skilled in neurologic rescue and intraarterial stroke therapy
   Familiar in neurologic imaging including CT, MRI
      Relatively few in numbers: 180 in U.S.
      Busy with other diagnostic tests, not present in lab every day
      Limited skills in guiding catheters and stent delivery
      Limited patient management skills
      Limited cardiac treatment skills

Interventional Radiology
   Greatest experience in peripheral interventions including great vessels
   Excellent clinical skills with time spent every day in the lab
   Cross training in other fluoroscopic treatment modalities
   Training in neuroanatomy and diagnostic angiograms, including neurorescue
   Access to MRA/MRI and CT angiography, which will replace standard angiography shortly
      Fair patient management skills
      Limited patient outpatient
      Limited cardiac treatment skills
      No or limited patient referral patterns
      Training and practicing physicians
         22,000 radiologists in U.S.
         2,500–3,000 practicing interventional radiologists
         200 IR fellows in training

Interventional Cardiology
   Greatest experience in cardiac management
   Excellent skills in guide catheter and small wire motions
   Large-number physician base
      18,000–20,000 cardiologists in U.S.
      5,500 practicing interventional cardiologists
      1,800 interventional cardiology fellows
   Very aggressive patient referral patterns
   Industry strongly sponsored
      Limited or no training in the cerebral anatomy and treatment of complications
      Limited equipment currently used in regards to DSA and peripherally adapted rooms
      Credibility damaged by being overaggressive in encroaching upon areas not related to the heart

Vascular Surgery
   Greatest experience in management of carotid occlusive disease
   Greatest experience in managing patients with above disease
   Excellent understanding of the pathology and disease process
   Excellent relationships with patients
   Excellent clinical referrals, especially from symptomatic patients
      Limited interventional background
      History of antagonistic feeling towards interventional procedures
      Limited angiographic equipment and fluoroscopy

CT, computed tomography; MRI, magnetic resonance imaging; MRA, magnetic resonance angiography; IR, interventional radiography; DSA, digital subtraction angiography.

Eastman and Cooley in the 1950s, intervention of the cervical carotid has remained in the surgical domain. Hence, they will not let it go to another specialty.

It was not until the introduction of iliac stent placement, and not until the vascular surgeons started doing their own iliac stents, that they realized the benefits of endovascular technique. Until then, interventional radiologists have traditionally met resistance in trying to introduce interventional techniques for the peripheral circulation. Now, with the overwhelming popularity of peripheral intervention among the cardiologists, many vascular surgeons feel threatened. Having ignored, or fought, the trend, many vascular surgeons are playing catch-up to learn endovascular skills. This trend has resulted in friction with many of their interventional radiology colleagues: Many diagnostic runoffs and interventions of the lower extremities are being performed by vascular surgeons as part of their training and revenue.

Many vascular surgeons have responded harshly to the current push for CAS. Obstacles to carotid stenting have included: establishing new hospital committees to review (disapprove) carotid stent protocols, delaying Institutional Review Board (IRB) committee approvals, and creating committees to review (disapprove) physician privileges. By not being part of the future, they have slowed carotid stenting; it is the author's opinion that CAS is approximately 4 years behind schedule. So, the questions remain: First, do surgeons have the skills to perform carotid stenting? I believe most do, but require basic training in catheter and guide-wire manipulation. Most require fundamental work in periphery, then renals or subclavians, and then carotids. It is a mistake for most to jump quickly to carotid intervention.

Second question, do we need to bring vascular surgeons into the field? Ironically, many cardiologists who faced the same criticism from radiologists earlier push this complaint. Again, in order for the field to receive greater acceptance and growth, it is important to establish pathways for vascular surgeons and other surgeons, such as those in neurosurgery.

Position of Interventional Cardiologists

With a large number of fellows and even larger number of actively practicing interventionalists, cardiologists are in a very strong position. They have excellent outpatient and inpatient referrals. Almost all patients undergoing surgical procedures require cardiac clearance. Hence, patients must come for various tests, such as electrocardiogram (EKG), cardiac echo, thallium stress test, and coronary angiography/PTCI. Once seen by a cardiologist, asymptomatic carotid disease can be screened by "drive-by" injections.

Many cardiologists appear overly confident that carotid stenting is simple, believing their coronary skills will translate into carotid success, especially because it is not a moving target. Most cardiologists have excellent catheter skills and combined with patient management, especially treating cardiac-related abnormalities during stent placement. Still, carotid intervention is a specialty not to be taken lightly. Hence, with patient referrals, which attracts many hospital administrators' attention, as well as clinical skills, what is to stop interventional cardiologists from dominating carotid stenting? As stated, cardiologists control 60–70% of carotid stenting. Will it increase to 80–90%?

FORECAST TRENDS (TABLE 7-2)

What do you expect the trend will be for CAS in your region? Will it grow 20% per year or 40% per year once established? What are the factors that will help accelerate or slow down its growth?

TABLE 7-2. FORECASTING TRENDS IN YOUR FIELD

Identify
  Customers
    Patients, referring physicians, third-party payers
  Competitors
    Region: other radiologists, cardiologists, vascular surgeons
    Within your own group
  Resources
    Internal/external
Patient issues
  Consumer orientation
  Patient education
  Aging population
Economic changes
  Managed care era
  Corporate involvement
  Reimbursement control
  Vertical integration

WHAT ARE MY GOALS?

Refer to Table 3.

ASK THE QUESTION: WHAT GOOD WILL THIS CHANGE DO FOR ME?

Why Form a Multispecialty Group in CAS?

This brings the important question, why would the three specialties try to form a multispecialty group? Looking at each group, we can analyze these gains and losses.

Radiology (Neuroradiology and Peripheral Trained)

- Survival: Radiologists can become part of team performing arterial interventions, which many have lost.
- With improved relations, they will obtain other vascular referrals, share call, have access to cutting edge innovations and equipment, and provide support to cardiology colleagues.
- Downside: They risk being replaced after teaching skills to others.

Vascular Surgery

- Retain carotid patient base, being able to provide both surgical as well as endovascular options.
- Learn fundamentals of interventional procedures and master carotid stent techniques.
- Gain credibility among their peers, which will increase potential referrals.
- Downside: risk of being overrun by cardiology colleagues.

TABLE 7-3. WHAT ARE MY GOALS?

Short-term goals (1–3 yrs)
  Influenced by professional and personnel interests
  Establish milestones for the group
   No. procedures performed
   No. patients treated
   Revenue generated/mo
   Recheck every 6 mo
Long-term objectives (5–10 yrs)
  Examples
   Establish stable relations with managed care organizations
   Become a major referral center
   Excel in teaching/research
   Acquire or merge with other centers
   Develop a regional cardiovascular center
Other goals
  Entrenchment
   Maintain current important role in endovascular procedures
  Market development
   Become more aggressive
   Increase endovascular procedures
  New service development
  Diversification

Interventional Cardiology

- Gain credibility within the hospital and community by having a multispecialty approach to a complex disease process, which may be essential in order to overcome the blockade placed against cardiologists in performing CAS.
- Gain credibility among industry, which is important in the determination of site selection for various carotid trials and registries.
- Having specialists in the diagnosis and management of neurologic diseases including providing expertise in neurorescue.
- Establishing the fundamental team for the next growth area of acute stroke intervention.
- Downside: loss of potential income from sharing revenue.

CREATE A PLAN

Create a multispecialty group. After assessing the environment and using the variables presenting in the terms of technological changes, patient issues, and economic, devise a plan. The plan should take into account desired market share, procedures desired, and revenue expected.

HOW TO CREATE A MULTISPECIALTY GROUP

Once the important decision has been made about the need to create a multispecialty group, various steps must be made:

1. Decide who you want to join your team. Much of this will be based upon your personal relationship with the other person. It will be important to choose a compatible partner who will be reliably involved in CAS for the long term.
2. Review the environment for establishing a carotid stent program.

   - How competitive is it in your area?
   - How receptive are your hospital administrators? How are the hospital finances and overall commitment to such a program?
   - What equipment will you need?
   - Do you have the ancillary services [nursing, intensive care unit (ICU), imaging, etc.]?
   - How are your chances and connections with industry in being able to get involved in clinical trials?

3. Nuts and bolts issues

   - Where are the cases going to be performed?
   - Who will be the primary operators?
   - Which research nurses will take charge?
   - If there are disputes, who will decide?
   - How are revenues and expenses divided?

4. Create various scenarios of your team and its dynamics and growth.

   - Optimistic scenario: You have good group relations, volume picks up immediately, and the creation of vascular institute with the various specialties becomes a possible reality.
   - Probable scenario: After initial thorny issues are resolved, patient volume is growing, slowly at first, but steadily. Many issues and decisions are made along the way with as few difficulties as possible.

5. What are your goals in starting a carotid stent team?

   - What are your revenue expectations?
   - How much cost are you willing to incur?
   - Do you plan on publishing your data and achieving regional or national prominence?
   - How active do you want to be in the team?
   - What will your partners, especially those who do not perform interventions, think of the plan?
   - What will your team members' partners feel about your plans?

CONCLUSIONS

Agree on the following:

- The old status quo was not beneficial for the sections and especially for patients.
- Clear understanding of others' perspectives
- Maintain good lines of communication.
- Common goal to advance the hospital and other sections
- For effective and efficient use of available resources, peripheral vascular disease will have to be treated by a team approach of interventional radiology, vascular surgery, and cardiology.

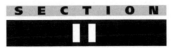

SECTION II

CAROTID ARTERY STENTING TECHNIQUES

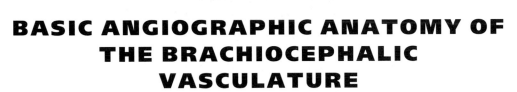

8

BASIC ANGIOGRAPHIC ANATOMY OF THE BRACHIOCEPHALIC VASCULATURE

NADIM AL-MUBARAK
JIRI J. VITEK

The knowledge of basic angiographic anatomy of the aortic arch and the brachiocephalic vasculature is an essential component of successful carotid artery access and the safe execution of the carotid artery stenting (CAS) procedure. In addition to being the standard method to assess the severity of carotid artery obstruction, brachiocephalic angiography uncovers unfavorable anatomical conditions that may increase the difficulty of the stenting procedure, such as dilated aortic arch, marked vessel tortuosities, heavy lesion calcifications, and filling defects indicative of thrombus within the lesion. The preprocedural identification of severe contralateral carotid artery stenosis and complete occlusion, as well as the status of the intracranial circulation (isolated hemispheres, collateral supply, severe distal obstructive disease), determines the most suitable technical approach to the carotid stenting procedure and aids the selection of the appropriate Anti-Embolization strategy. The benefits of prestenting brachiocephalic angiography are summarized in Table 8-1. The objective of this chapter is to discuss the basic radiographic anatomy of the aortic arch, the aortic arch vessels, and the intracranial vasculature relevant to the development and treatment of obstructive carotid artery disease. Detailed catheterization and angiographic techniques will be discussed later in chapter 9.

NORMAL ANATOMY OF THE AORTIC ARCH

In our practice, aortic arch angiography is performed when severe ostial stenosis of an arch vessel is suspected or when difficulty accessing the carotid arteries is encountered. This is usually performed with a curved 5F Pigtail catheter in the left oblique projection (40 to 50 degrees) using digital subtraction angiography (DSA) and a high-pressure automatic injector (40 mL of 60% diluted contrast medium at 20 mL per second). The tip of the catheter is positioned in the ascending aorta above the aortic valve to achieve optimal mixture of the contrast medium with the blood prior to reaching the aortic arch (Fig. 8-1). In children and young adults, the aortic arch is a symmetrically curved vascular structure that courses from the right anterior to the left posterior mediastinal compartment prior to its transition into the descending thoracic aorta (Fig. 8-1). Therefore, the aortic arch and its branches are best displayed in the left anterior oblique projection. Three main vessels originate from the aortic arch, including (from right to left) the brachiocephalic artery (innominate artery), the left common carotid artery (CCA),

TABLE 8-1. ADVANTAGES AND DISADVANTAGES OF BRACHIOCEPHALIC ANGIOGRAPHY

Advantages of the initial brachiocephalic angiography
1. The standard for the severity assessment of carotid artery stenosis
2. Uncovers unfavorable anatomies that may complicate the carotid stenting procedure (e.g., dilated aortic arch, marked tortuosity, heavy lesion calcifications, and filling defects within the lesion)
3. Preprocedural knowledge of the contralateral carotid stenosis/occlusion and the status of intracranial circulation (isolated hemisphere, collateral supply) may influence the technical approach and the choice of the Anti-Embolization device
4. Reliable demonstration of severe distal and intracranial ICA stenosis
5. In case of an intraprocedural neurological event, the postprocedure intracranial angiogram can be compared with the baseline preinterventional study

Disadvantages of brachiocephalic angiography
1. Contrast-induced acute tubular necrosis
2. Risk of neurological events

With present techniques and in experienced hands, these risks are very small (0.1–0.2%)

ICA, internal carotid artery.

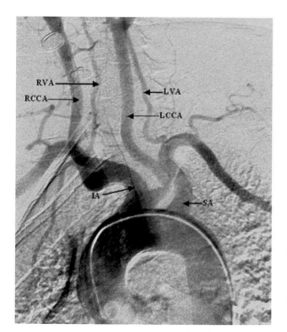

FIGURE 8-1. Angiography of the aortic arch and the aortic arch vasculature in a young patient. In this case, the left common carotid artery (LCCA) originates from the innominate artery (IA). SA, subclavian artery; LVA, left vertebral artery; RVA, right vertebral artery; RCCA, right common carotid artery.

and the left subclavian artery (Fig. 8-1) (1). The origins of the brachiocephalic arteries are nicely aligned in straight lines and course superiorly. The innominate artery divides shortly after its origin into the right CCA and the right subclavian artery (SA), which gives rise to the right vertebral artery (VA). The left SA gives rise to the left VA. Aging and the atherosclerotic degenerative process elongate the aortic arch and displace the aortic knob more superiorly and posteriorly, shifting the ostia of brachiocephalic arteries (Fig. 8-2), an important anatomical finding that needs to be considered when accessing the carotid artery with a catheter in the elderly patient. In young adults, the ostium of the left CCA is located between the ostium of the left SA and the innominate artery, and the vessel courses superiorly. With aging, the ostium shifts posteriorly and the artery elongates, courses to the left, and can form a sharp superior turn (Figs. 8-2, 8-3). This vascular arrangement can make selective catheterization of the left CCA very difficult (see chapter 9).

Congenital variations and anomalies of the aortic arch vessels occur in 30% of the cases, the majority of which are minor anatomical variations (1–3). The most common anomaly is the joint origin of the left CCA with the innominate artery. The second is the left CCA originating from the innominate artery itself (Figs. 8-1, 8-4). In this instance, the left CCA may originate close to the aortic arch, deeply resembling a *truncus bicaroticus* (Fig. 8-4). Other anomalies of the aortic arch and the origins of the brachiocephalic arteries are rare, with the most common being anomalous origin of the right SA (1%) and direct origin of the left VA (8%) from the aortic arch (Fig. 8-5). In the first case, the right CCA is the first vessel to originate separately from the proximal aortic arch, and the right SA originates separately distal to the left SA.

As already stated, aging and the atherosclerotic process elongate and distend the aortic arch, shifting the ostia of the brachiocephalic arteries (Figs. 8-2, 8-3). As the aortic knob is displaced more superiorly and posteriorly, the innominate artery and left CCA origins and their proximal segments sharply tilt from right to left, increasing the disadvantageous angulations for selective cannulation. Deep advancement of the catheter into the carotid arteries can be challenging or impossible if the innominate artery or the left CCA are sharply tilted to the left, or if the proximal segments of these vessels are very tortuous (Fig. 8-6). Statistically noting, there are more failures to selectively catheterize the left CCA than the right.

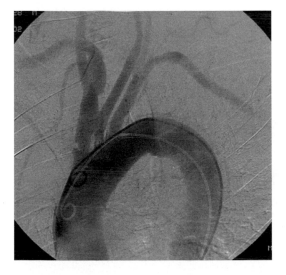

FIGURE 8-2. Aortic arch angiography in an elderly patient. The aging and atherosclerotic degenerative processes elongate the aortic arch and displace the aortic knob more superiorly and posteriorly, shifting the ostia of the brachiocephalic arteries. The ostium of the left common carotid artery (CCA) shifts posteriorly and the artery elongates and courses to the left, forming a sharp superior turn. The proximal segments of the left CCA and innominate artery (IA) have mild stenoses.

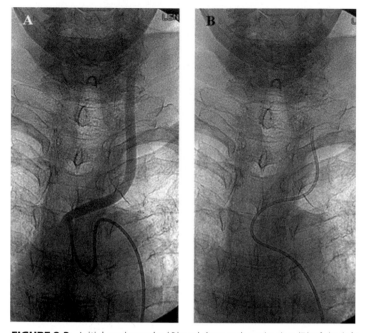

FIGURE 8-3. Initial angiography (**A**) and deep catheterization (**B**) of the left common carotid artery (CCA) in an elderly patient. The origin of the CCA is sharply angulated.

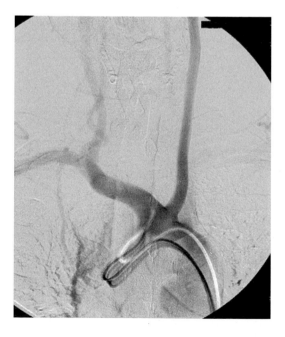

FIGURE 8-4. *Truncus bicaroticus*. The innominate and the left common carotid artery share a common origin.

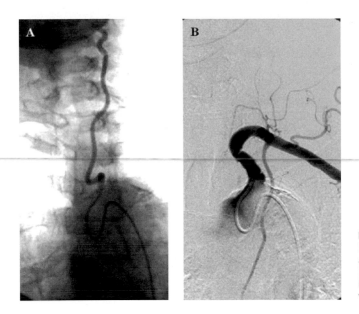

FIGURE 8-5. Direct origin of the left vertebral artery (VA) from the aortic arch. **A:** The left VA is cannulated directly from the aortic arch. **B**: subclavian artery angiography with absent VA.

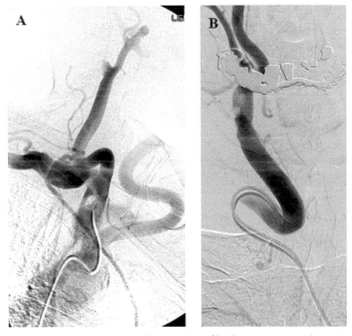

FIGURE 8-6. Severe proximal tortuosities of both common carotid arteries (CCA) (**A** and **B**). In (**B**), the origin of the left CCA is sharply tilted. This anatomy is disadvantageous for selective cannulation of any of the CCA, and deep advancement of the catheter into these arteries can be very challenging or impossible.

THE CAROTID ARTERIES

In the majority of cases, the CCA typically bifurcates at the C3-4 level into the internal carotid artery (ICA) and external carotid artery (ECA) with both carotid bifurcations located at the same level (4). In some instances, the bifurcation is located at C2 or higher, deep underneath the mandible, a position that makes it inaccessible to the standard carotid endarterectomy (CEA), mandating an extensive surgical mobilization of the mandible in order to expose the stenotic segment. Bifurcations within the upper thoracic or lower cervical levels are very rare.

The CCA usually has no significant branches. The proximal segment of the ICA dilates, forming the carotid bulb where the carotid sinus is located (5) (Fig. 8-7). The atherosclerotic process typically involves the carotid artery bifurcation and the proximal cervical segment of the ICA. Within the carotid bifurcation, the origin of the ICA usually points medially and posteriorly. The origin of the ECA points towards the anterior-lateral direction. For these anatomical reasons, the best views to separate both origins are the ipsilateral oblique and the straight lateral projection (Fig. 8-7). Occasionally, the bifurcation is congenitally overrotated, i.e., in the lateral projection, the ICA and ECA are superimposed. In this arrangement, the best projection to separate the ICA and ECA is the contralateral oblique or anterior-posterior (AP) projections.

The ICA can present with kinks, coils, and tortuosities (Fig. 8-8) (6). Coils and tortuosities are congenital; kinks are usually related to the aging process (6). The aging process, atherosclerotic vascular changes, and shortening of the cervical spine can exaggerate all of these anatomies. Kinks can turn into significant stenotic lesions with hyaline-wall degeneration. All of these conditions are prone to produce spasm when entered with a guide wire or catheter. The cervical segment of the ICA does not have any branches. In rare exceptions, the occipital or ascending pharyngeal artery may originate from this artery or replace it (Fig. 8-9). It should be noted that especially in women, the cervical segment of the ICA

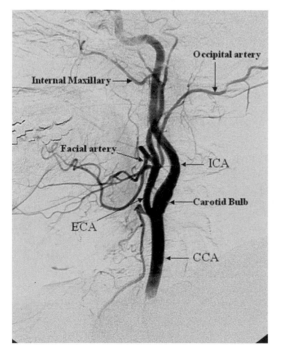

FIGURE 8-7. Normal carotid artery bifurcation. CCA, common carotid artery; ICA, internal carotid artery; ECA, external carotid artery.

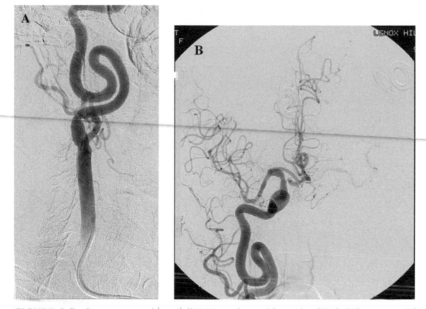

FIGURE 8-8. Severe tortuosities of the internal carotid arteries (ICA); (**A**) extracranial segments and (**B**) distal and intracranial segment of the ICA.

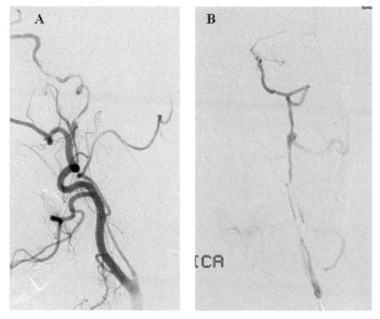

FIGURE 8-9. Anomaly of the internal carotid artery (ICA). In this case, the ICA is replaced by the ascending pharyngeal artery.

could be involved with fibromuscular dysplasia, a condition that is very prone to vascular spasm (Fig. 8-10) (7). The cavernous segment of the ICA can be straight or very tortuous (Fig. 8-8B). Rarely, the primitive trigeminal artery originates at this level, supplying the upper third of the basilar artery (Fig. 8-11).

The intracranial segment of the ICA is divided into the clinoidal and the supraclinoidal segments (5). The ophthalmic artery is the first intracranial branch of the ICA from within the clinoidal segment (Fig. 8-12). The posterior communicating and the anterior choroidal arteries originate more distally (Fig. 8-12). The posterior communicating artery can be either absent or well developed to such a degree that it exclusively supplies the posterior cerebral artery. The supraclinoidal segment terminates in the bifurcation where the ICA divides into the larger middle cerebral artery (MCA) and a smaller anterior cerebral artery (ACA). The horizontal segments of both ACAs (A1 segments) can communicate across the midline through the anterior communicating artery (Fig. 8-13). The horizontal segment of the MCA (M1 segment) terminates within the trifurcation in the proximal sylvian fissure. Distal branches of the MCA are the ascending frontoparietal artery, parietal artery, and anterior temporal artery.

The ECA carries blood supply to the facial and meningeal structures (8). It can also become an important source of blood supply to the brain when the ICA is significantly stenosed or completely occluded (mainly via the ophthalmic artery). The ECA-to-VA anastomosis via the occipital artery is not uncommon, and ECA-to-VA steal is not uncommon when the proximal SA is stenosed or occluded.

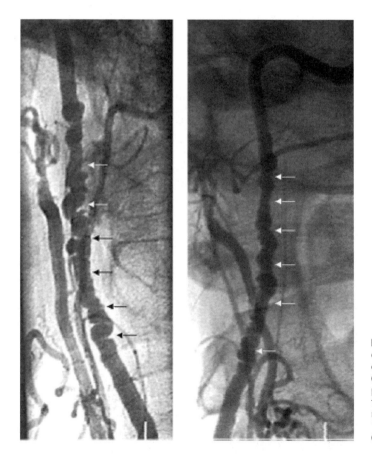

FIGURE 8-10. Fibromuscular dysplasia of the cervical internal carotid artery. The angiograms (**A** and **B**) show the typical appearance of multifocal stenoses that alternate with areas of mural dilatations, called the "string of beads" appearance (*arrows*).

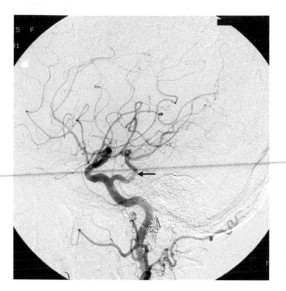

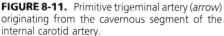

FIGURE 8-11. Primitive trigeminal artery (*arrow*) originating from the cavernous segment of the internal carotid artery.

THE VERTEBRAL ARTERY SYSTEM

The VAs are the first branches originating from the subclavian arteries, entering the foramen transversariums at C-6, and traversing the dura mater through the atlantooccipital membrane above the posterior arch of the atlas (9). In approximately 6% to 8% of the cases, the left VA originates directly from the aortic arch (Fig. 8-5). In 35% of the cases, the left VA is of the same size or larger than the right one. The VA is divided into intracranial and extracranial cervical segments. The basilar artery (BA) is formed by the fusion of the intracranial segments of both VA at or near the level of the pontomedullary sulcus and gives rise to the intracranial posterior circulation (Fig. 8-14) (9).

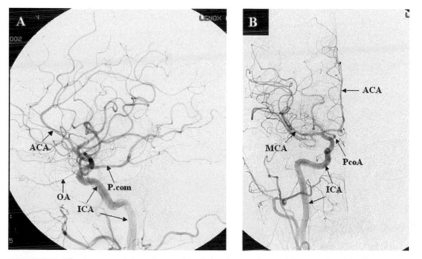

FIGURE 8-12. Intracranial angiography of the internal carotid artery (ICA) in the antero-posterior (**A**) and lateral (**B**) projections. OA, ophthalmic artery; P.com, posterior communicating artery; A.com, anterior communicating artery; MCA, middle cerebral artery; ACA, anterior cerebral artery.

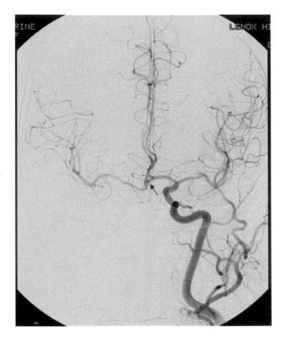

FIGURE 8-13. The horizontal segments of both anterior cerebral arteries (ACA) (A1 segments) communicate across the midline to form the anterior communicating artery (*arrow*). The right internal carotid artery (ICA) is completely occluded with cross-filling of the right intracranial vessels and visualization of both the right middle cerebral artery (MCA) and right external carotid artery (ECA).

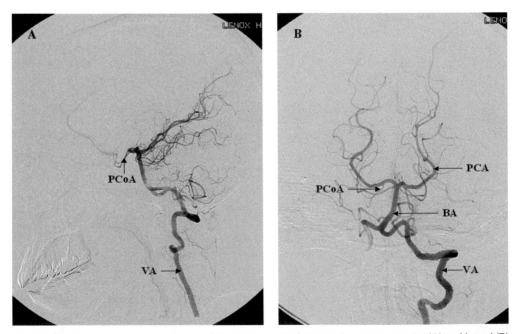

FIGURE 8-14. Intracranial angiography of the posterior circulation in the anteroposterior (**A**) and lateral (**B**) projections. VA, vertebral artery; BA, basilar artery; PCA, posterior cerebral artery; PCoA, posterior communicating artery.

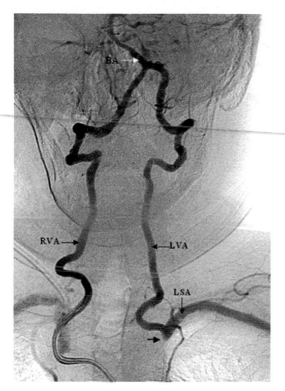

FIGURE 8-15. Angiographic demonstration of subclavian steal syndrome. The right vertebral artery (RVA) is selectively catheterized and the blood flow is diverted via the basilar artery into the left vertebral artery (LVA), where the flow is reversed and diverted to the left subclavian artery (LSA), which is completely occluded at its origin (*arrow*).

The cervical segments of the VA are best displayed in the ipsilateral oblique or lateral projection. Selective catheterization of the VA may result in spasm if the catheter is placed too distal within the artery or if the contrast jet is directed to the vessel wall. A careful test injection immediately following the catheter placement will verify the blood flow status in the VA. If the flow is compromised, the angiographic injection should be expeditiously completed. If the patient becomes symptomatic, the catheter is withdrawn, and a nonselective injection with the catheter positioned within the SA is performed.

The atherosclerotic process typically involves the origin of the VA. Therefore, angiographic assessment of the VA should begin with ipsilateral SA angiography. The VA origin is best demonstrated in the contralateral cranial oblique projection. Intracranial angiography is performed after selective catheterization of the VA using the standard AP with the petrous ridges projected above the orbital roofs and lateral projections (Fig. 8-14). In cases where the SA is completely occluded, the vertebral basilar system functions as a collateral circulation to the distal SA with reversal of the blood flow within the ipsilateral VA, leading to the clinical entity of "subclavian steal syndrome" (Fig. 8-15).

CIRCLE OF WILLIS

The intracranial brain vasculature is divided into an anterior brain circulation consisting of both the ICA and their branches, and a posterior brain circulation consisting of the vertebrobasilar system. The two vascular territories are interconnected by the anterior communicating artery (ACoA) and two posterior communicating arteries (PCoA) to form a complete vascular circle, the "Circle of Willis," located at the base of the brain and providing an important

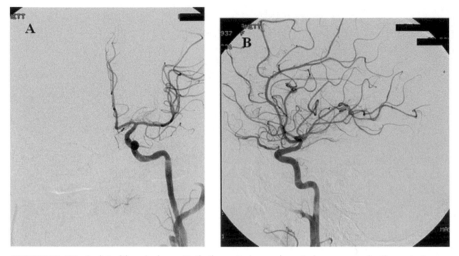

FIGURE 8-16. Isolated hemisphere: Both the anterior and posterior communicating arteries are absent, and the left hemisphere is solely dependent on the left internal carotid artery (**A**: Anterior-posterior projection; **B**: Lateral projection).

collateral pathway between the proximal segments of the intracerebral arteries (ACA, MCA, PCA, and BA) (Figs. 8-12, 8-14). The ACoA is 1 to 2 mm in length and connects the two horizontal segments of the ACA. The PCoA arises from the clinoid segment of the intracranial ICA and connects the latter with the posterior circulation on each side. This collateral channel can readily compensate for any occluded ICAs or VAs (Fig. 8-13).

The circle of Willis is not always well developed, and a complete circle is present in only 50% to 60% of the population. Variations in presence or absence of the ACoA or PCoA are very frequent. Both the ACoA and PCoA can be hypoplastic or completely absent, in which case the hemispheric blood supply can be completely isolated and depends only on the ipsilateral ICA, termed the "isolated hemisphere" (Fig. 8-16). In these cases, even a short, temporary occlusion of the ICA can result in significant clinical consequences.

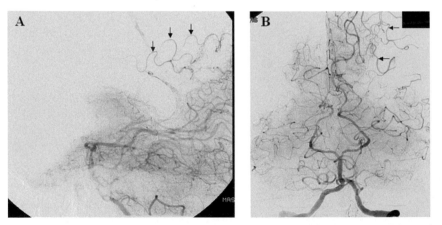

FIGURE 8-17. Leptomeningeal anastomoses: small branches of the anterior, middle, and posterior cerebral arteries are connected within the pia mater and can supply peripheral branches of these vessels through retrograde flow. **A** and **B**: anteroposterior and lateral projections with a catheter injection within the left vertebral artery.

A less pronounced collateral blood supply to the brain can develop through the lepto-meningeal anastomoses, where small branches of the anterior, middle, and posterior cerebral arteries are connected within the pia mater and can supply peripheral branches of these vessels through retrograde flow (Fig. 8-17). This collateral system functions much better in early life than in advanced age, and when present, it is usually insufficient to maintain viable blood supply to the cerebral hemisphere for a longer period of time when the ipsilateral ICA is temporarily occluded. Reversal of the flow within the ipsilateral ophthalmic artery and other connections from the ECA can also provide collateral blood supply and may contribute to better tolerance to the ICA occlusion.

REFERENCES

1. Zamir M, Sinclair P. Origin of the brachiocephalic trunk, left carotid and left subclavian arteries from the arch of the human aorta. *Invest Radiol* 1991;26:128–133.
2. Edwards JE. Anomalies of the derivatives of the aortic arch system. *Med Clin North Am* 1948;32: 925–949.
3. Vitek JJ. Femoro-cerebral angiography Analysis of two thousand consecutive examinations, special emphasis on carotid arteries catheterizations in older patients. *Am J Roentgenol* 1973;118:633 647.
4. William PL, ed. Carotid system in arteries. In: *Gray's anatomy*, 38th ed. New York: Churchill Livingstone, 1995:1513–1523.
5. William PL, ed. Internal carotid artery. In: *Gray's anatomy*, 38th ed. New York: Churchill Livingstone, 1995:1523–1529.
6. Vannix RS, Joergenson EJ, Carter R. Kinking of the internal carotid artery. Clinical significance and surgical management. *Am J Surg* 1977;134:82–89.
7. Osborn AG. *Diagnostic cerebral angiography*. Philadelphia: Lippincott Williams & Wilkins, 1999.
8. Lasjaunias PL, Choi IS. The external carotid artery: functional anatomy. *Riv Neuroradiol* 1991;4(Suppl 1):39–45.
9. Parent A. The vertebral basilar system. In: *Carpenter's human neuroanatomy*, 9th ed. Media: Williams and Wilkins, 1996:113–119.

CAROTID ARTERY ACCESS TECHNIQUES

NADIM AL-MUBARAK
JIRI J. VITEK
SRIRAM S. IYER
GARY S. ROUBIN

The safe and expeditious guide catheter or sheath placement within the common carotid artery (CCA) is a key step and a prerequisite for successful carotid artery stenting (CAS). To access the carotid artery, experienced operators have practiced a variety of techniques (1–3). With experience, carotid artery access is successfully achieved in the majority of cases. Catheter access difficulties, mostly resulting from extensive atherosclerotic process, anatomical variations, and/or vascular tortuosities occur in approximately 5% of the patients. The ability to recognize the various "difficult-to-access" situations and the application of appropriate access strategy in these cases constitutes an important part of the learning process of the interventionist pursuing safe CAS (1,2). In this chapter, we describe our approach for successful carotid access techniques and discuss technical pearls helpful in approaching carotid access difficulties and challenges.

ANATOMICAL CONSIDERATIONS

As already described in the previous chapter, the aortic arch in children and young adults is a symmetrically curved vascular structure tilted from the right anterior to the left posterior upper mediastinal compartment. The origins of the brachiocephalic arteries are aligned in straight lines and course superiorly (Fig. 9-1A). Aging and the atherosclerotic degenerative process elongate the aortic arch, displacing the aortic knob more superiorly and posteriorly and thereby shifting the ostia of the brachiocephalic arteries (Fig. 9-1B). Because of this anatomical distortion, it is more difficult to selectively catheterize these vessels and advance the catheter deep into the carotid arteries (Fig. 9-2A–C) (4). In young adults, the left CCA courses superiorly, but with aging, it can elongate and courses to the left with a sharp superior turn. The brachiocephalic arteries start to tilt from the right to the left, further increasing the disadvantageous angulations for selective catheterization (Fig. 9-1B, 9-2A). This vascular arrangement can make selective catheterization of the left CCA very difficult. If the origin of the innominate artery is well bellow the level of the aortic knob, if the innominate artery is tilted to the left, and if the proximal right CCA is tortuous, it might be impossible to selectively advance the catheter deep into the right CCA (Fig. 9-1B, 9-2). With aging and atherosclerotic elongation of the aortic arch, one has to remember that the

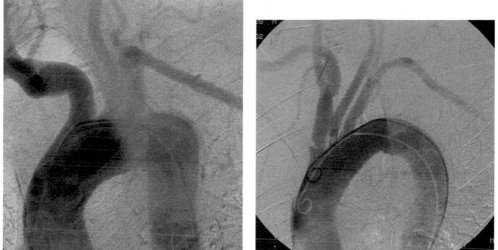

A   B

FIGURE 9-1. A: normal aortic arch in a young patient. **B**: age-related elongation of the aortic arch. Aging and the atherosclerotic degenerative process elongate the aortic arch and displace the aortic knob more superiorly and posteriorly, shifting the ostia of the arch arteries, which in this case tilt from the right to the left forming sharp angulations that are disadvantageous and may make selective catheterization of these vessels very difficult.

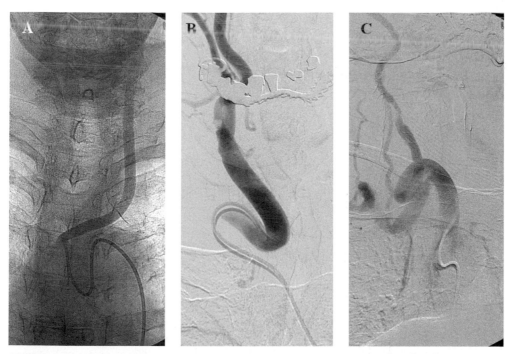

FIGURE 9-2. Proximal angulations/tortuosities of both the left (**A**) and the right (**B** and **C**) common carotid arteries (LCCA and RCCA, respectively). These tortuosities make it difficult to selectively advance the catheter deep into the common carotid artery.

ostium of the left CCA is displaced posteriorly, and the origins of the brachiocephalic arteries form a triangle when looking at the top of the aortic arch. Statistically, there are more failures to selectively catheterize the right CCA compared with the left.

Anatomical distortion of the aortic arch and the arrangement of the brachiocephalic arteries may also result from congenital anomalies. The most common congenital anomaly is the joint origin of the left common carotid and innominate arteries. The second is the left CCA originating from the innominate artery itself. In this instance, it can originate close to the aortic arch, but also deeper, resembling a truncus bicaroticus.

CAROTID ARTERY ACCESS

Femoral arterial access is the preferred approach. In the authors' opinion, direct percutaneous puncture of the CCA for the purpose of stenting is significantly disadvantageous. The frequent need for general anesthesia, the proximity of the access site to the atherosclerotic lesion, the risk of local hematoma with the possible compression of the trachea, and the need for compressing the stented vessel for hemostasis after the procedure is completed are some of the reasons why the direct-carotid-stick approach should be avoided (3). The brachial/radial arterial access can be utilized as an alternative in patients with severe peripheral arterial disease where the femoral artery access is not possible (5–7).

The techniques of guide sheath placement into the CCA consists of two main steps; the first step is selective catheterization of the carotid artery with a 5F catheter that is deeply advanced into the ipsilateral external carotid artery (ECA) over a hydrophilic-coated, angled-tip 0.038-inch guide wire (Glidewire, Boston Scientific Inc. Watertown, MA) (Figs. 9-3–9-8) (1,2). From this position, the 5F catheter–Glidewire combination will provide a platform for the guide sheath advancement into the CCA, either over the 5F catheter–guide

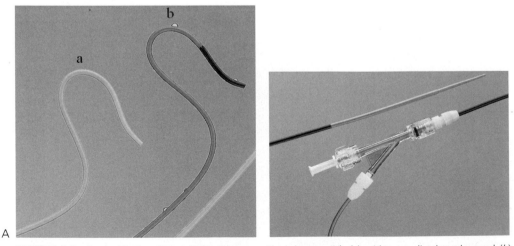

A   B

FIGURE 9-3. A: the Vitek catheter (VTK, Cook Inc. Bloomington, IN); (*a*) without a distal marker and (*b*) with a radio-opaque marker at the catheter tip. **B**: the guide sheath tip and the proximal end with an open-ended Tuohy-Borst adapter and the side arm (Shuttle, Cook Inc., Bloomington, IN).

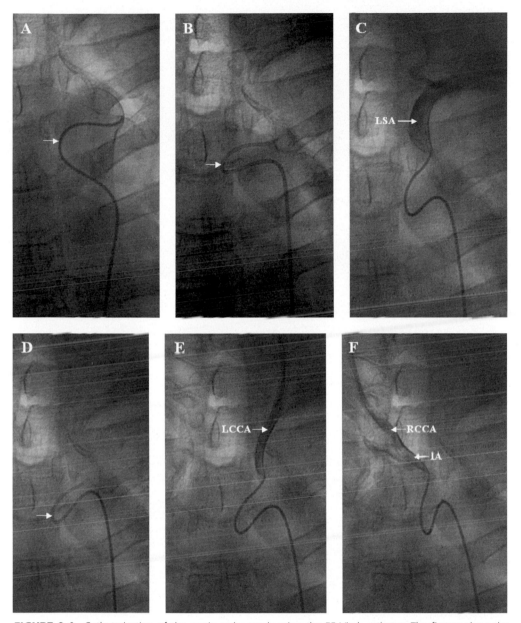

FIGURE 9-4. Catheterization of the aortic arch vessels using the 5F Vitek catheter. The figures show the catheter positions and shapes within the aortic arch during the catheterization procedure with test injections displaying the individual arteries. **A**: the starting position of the brachiocephalic arteries catheterization using the Vitek catheter; in the anteroposterior fluoroscopic projection, the catheter is placed in the upper thoracic aorta retaining its double curve with the tip pointing up to the left side of the patient. A gentle slow advancement of the catheter retaining its curved shape (**B**) engages it sequentially into the left subclavian artery (LSA) (**C**), the left common carotid artery (LCCA) (**E**), and the innominate artery (IA) (**F**). RCCA, right common carotid artery. **D**: gentle advancement of the catheter from the subclavian artery (SA) position to the LCCA.

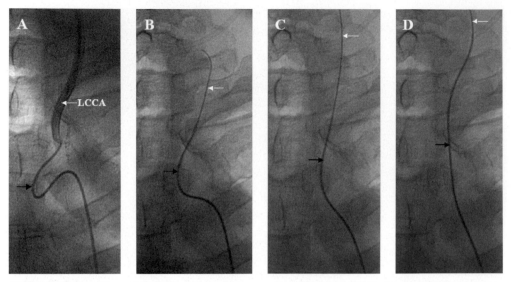

FIGURE 9-5. Selective catheterization of the left common carotid artery (CCA) using the 5F Vitek catheter. **A**: the left CCA is first engaged with the catheter. The angled-tip Glidewire *(white arrow)* is then advanced into a stable position within the CCA (**B** and **C**). The catheter *(black arrow)* is then advanced over the Glidewire into the distal CCA (**C** and **D**). Note that as the catheter is advanced into the CCA, the curve loses its shape.

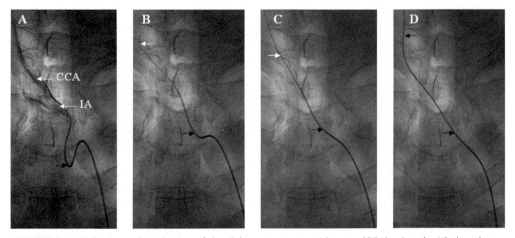

FIGURE 9-6. Selective catheterization of the right common carotid artery (CCA) using the Vitek catheter. **A**: The innominate artery is first engaged with the Vitek catheter in the manner described above. Slight medial rotation of the catheter within the innominate artery directs the tip into the right common carotid artery. The 0.038-inch Glidewire is then advanced into a stable position within the CCA *(white arrows* in **B** and **C**). The catheter *(black arrow)* is then advanced into the CCA over the Glidewire (**D**). Note that as the catheter is advanced into the CCA, the curve loses its shape.

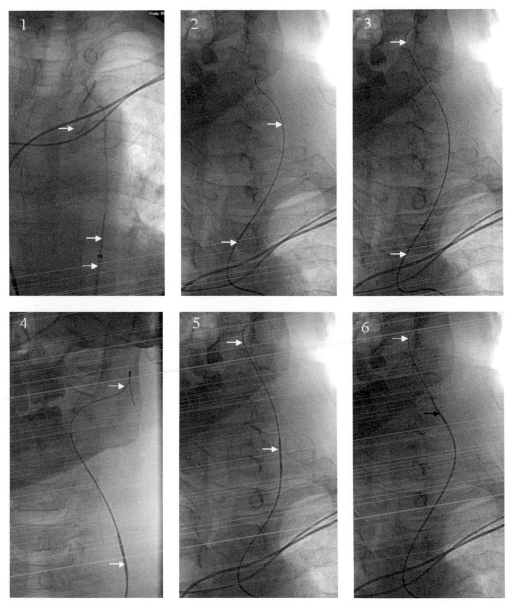

FIGURE 9-7. Guide sheath placement within the common carotid artery (CCA). (*1*) In the first step, the guide sheath *(bottom arrow)* is positioned in the upper descending aorta, and a 125-cm long Vitek catheter *(top arrow)* is introduced through the sheath to selectively catheterize the CCA (here the left CCA). The 0.038-inch Glidewire *(middle arrow)* is visible within the Vitek catheter. In steps *2* through *6*, the Glidewire *(top arrow)* is advanced into the external carotid artery (ECA), followed by the Vitek catheter *(bottom arrow)*. Once a stable position of the Glidewire–Vitek catheter assembly *(top arrows)* is achieved (*6*), the shuttle sheath *(bottom arrow)* is advanced into the distal position within the CCA (*7–9*). The Vitek catheter and the Glidewire are then removed (*10* and *11*). The guide sheath *(black arrow)* is carefully back-flushed and carotid angiography is performed (*12*). (*Continues.*)

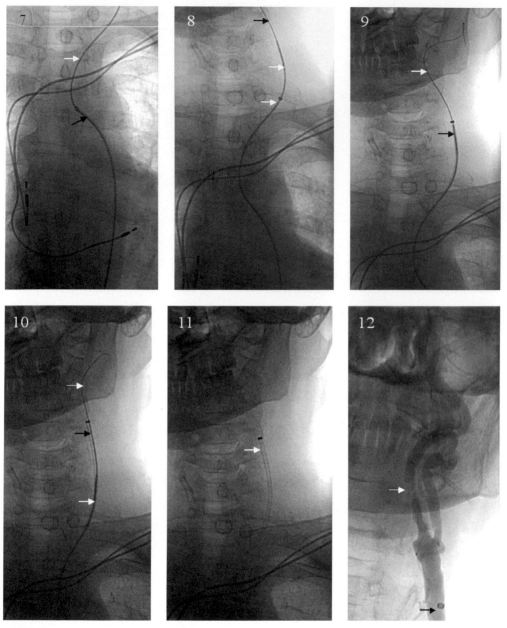

FIGURE 9-7. (Continued.)

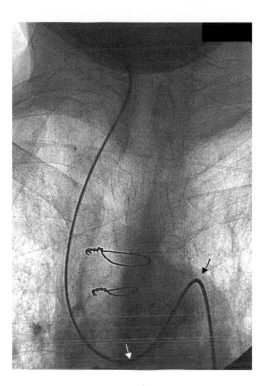

FIGURE 9-8. The formation of a "favorable" curve between the aortic arch and left upper thoracic aorta *(arrows)* is utilized to support the advancement of the Vitek catheter into the respective common carotid artery.

wire combination or after placement of a bare extra-support guide wire through the 5F catheter in the second step of the carotid access technique (Fig. 9-7). In the majority of cases, the successful carotid access is dependent upon the successful and secure placement of the 5F catheter within the ipsilateral ECA. Failures to position the guiding sheath after successful placement of the 5F catheter into the ECA are very rare.

CATHETERIZATION OF THE CAROTID ARTERIES

In the vast majority of patients, a 5F double-curve Vitek-catheter (VTK, Cook Inc. Bloomington, IN) (Fig. 9-3A) is adequate to access the carotid arteries. We also prefer this catheter for the performance of the diagnostic cervicocerebral angiography (Figs. 9-4–9-6). The distal curve of this catheter is opened, and the tip, when located in the aortic arch, is pointing upwards (Figs. 9-3A, 9-4A). This facilitates the advancement of the 0.038-inch Glidewire, even into the severely tortuous arteries.

The catheterization procedure is carried out in the anteroposterior or the left oblique fluoroscopic projection. At the beginning of the procedure, the catheter is placed in the upper thoracic aorta, retaining its double curve with the tip pointing up to the left shoulder of the patient (Fig. 9-4A). From this position, gentle and slow advancement of the catheter retaining its curved shape (Fig. 9-4B) engages it sequentially into the left subclavian artery (Fig. 9-4C), the left CCA (Fig. 9-4E), and the innominate artery (Fig. 9-4F). Slight rotation of the catheter within the innominate artery helps to direct the catheter tip into the right CCA or the right subclavian artery (Fig. 9-6A). If the catheter does not retain its shape or if it folds or twists to the right, it is repositioned, and the engagement maneuver is repeated. The Glidewire can be used to reshape and/or reposition the catheter.

After engagement of the target vessel, the Glidewire is advanced into a stable position within the distal CCA followed by the Vitek catheter (Figs. 9-5, 9-6). To accurately direct the Glidewire into the vessel, the catheter may be gently rotated, pushed forward, or slightly retracted. Medial rotation of the Glidewire tip while the catheter is in the innominate artery will direct it into the right CCA (Fig. 9-6B). Road mapping can often be useful. If the wire starts to "slip back," it is readvanced further cephalad. The wire should always enter into the artery first followed by the catheter, never the catheter alone. Successful advancement of the catheter over the wire is achieved by holding the Glidewire in position with the right hand while sliding the catheter slowly forward with the left hand, maintaining the wire position within the distal carotid artery. In the very angulated origins, this maneuver is performed very slowly using push-pull and rotational maneuvers, taking advantage of the pulsating blood flow and the formation of a favorable supporting curve between the aortic arch and left upper thoracic aorta (Fig. 9-8). A deep inspiration by the patient can often be helpful.

Once the tip of the catheter is within the CCA, the Glidewire is removed, the catheter is carefully flushed, and carotid bifurcation angiogram is performed to display an "open" carotid bifurcation. This is usually the ipsilateral oblique (30 degrees to 40 degrees) or lateral projection, but some modification may be required. Occasionally, some modifications of the projections may be required, especially if the bifurcation is congenitally overrotated. Control angiogram is then used to guide the Glidewire placement and subsequently the 5F catheter into the ECA. It is very important to carefully backflush the catheter each time the Glidewire is removed to prevent air embolism. Small test injections are used to confirm the catheter position and exclude catheter-induced dissections or flow impairment. A hand injection using a 6-cc control syringe with injection speed adjusted to the blood flow within the carotid artery is used (no more than 4-cc of 50% diluted contrast per injection). In distended and elongated aortic arches, the origin of the left CCA migrates posteriorly. In this situation, the 5F catheter can be rotated within the aortic arch so that the tip of the catheter is located more posteriorly. In the extremely dilated aortic arch, a sidewinder larger-curved catheter (Simmons-3, Cook Inc., Bloomington, IN) is used in a similar fashion to the Vitek catheter.

GUIDE SHEATH PLACEMENT

A 6F/90-cm guide sheath (Shuttle, Cook Inc., Bloomington, IN) (Fig. 9-3B) is preferred to a guide catheter. The sheath is thin-walled, kink and pressure-resistant, and is very flexible. A 7F sheath is seldom used: (i) when a larger-profile interventional device is used (such as a larger profile, self-expanding stent catheter or balloon expandable stents used for innominate or left CCA ostial lesions), and (ii) for better stability of the sheath in the CCA when the aortic arch is elongated or CCA is significantly tortuous. An inner dilator, a straight tip introducer, and hydrophilic coating facilitate its smooth introduction and advancement into the femoral and carotid arteries even in the tortuous vasculature. The sheath has an open-ended Tuohy-Borst adopter with a manually adjustable valve that permits unimpeded catheter or guide wire introduction. A side arm allows flushing and contrast injection as well as continuous intraarterial blood pressure monitoring.

Once the 5F catheter is placed in a secured position within the ipsilateral ECA, the guide sheath placement within the CCA can successfully be achieved in the vast majority of the cases. Failures to position the guide sheath in these situations are rare. With the 5F catheter in the ECA, two approaches are utilized to complete the guide sheath placement. This depends on whether cervicocerebral angiography preceded the sheath placement during the same setting or not.

If the cervicocerebral angiography was performed during the same setting, the target vessel to be treated (as indicated by the prior noninvasive testing) is cannulated as the last one. Following the standard angiography of this vessel, the Vitek catheter (100 cm) is advanced over the Glidewire into the ipsilateral ECA as previously described. The Glidewire is then replaced with an extra-stiff 0.038-inch exchange-length guide wire (Amplatz wire, Cook Inc, Bloomington, IN) and the Vitek catheter is removed. The guide sheath is then introduced through the common femoral artery and advanced into the CCA over the Amplatz wire until the guide sheath tip is located just below the stenotic lesion. The Amplatz wire and the sheath introducer are then removed. The guide sheath is carefully back-flushed.

If the diagnostic angiography has previously been performed and the carotid anatomy is well delineated, the stenting procedure is began by advancing the guiding sheath into the descending thoracic aorta with the sheath tip positioned just a short distance below the origin of the left subclavian artery. The inner sheath dilator is then removed, the sheath is flushed, and a 125-cm 5Fr Vitek catheter (VTK, Thorocon NB 125-cm, Cook Inc., Bloomington, IN) is introduced into the sheath. Care must be taken not to advance the shuttle sheath too close to the aortic arch, as this may compromise the operator's ability to maneuver the Vitek catheter (Fig. 9-7, step 1). Using the technique described earlier, the target carotid artery is accessed with a 125-cm Vitek catheter that is advanced into a secure position within the ipsilateral ECA over a 0.038-inch Glidewire (Fig. 9-7, steps 1–6). The Shuttle sheath is then advanced into the CCA over the Glidewire–Vitek catheter assembly (Fig. 9-7, steps 7–11). This can be best achieved by holding the Glidewire–Vitek catheter assembly in position using the right hand and advancing the sheath using the operator's left hand. In cases where the innominate artery or the left CCA sharply unfold from the aortic arch, and/or moderate to severe carotid tortuosities exist, the Glidewire is exchanged to a 0.038-inch extra-support wire (Amplatz guide wire) prior to the sheath advancement. In the majority of cases, the sheath can be advanced over the Vitek catheter–Glidewire combination without the need for an Amplatz wire. If the advancement of the sheath over the Vitek catheter is not smooth—i.e., the operator senses that any further push on the guide sheath is met with resistance, would be counterproductive, and may result in the prolapse of the entire system out of the carotid artery, the Vitek catheter is exchanged for the inner introducer of the sheath (over the Amplatz wire), and the sheath advancement into the common carotid artery is reattempted.

One should be aware that when placing the guide sheath into the CCA, particularly if the carotid artery is tortuous, the vessel can be displaced upward and kinks can be formed in the internal carotid artery, occasionally simulating vascular spasm. These kinks disappear once the sheath is withdrawn (see Chapter 12).

SOLVING DIFFICULT ACCESS PROBLEMS

With experience, 95% of the carotid arteries can be accessed using the techniques described above. Difficulties in accessing the carotid arteries with this technique may ensue when severe vascular tortuosities exist and/or when the origin of the vessel is sharply angulated (Fig. 9-2). In these situations, the Glidewire may not advance into the carotid artery without "kicking" the Vitek catheter back into the aorta. Less commonly, difficulties occur when the Vitek catheter does not advance into the carotid artery after a distal Glidewire position is secured. In these cases, an alternative access strategy is utilized.

The first step in overcoming any carotid access difficulty is identifying the source. The goal of any alternative access maneuvers is to achieve a secure position of a 5F or 4F catheter with or without an extra-stiff 0.038-inch guide wire within the ipsilateral ECA. Once this is achieved, the currently available, highly trackable, hydrophilic-coated guide sheaths are capable of negotiating extreme tortuosities. Failures to advance the sheath after the 5F catheter is secured within the ECA are very rare.

It should be noted that severe tortuosities and atherosclerosis not only make the carotid artery access difficult, but also increase the risk for embolic neurological events and therefore may represent a contraindication for CAS. In these situations, the operator judgment is critical to avoid complications. Because there are reasonable alternative therapies, the operator should be prepared to abandon the procedure and consider elective carotid endarterectomy (CEA) or continuing medical management. It must be emphasized that failure to complete the procedure is acceptable but an avoidable complication is not.

Difficulties in advancing the Glidewire may result from an unstable Vitek catheter position and resultant inability to provide a stable platform for the Glidewire advancement. In these instances, a "softer" 0.035-inch Glidewire (instead of the 0.038-inch) may successfully negotiate vascular tortuosities. If this is unsuccessful, then a large-curve catheter (Simmons-3, Cook Inc. Bloomington, IN) is used to engage the carotid artery and provide a stronger basis for the Glidewire advancement. This catheter is maneuvered in a similar fashion to the Vitek catheter. This is especially helpful in a large dilated aortic arch or sharply angulated origins of the brachiocephalic arteries. In either case, rapid torqueing of the Glidewire helps forward movements.

In cases where the Vitek catheter does not advance after the regular Glidewire is placed within the distal ECA, the regular Glidewire is exchanged for a 0.038-inch super-stiff Glidewire and the catheter advancement is reattempted. During the wire advancements and exchanges, it is important to gently ease back on the catheter curve in the aortic arch in order to prevent the stiff wire from prolapsing the catheter back into the ascending aorta. Additional techniques such as slow catheter pushback and torqueing maneuvers during these attempts may facilitate the catheter advancement. If the Vitek catheter does not fully advance into the ECA, a regular exchange-length Glidewire is first positioned within the ECA. The Vitek catheter is then exchanged to a 4F glide catheter that is advanced into the ECA. The Glidewire is then replaced with an extra-support wire (such as the 0.038-inch Amplatz wire, Cook Inc, Bloomington, IN), and the sheath placement is completed.

CAROTID ACCESS IN THE PRESENCE OF COMMON CAROTID ARTERY LESIONS OR AN OCCLUDED EXTERNAL CAROTID ARTERY

Guide sheath placement into the CCA may present special challenges when the ECA is occluded, when a critical lesion is situated below the carotid bifurcation, or when there is a critical ostial CCA stenosis. Careful attention must be paid to avoid crossing the lesion with a 0.038-inch Glidewire, as this may disrupt the atherosclerotic plaque material, leading to embolic events. When possible, the 5F Vitek catheter is advanced over the 0.038-inch Glidewire in the usual fashion, with the tip of the Glidewire carefully kept below the lesion. In the nontortuous anatomy, the guide sheath can be advanced and positioned within the CCA over the Glidewire–Vitek catheter combination located proximal to the carotid lesion and without additional maneuvers. If vascular tortuosities exist, the Glidewire is first exchanged for a 0.038-inch Amplatz wire, the tip of which is shaped into a "pigtail," which prevents it from crossing the lesion and serves as an anchor. The guiding sheath is then advanced into the CCA. If the proximal CCA is very tortuous or angulated and more support is needed, the Amplatz wire may have to be placed more distally. In this situation, the Glidewire and the 5F catheter are first carefully advanced through the lesion. In the presence of a CCA ostial lesion, the origin of the CCA should be first dilated to allow sheath access. The bifurcation is stented first, and the ostium treated with a balloon-expandable stent on the way out.

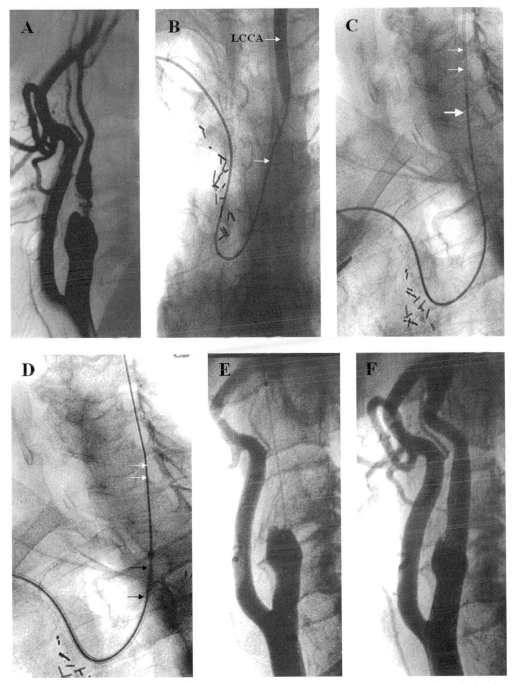

FIGURE 9-9. Guide sheath placement via the brachial artery approach. **A**: diagnostic angiogram showing the carotid lesion to be treated. **B**: The left common carotid artery (CCA) is catheterized using the Simons-3 catheter *(bottom arrow)*. **C**: The catheter *(thin arrows)* is positioned distal in the CCA, and an Amplatz guide wire *(thick arrow)* is being advanced. **D**: The guide sheath *(black arrows)* is being advanced over the Simons-3 catheter/Amplatz guide wire assembly *(white arrows)*. **E**: carotid angiogram with the distal balloon occlusion system. **F**: final angiogram after successful stenting.

BRACHIAL ARTERY APPROACH

Carotid stenting is technically applicable to a variety of patients, including those with severe peripheral artery disease in whom the vascular access through the femoral artery is not possible—as in patients with severe occlusive iliac disease, aortic occlusion, or morbid obesity. The brachial/radial artery may be successfully used as an alternative route even in the more complex carotid intervention with distal protection (5–7) (Fig. 9-9). In this situation, the vascular access is obtained via the right brachial artery. A 5F large double-curve catheter (Simmons-3, Cook Inc, Bloomington, IN) is advanced into the aortic arch over a 0.038-inch Guidewire, and the target CCA is cannulated (Fig. 9-9). The Simmons catheter is then advanced into the ECA over the Glidewire, which is then exchanged to an extra-support straight-tip Amplatz wire. Following removal of the Simmons-3 catheter, the guide sheath is advanced into the CCA and positioned below to the bifurcation.

Utilizing the brachial approach, some operators have used a 5F internal mammary artery catheter to access ipsilateral and contralateral CCA (5). We find the Simmons-3 catheter to be more suitable for canalizing any of the carotid arteries via the brachial approach especially in the presence of tortuous carotid anatomy. If difficulties in advancing the Simmons-3 catheter into the ECA over the regular Glidewire are encountered, a super-stiff 0.038-inch Glidewire is used.

REFERENCES

1. Al-Mubarak N, Roubin GS, Iyer SS, et al. Techniques of carotid artery stenting: the state of the art. *Sem Vasc Surg* 2000;13:117–129.
2. Vitek JJ, Roubin GS, Al-Mubarak N, et al. Carotid artery stenting: technical considerations. *Am J Neuroradiol* 2000;21:1736–1743.
3. Diethrich EB, Ndiaye M, Reid DB. Stenting in the carotid artery: initial experience in 110 patients. *J Endovasc Surg* 1996;3:42–62.
4. Vitek JJ. Femoro-cerebral angiography: analysis of 2,000 consecutive examinations with special emphasis on carotid arteries catheterizations in older patients. *Am J Roentgenol Radium Ther Nucl Med* 1973;118:633–647.
5. Al-Mubarak N, Vitek JJ, Iyer SS, et al. Carotid stenting with distal-balloon protection via the transbrachial approach. *J Endovasc Ther* 2001;8:571–575.
6. Sievert H, Ensslen R, Fach Merle H, et al. Brachial artery approach for transluminal angioplasty of the internal carotid artery. *Cathet Cardiovasc Diag* 1996;39:421–423.
7. Castriota F, Cremonesi A, Manneti R, et al. Carotid stenting using radial artery access. *J Endovas Surg* 1999;6:385–386.

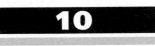

PROCEDURAL TECHNIQUES

SRIRAM S. IYER
NADIM AL-MUBARAK
JIRI J. VITEK
GARY S. ROUBIN

The efficacy of carotid artery stenting (CAS) in preventing stroke is dependent on the ability of the operator to produce complication-free results. These can be achieved by the careful attention to patient selection and meticulous techniques (1–5). The recent introduction of Anti-Embolization devices that are designed to capture embolic matter released during the carotid intervention before it reaches the brain has added an important dimension to the performance of safe carotid stenting (6–11). This chapter provides a step-by-step approach to the clinical and technical aspects of the carotid stenting procedure that will ensure safe outcomes.

CONSIDERATIONS FOR SAFE CAROTID ARTERY STENTING

Although carotid angioplasty was performed in the early 1980s, two important and potentially disastrous complications limited the subsequent growth of this treatment (1–5). These include (a) acute closure of the treated vessel, and (b) distal embolization of plaque material during the intervention (7,11). With the introduction of the intravascular stent technology and its subsequent rapid maturation, the problem of acute closure has been effectively resolved. The current source of major complications during CAS is related to the universal problem of distal embolization (7,11). Hence, enhancing the safety of CAS is dependent on the effective reduction of the embolic risk during the intervention. The first steps towards achieving this goal are the appropriate patient and lesion selection and meticulous interventional techniques. Our advanced understanding of a number of factors that impact the clinical outcomes of CAS has significantly contributed to the reduction in the risk of embolic neurological complications associated with the procedure (1). The patient and lesion selections have been modified based on the analysis of complications observed in different subgroups of patients (Table 10-1). Advanced age has been the most important predictor of procedural neurological complications, as evidenced in the outcomes of patients older than 80 years (12). Patients with comorbidities, especially those with severe untreated hypertension and patients with recent major stroke, are also at increased risk for embolic neurological complications. Those with significant brain atrophy resulting in dementia and advanced Alzheimer's and patients with extensive lacunar infarctions do not tolerate carotid stenting well and should not be considered for this treatment. Those patients with severe renal impairment (creatinine >3 to 3.5 mg) precluding safe use of iodinated contrast agent and patients who are unable

TABLE 10-1. CLINICAL AND ANATOMICAL RISK FACTORS FOR EMBOLIC EVENTS DURING CAS

Patients at increased risk for embolic neurological complications
Clinical factors
  1. Advanced age (>80 yrs)
  2. Recent major stroke
  3. Cerebral atrophy/dementia
  4. Unstable neurological symptoms (recent TIA or stroke)
Anatomical factors
  1. Severely tortuous, calcified, and atherosclerotic aortic arch/arch vessels
  2. Severe tortuosities distal to the bifurcation
  3. Coexisting proximal common carotid artery lesions
  4. Total occlusion or long subtotal occlusions ("string sign lesions")
  5. Severe concentric calcification
  6. Angiographic evidence of a large thrombus
Patients at lower risk for embolic neurological complications
Clinical factors
  1. Age ≤ 80 years
  2. Less severe stenosis (within the AHA guidelines)
Anatomical factors
  1. Straight, noncalcified aortic arch vessels
  2. Nontortuous bifurcation
  3. Absence of kinks, loops, bend points at lesion site
  4. Short lesions
  5. Prior CEA

CAS, Carotid artery stenting; TIA, transient ischemic attack; AHA, American Heart Association; CEA, carotid endarterectomy.

to tolerate appropriate doses of antiplatelet agents should also be excluded from this treatment.

On the other hand, analysis of our learning curve also showed that a number of higher-risk situations for carotid endarterectomy (CEA) represent ideal indications for CAS (1). These include restenosis after CEA, radiation-induced carotid stenosis with or without radical neck surgery, contralateral carotid occlusion, and obstructive carotid lesions located in the distal internal carotid artery (ICA) or involving high retromandibular carotid bifurcation. Female gender, coronary artery disease, diabetes mellitus, the presence of severe bilateral carotid artery stenoses or contralateral carotid occlusion, and lesion ulcerations do not seem to influence the incidence of neurological complications during CAS. In general, it should be noted that systemic factors and comorbidities increase the risk of CEA, whereas local anatomical factors increase the risk of CAS.

At the beginning of our experience, our only contraindication for CAS was pedunculated thrombus at the lesion site (Fig. 10-1) (13). Subsequent analysis of our outcomes revealed that lesion severity (more than or equal to 90% diameter obstruction) and lesion length, as well as multiplicity of the lesions, were also associated with a high embolic risk. Recognition of factors associated with a higher risk for embolic neurological events during CAS prompted us to modify our techniques and patient selection for this treatment. We have since completely abandoned recanalization of the occluded ICA, not only because of the high risk for embolic neurological complications, but also because of the increased risk of intracerebral hemorrhage. The patients with the highest risk for neurological complications are those with severely tortuous, calcified, and atherosclerotic carotid arteries and carotid artery lesions (Fig. 10-1). Severe kinks, tortuousities, and angulated take-offs of the ICA bring significant technical difficulties to the procedure, and these patients are at high risk for embolic complications. A complete risk assessment for the individual patient should precede the carotid

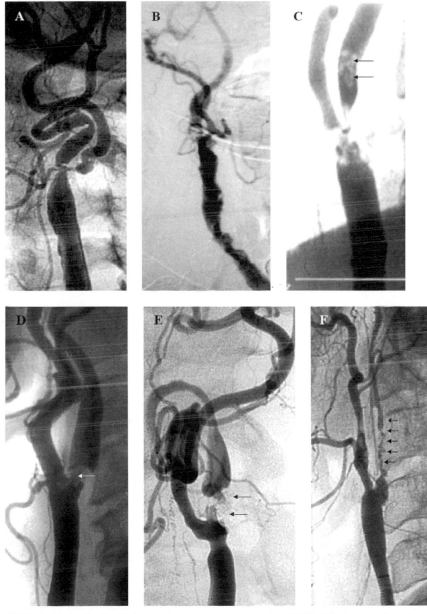

FIGURE 10-1. Unsuitable lesions for carotid artery stenting (CAS). (**A**): Angulated origin of the internal carotid artery (ICA). (**B**): Diffuse atherosclerosis of the ICA and the common carotid artery (CCA). (**C**): Pedunculated thrombus. (**D** and **E**). Heavy lesion calcifications. (**F**): Subtotal occlusion "string sign."

stenting procedure. Those patients found to be at high risk for complications should be considered for medical or surgical alternative treatments as applicable.

RATIONALE FOR ANTI-EMBOLIZATION

Despite the advanced stenting techniques, optimal antiplatelet therapy, and appropriate patient selection, embolic neurological events occur invariably during CAS (1–5). Obstructive carotid artery lesions are known to contain friable thrombotic and atherosclerotic components that can embolize during the intervention and are responsible for the majority of the neurological events during CAS. This has been demonstrated in an *ex vivo* human carotid artery model by Ohki et al. (14), as well as transcranial Doppler studies performed during CAS (15). Embolization can be aggravated by aggressive guide wire manipulation, balloon dilatation (particularly by large diameter balloons), and stent deployment (15). The development of Anti-Embolization strategies that reliably capture embolic matter released during the carotid intervention, preventing them from reaching the brain, has been a major technical breakthrough (7). A number of protection strategies have recently been introduced into the carotid stenting procedure and are currently being evaluated for their efficacy in minimizing the risk of embolic neurological events. Preliminary clinical results with these devices have been encouraging and indicate that these strategies are associated with a low incidence of embolic neurological events, particularly a very low incidence of major disabling stroke (6–11). Although this chapter discusses the "protected" and "nonprotected" techniques, it is our current practice to use Anti-Embolization protection in all carotid stent cases.

CLINICAL PROTOCOL AND PERIPROCEDURAL CARE

Careful attention to the periprocedural clinical care is critical for a safe carotid stenting procedure (Table 10-2). In our practice, patients with noninvasive evidence of severe carotid artery stenosis present to the angiographic suite on the same day of the procedure and are consented for both brachiocephalic angiography and stent placement, which is then completed during the same setting if the lesion proves to be of significant severity and is anatomically suitable for intervention. All patients are evaluated by a neurologist to document the preprocedural neurological status and to assess a baseline National Institutes of Health Stroke Scale (NIHSS) and other functional scales. Symptomatic patients with previous stroke, transient ischemic attack (TIA), or amaurosis fugax and those with an abnormal neurological examination would have a computed tomography (CT) scan or magnetic resonance imaging (MRI) of the brain to document baseline presenting changes. Prior to the stenting procedure, all patients undergo complete brachiocephalic angiography if it has not been done recently. Great emphasis is placed on optimal antiplatelet therapy before and after CAS. The low rates of acute and delayed stent thrombosis and poststenting embolic events are predicated upon correct and compulsive doses of adjunctive antiplatelet agents, e.g., a combination of aspirin and clopidogrel. Patients are started on antiplatelet therapy that includes aspirin 325 mg daily and clopidogrel (Plavix) 75 mg twice a day preferably for a minimum of 1 week prior to the procedure. Alternatively, a loading dose of clopidogrel (450 mg) in addition to 650 mg of aspirin is administered at a minimum of 4 hours before the procedure. Angiography and stenting is performed via the femoral approach using local anesthesia at the puncture site. Neurological status, electrocardiogram, heart rate, and blood pressure are monitored throughout the procedure. Bradyarrhythmias are not uncommon during predilatation and

TABLE 10-2. CLINICAL AND PROCEDURAL PROTOCOL

Premedications
  ASA: 325 mg po qd × 3 d
  Clopidogrel: 450 mg po loading, then 75 mg qd × 30 d
Preprocedure
  Noninvasive assessment of carotid stenosis (carotid duplex
    ultrasound, carotid MRA)
  Basic laboratory tests including renal function, coagulation
    profile, and blood counts
  CT scan/MRI of the brain in patients with prior neurological
    symptoms
  Neurological examination to document any preinterventional
    deficits
  Informed written consent
  Appropriate hydration
Procedure
  No sedation
  Head restrained in a specially designed head cradle
  4-vessel angiography
  Squeezing toy in contralateral hand
  Careful monitoring of hemodynamics and cardiac rhythm
  Intravenous atropine prior to the balloon deflation
  Stent only one side if bilateral disease
  Postprocedural neurological examination
Postprocedure and after discharge
  Hemodynamic monitoring
  Aim for early ambulation (use vascular closure device if feasible)
  ASA 325 mg qd indefinitely
  Clopidogrel 75 mg qd for 30 d
  Carotid ultrasound within 24 hrs (baseline), then at 6 mo, and
    annual

ASA, aspirin, po, by mouth; qd, every day; MRA, magnetic resonance
angiography; CT, computed tomography; MRI, magnetic resonance
imaging.

stent postdilatation, especially when the stenosis involves the ostium or the bulb of the ICA. Bradycardia and asystole usually recover spontaneously after balloon deflation and can be effectively avoided by the intravenous preadministration of 1 mg of atropine prior to the first balloon inflation. Temporary cardiac pacing is available if required, but its utilization in our experience has been extremely rare. Modest fall in blood pressure requires no specific intervention. In order to constantly monitor the neurological status and the effect of distal embolization during the intervention, a squeezing toy is placed in the patient's contralateral hand (16).

Occasionally, vascular spasm may develop in the ICA especially after placement of an extra support wire that straightens a tortuous artery or when an Anti-Embolization device is utilized. This condition can be treated with intraarterial nitroglycerine (100 to 200 mg) and usually resolves within a short time. Rarely, loss of consciousness can occur during the balloon inflation, especially if the ipsilateral hemispheric blood supply is isolated or if the contralateral carotid artery is occluded. These patients recover immediately after the balloon is deflated and the blood flow is restored. Although hypotension is not unusual in the immediate postprocedural period, it should be emphasized that other potential causes of hemodynamic instabilities, such as retroperitoneal bleed related to vascular access, should be considered and carefully excluded. Patients are typically ambulated within 2 to 4 hours after treatment (early ambulation—after 2 hours—when a vascular sealing device is used). A neurologist evaluates all patients within 24 hours following the procedure. Selected patients with low risk for neurological events can be discharged safely on the same day following an observation period of 4 to 6 hours (17).

TECHNIQUE

The carotid stenting procedure begins with the arterial access and the safe placement of vascular guiding sheath within the common carotid artery (CCA). The techniques of the guiding sheath placement have been discussed in the previous chapter. This chapter discusses the various details of the carotid stenting procedure after the guiding sheath is successfully positioned within the CCA (Table 10-3).

CROSSING THE LESSION

Appropriate angulations are first selected and baseline presenting angiograms are acquired. Optimal angulation for performing the intervention need not be identical to the one displaying the stenosis with its maximum severity. The presenting angiograms are obtained when quantitative carotid angiography (QCA) is required to ascertain the severity of the stenosis. The interventional projection should optimally separate the ICA and external carotid artery (ECA) and clearly display bony landmarks (Figs. 10-2, 10-3). The operator should have a clear mental image of the lesion location in relationship to the bony landmarks, as this will facilitate accurate stent placement, particularly in tortuous arteries where the arterial segment of the lesion may have been distorted by the guide wire. The technique of guide wire placement depends on whether the procedure is planned with or without an Anti-Embolization device.

Crossing the Lesion Without an Anti-Embolization Device

Guide wires ranging from soft coronary 0.014-inch to 0.018-inch stiff wires are used during various stages of the procedure. Guide-wire selection depends on the lesion severity, location,

TABLE 10-3. THE 10 STEPS OF CAROTID ARTERY STENTING

1. Vascular access (femoral approach is preferred)
2. Guiding sheath placement
3. Angiographic assessment including intracranial angiography
4. Crossing the stenosis (placement of the Anti-Embolization device)
5. Lesion predilatation
6. Stent deployment
7. Stent postdilatation
8. Removal of the Anti-Embolization device
9. Final angiographic assessment
10. Guiding sheath removal and hemostasis

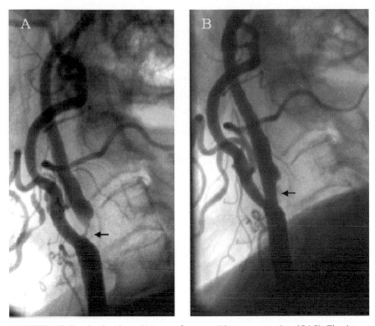

FIGURE 10-2. Optimal angiograms for carotid artery stenting (CAS): The interventional projections should optimally separate the internal and external carotid arteries and clearly display the bony landmarks that would guide the stent deployment.

length, angulation, and the anatomy of the bifurcation. After appropriate shaping of the guide-wire tip, the stenotic lesion is crossed with a steerable 0.014-inch guide wire. After crossing the stenosis, the tip of the wire is placed close to the skull base. At all times, the operator and the assistant must exercise full guide-wire control and should be aware of the position of the distal wire tip. Visibility of the opaque wire tip is maintained throughout the procedure to avoid inadvertent distal wire movement and vascular dissections or spasm. This will minimize the risk of wire-induced dissection, spasm, and perforations. When a 0.014-inch coronary wire is used as the initial wire, it can be exchanged for the 0.014-inch extra-support wire before stent placement. It is easier to advance and accurately place the stent over the stiffer, more robust guide wire as it straightens the ICA, facilitating the delivery and deployment of the stent. Currently, almost all self-expanding stents (both nitinol and non-nitinol) are 0.014-inch compatible, rendering the use of 0.018-inch guide wires obsolete.

Crossing Lesions with Anti-Embolization Devices

All currently available distal protection devices are developed in a 0.014-inch wire system. After the Anti-Embolization device is prepped, the wire tip is shaped appropriately, and the device is negotiated through the stenosis. The device has to be placed more than or at 2-cm cephalad to the stenosis. If the protection device is placed very close to the stenosis, there will not be adequate room to accommodate the tip of the stent delivery system, and satisfactory coverage of the lesion with the stent will not be possible.

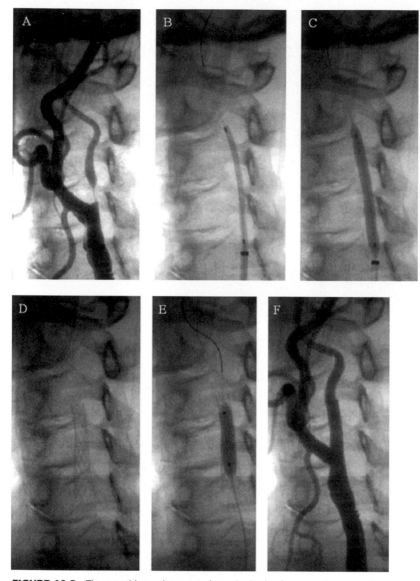

FIGURE 10-3. The carotid stenting procedure. **A**: Optimal prestenting carotid angiogram. The internal and external carotid arteries are well separated and the bony landmarks are displayed. **B** and **C**: Owing to the preocclusive lesion severity, a gradual step up in the balloon size is made to minimize plaque disruption and distal embolization. Predilatation is first performed using a 2 × 40-mm balloon (**B**). A second dilatation using a 4 × 40-mm balloon then followed (**C**). **D**: The stent is deployed. **E**: During the postdilatation, a single inflation is peformed using a 5-mm balloon that is limited to the lesion site within the stent avoiding the stent edges. **F**: Final carotid angiography.

ANTI-EMBOLIZATION DEVICES

Anti-Embolization devices can be classified into two groups: occlusion systems and filters (Fig. 10-4). Several of these devices have been approved for public use in Europe and are expected to be approved soon in the United States:

1. Distal occlusion balloon (Figs. 10-4A and 10-5): In this system, a low-pressure balloon mounted on a hollow guide wire occludes the ICA distal to the stenosis to be treated. The balloon guide-wire system is used to cross the obstructive lesion and the distal balloon—sized to the distal ICA—is positioned more than or at 2 cm within the ICA and then inflated. This guide wire is used to deliver interventional equipment. The blood flow is diverted into the ECA, which remains patent throughout the procedure. The stenting procedure is then carried out. Following the intervention, the blood within the ICA proximal to the occlusion balloon is aspirated to remove the trapped embolic material prior to the deflation of the occlusion balloon.

    Even in the hands of an experienced operator, the time that an Anti-Embolization device is placed within the ICA averages about 7 to 10 minutes. In contrast to the

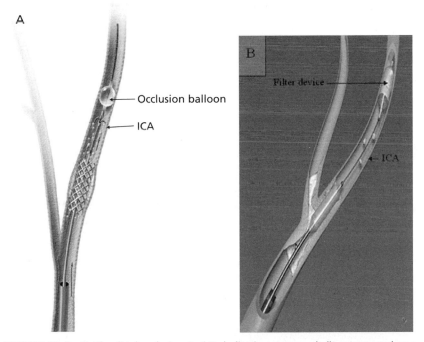

FIGURE 10-4. A: The distal occlusion Anti-Embolization system: a balloon mounted on a hollow guide wire occludes the internal carotid artery (ICA) by more than or equal to 2 cm distal to the stenosis to be treated. The balloon guide-wire system is used to cross the obstructive lesion and to deliver interventional equipment. The blood flow is diverted into the external carotid artery, which remains patent throughout the procedure. At the end of the intervention, the blood within the ICA proximal to the occlusion balloon is aspirated to remove the trapped embolic material prior to the final deflation. **B:** The filter Anti-Embolization system is a temporary intravascular filter that is designed to capture atheromatous material released during the carotid intervention. The filter (either mounted on a guide wire or delivered over the wire) is first placed within the distal ICA (more than or equal to 2 cm cephalad to the lesion), and the stenting procedure is completed. The filter is then completely retrieved at the end of the procedure using a dedicated retrieval catheter. (*Continues.*)

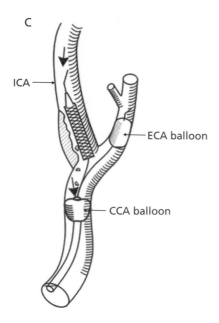

FIGURE 10-4. (*Continued.*) **C:** The Parodi Anti-Embolization system: Using this system, distal protection is conferred by simultaneous inflation of two balloons within the CCA and the ECA. This dual inflation reverses blood flow within the index carotid artery into a second lumen within the guiding catheter that drains into the low-pressure contralateral femoral vein. Emboli released during the intervention travel into the direction of the flow.

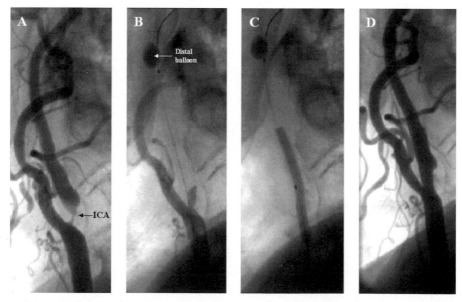

FIGURE 10-5. Carotid artery stenting (CAS) with theGuardWire Anti-Embolization system: (**A**) prestenting angiograms; (**B**) carotid angiograms after inflating the occlusion balloon. Complete occlusion of the internal carotid artery (ICA) is demonstrated: (**C**) predilatation and (**D**) in final poststenting angiograms.

intravascular filters, the distal occlusion balloon does not allow flow into the distal vascular bed during the stenting procedure. Therefore, and before selecting an occlusion balloon as the Anti-Embolization device during CAS, it is important to verify the competency of the circle of Willis. Hence, the value of an optimally performed and interpreted brachiocephalic angiography cannot be overstated. If the contralateral carotid artery is occluded and flow to that hemisphere is maintained by crossover collaterals from the index carotid artery, in cases of "isolated hemisphere" (hemisphere relies solely on the ipsilateral carotid artery for supply; absent or inadequate collaterals from the vertebral arteries and contralateral carotid), and when the ipsilateral ECA-ICA or ECA-vertebral artery (VA) collateral circulation is well developed, then Anti-Embolization protection using the distal balloon occlusion is not a suitable option because of the poor intolerance for the total ICA occlusion (see Chapters 13 and 15). (18).

2. Intravascular filter (Figs. 10-4B and 10-6): In this Anti-Embolization strategy, a temporary intravascular filter designed to capture atheromatous material released during the carotid intervention is first placed within the distal ICA, and the stenting procedure is completed. The filter is then completely retrieved at the end of the procedure. The basic application of the currently available systems is identical. These systems are typically composed of three major components: the filter guide wire, a delivery catheter, and a retrieval catheter. The filter assembly is located at the distal end of a 0.014-inch guide wire that is used to cross the lesion and deliver balloon and stent catheters (Fig. 10-6). The filtration element has a self-expanding mechanism, proximal entry ports, and multiple distal perfusion pores (100 to 150 μm in size) that allow blood flow to the cerebral circulation while capturing released debris. The filter is sized to the selected distal ICA segment (4 to 6 mm). Filter deployment and retrieval are performed using dedicated catheters. At the commencement of the interventional procedure, the filter system, loaded

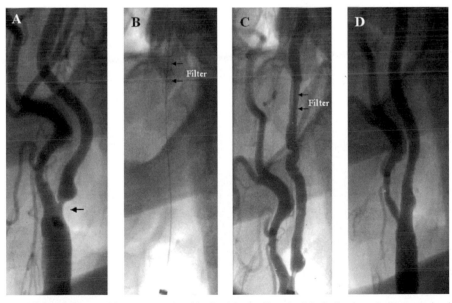

FIGURE 10-6. Carotid artery stenting (CAS) with the filter Anti-Embolization. **A**: Preprocedural angiography. **B**: The intravascular filter is placed in the distal internal carotid artery (ICA). Visible are the Nitinol filter expansion arms (*arrows*). **C**: Carotid angiography after the filter deployment. Flow through the filter is preserved. **D**: Final angiography.

into the delivery catheter, is advanced through the guiding sheath and across the target lesion into the distal ICA. The delivery catheter is withdrawn, and as it is withdrawn, the filter is deployed. In some filter systems, the lesion is first crossed using a bare 0.014-inch guide wire, and the filter system is then delivered "over the wire" into the distal ICA. After the delivery catheter is removed, an angiogram is obtained to document blood flow through the filter and device placement distal to the target lesion (Fig. 10-6C). After completing the stenting procedure, the entire device is then removed from the patient using a dedicated retrieval catheter with the captured emboli contained in the filtration element. In cases where the filter delivery system is not able to cross the lesion on the initial attempt owing to lesion severity or vessel tortuosities, a gentle predilation (using a 2-mm balloon), or a side-wire "buddy wire" is used to facilitate the system advancement.

Filter devices have the advantage of maintaining blood flow during the procedure while providing distal antiembolic protection, which makes them suitable in patients with poor collateral circulation (incomplete circle of Willis). Although the large crossing profile of the early generation filters has made them difficult to negotiate through high-grade stenoses and in certain anatomical situations, such as severely calcified lesions and markedly tortuous ICA, most of these difficulties have recently been overcomed by the introduction of the new generation "low-profile" and/or over-the-wire filter systems.

3. Proximal occlusion with flow reversal (Parodi Anti-Embolization system): In this system, distal protection is conferred by simultaneous inflation of two balloons within the CCA and the ECA (Figs. 10-4C, 10-7). This dual inflation reverses blood flow within the index carotid artery into the guiding catheter, which drains into the contralateral femoral

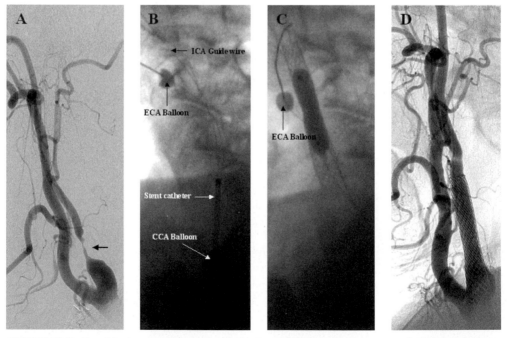

FIGURE 10-7. Carotid artery stenting (CAS) with the Parodi Anti-Embolization system. **A**: Presenting angiograms. **B**: Two balloons are inflated within the common carotid artery (CCA) and the external carotid artery (ECA). A stent is being advanced. **C**: Postdilatation of the stent with the ECA balloon visible. **D**: Final angiograms after removal of the occlusion balloons.

vein. Emboli released during the intervention travel in the direction of the flow. Two important features differentiate this proximal occlusion system from the other Anti-Embolization systems: (a) the protective effect can be activated prior to crossing the ICA stenosis, and (b) the carotid angioplasty and stenting procedure can be performed using standard low-profile coronary balloons and wires. In tortuous anatomy, a fair bit of wire manipulation can be anticipated. The advantage of a system that protects the distal bed from embolization during all stages of the procedure is obvious. Because flow reversal is an integral part of the protection mechanism with this system, intracranial anatomy that is not suitable for the distal occlusion balloon (poor collateral circulation) will also be unsuitable for proximal occlusion. With this system, forceful injection of contrast or saline through the sheath must be avoided, as it might lead to intracranial embolization.

LESION PREDILATATION

For predilatation of the stenosis, we routinely use a monorail (or an over-the-wire) 0.014-inch compatible balloon, and we prefer low-profile coronary balloons (Fig. 10-3B, 10-3C). These balloons "rewrap well" without residual wings, reducing the risk of trauma to the plaque during balloon withdrawal. Inflation pressures of 8, 10, and 16 atmospheres are used, and the balloon must be slowly and fully deflated before it is withdrawn. If the stenosis is preocclusive, we prefer to gradually step up the balloon size to minimize plaque disruption and distal embolization. In these situations, a predilatation is first performed using a 2 × 40-mm balloon (Fig. 10-3B). This is then followed by a second dilatation using a 4 × 40-mm balloon (Fig. 10-3C). In rare cases, mainly in heavily calcified lesions, if the stent does not easily pass through the stenosis after predilatation with the 4-mm–diameter balloon, a 5-mm balloon is used for additional predilatation. A long balloon (40 mm in length) is generally preferred to achieve balloon stability during the inflation and avoid the "watermelon seed effect." The balloon length can also guide selection of the appropriate stent length. If the operator anticipates a need for an extra-support guide wire (i.e., based on the presence of severe vessel tortuosities, angulations, and heavy calcifications), an over-the-wire balloon is used for the first predilation, and the soft wire is exchanged to an extra-support wire prior to the second upsized balloon dilatation. Again, the tip of this wire should always be visibly located close to the skull base and should be passed through all ICA kinks and tortuosities. In cases where the stenosis is smooth, not subocclusive, and the ICA is not very tortuous, the 0.014-inch support wire can be used as the primary wire to cross the stenosis. Prior to stenting, a control arteriogram is performed to reestablish the relationship of the stenosis to the bony landmarks.

Cases with Anti-Embolization Devices

Because all current Anti-Embolization devices are 0.014-inch guide wire–based systems, our current practice is to use 0.014-inch–compatible coronary balloons for predilatation, preferably a monorail system. Balloon catheter exchanges with the monorail systems are not only faster compared to over-the-wire systems, but also the entire system is more stable, as the operator has full control over both the guide wire carrying the Anti-Embolization device and the balloon. Such stability is very important, as it minimizes the vertical movements of the Anti-Embolization device and reduces the chance of spasm and/or dissection.

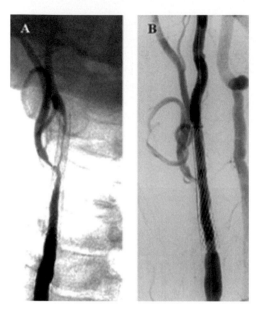

FIGURE 10-8. Carotid in-stent restenosis. **A**: Preintervention angiogram. **B**: Final carotid angiography after multiple balloon dilatations.

Rationale for Predilatation

Experimental work of Ohki et al. (14), as well as our clinical observation, has demonstrated that more embolic debris can be released with primary stenting without predilatation and during lesion dilatation with large peripheral (0.035-inch–compatible) balloons that form traumatic wings during the first deflation. From our experience, primary stenting without predilatation is associated with more "scissoring effect" of the stent struts on the plaque during the latter postdilatation with greater risk of embolization. Balloon predilatation creates a small passage within the lesion to facilitate stent delivery without forceful crossing, which can cause major occlusive dissections in the ICA. A cutting balloon has also been successfully used to treat carotid in-stent restenosis.

In cases where in-stent restenosis is approached, the treatment is achieved by applying multiple balloon dilatations within the stent using a larger diameter balloon (5 or 5.5-mm balloon) (Fig. 10-8). Rarely, a second self-expanding stent is necessary to obtain a sustained wide lumen, such as in cases of in-stent restenosis due to compression of the balloon-expandable stent (Fig. 10-9).

STENTING

At the beginning of our experience, we used balloon-expandable stents to treat carotid stenosis (13). Following the observations of external compression and deformation of these stents (Fig. 10-9), we started to use self-expanding stents, at first the Elgiloy tracheobronchial Wallstent (Boston Scientific Inc., Maple Grove, MN), and later Nitinol stents as well (19).

At the present time, the only indications for using balloon-expandable stents in the carotid circulation are: (a) to treat ostial common carotid artery stenoses (Fig. 10-10), (b) to treat distal cervical ICA stenoses within the distal (or intracranial) ICA segments, as the stiff self-expanding stent delivery systems may potentially damage these segments owing to the sharp bends, and (c) when the self-expanding stent cannot be advanced through the

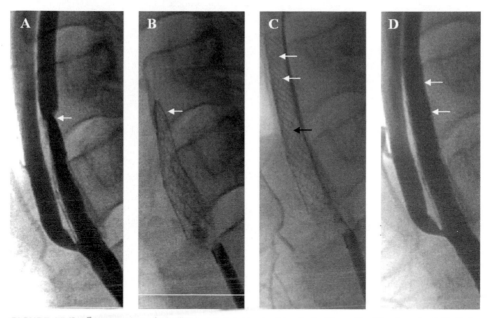

FIGURE 10-9. Compression of a balloon-expandable stent treated with a self-expanding stent. **A:** Preintervention carotid angiogram with the stenosis (*white arrow*) of the internal carotid artery (ICA) resulting from deformation of the distal edge of the balloon-expandable stent. **B:** Deformation of the distal edge of the balloon-expandable stent. **C:** The balloon-expandable stent has been dilated and a self-expanding stent (*arrows*) has been deployed. **D:** Final angiographic results with no residual stenosis.

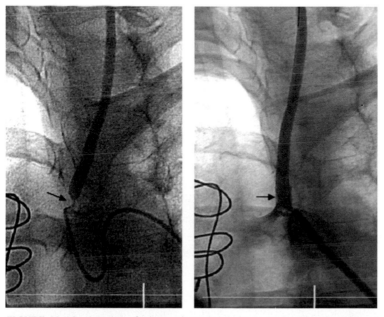

FIGURE 10-10. Stenting of a lesion that is located at a curve within the proximal internal carotid artery (ICA) using a self-expanding nitinol stent. The nitinol stent conforms very well to the ICA curve.

stenosis despite adequate balloon predilatation (usually because of calcified stenoses and/or high tendency of the lesions to recoil). In these instances, a 4- to 6-mm balloon-expandable stent is first deployed at the bifurcation to prevent recoil at the lesion site and to permit the passage of the self-expanding stent, which then functions as the definitive stent. Late compression of the balloon-expandable stent is prevented by the constant radial force exerted by the self-expanding stent.

Stent Diameter

The unconstrained diameter of the self-expanding stent to be deployed should be at least 1 to 2 mm larger than the largest vessel segment to be covered by the stent, almost always the CCA. We prefer a 10-mm–diameter stent in all cases. A large stent—sized to the CCA—would have large area coverage within the ICA lesion, effectively trapping the plaque material against the arterial wall and reducing the possibility of embolization during the postdilatation.

Stent Length

The stent is deployed to cover the whole carotid lesion that is typically located at the origin or the very proximal segment of the ICA (Figs. 10-2, 10-3). Complete coverage of the lesion is achieved by placing the stent across the carotid bifurcation into the CCA across the origin of the ECA (Figs. 10-2, 10-3). If a Wallstent (Boston Scientific Inc.) is used, a 20-mm length is selected. The true length of a 20-mm–long Wallstent is obtained only when the stent is expanded to the full diameter (10 mm). Because there is a size difference between the ICA and the CCA, the first being 5 to 6 mm and the latter 7 to 9 mm, the Wallstent does not expand to the full 10-mm diameter and therefore does not shorten to 20 mm in length. Instead, the final deployment length approximates 30 to 40 mm.

If a nitinol stent is selected, a 30- or 40-mm–long stent (10 mm in diameter) is typically required to completely cover the lesion. Despite the size difference between the ICA and the CCA, a nitinol self-expanding stent does not foreshorten, and therefore it retains the true length when deployed. Because there is no appreciable change in the length of the nitinol stent after deployment, these stents can be more precisely placed using the distal and proximal markers. Some manufacturers have recently introduced tapered stent designs that adapt to the deferential size between the ICA and the CCA (ACCULINK from Guidant Inc., Indianapolis, IN and Xact stent from MedNova, Galway, Ireland).

Stent Deployment

The stent is deployed using the vertebral bodies as landmarks (Fig. 10-2). Road mapping can also be helpful. An important technical pearl is to release 2 to 3 mm of the stent, adjust stent placement if needed, then wait for the stent to expand fully and stabilize against the vessel wall before the final full release. These stents have a tendency to "jump" distally if the stent is released too fast. The operator has to compensate for this tendency by slow deployment. The proximal end of the stent rests in the CCA, hence a 10-mm–diameter stent is preferred. On rare occasions, the stent is placed exclusively in the ICA. In these cases, a 6-mm or 8-mm–diameter stent is selected.

Placement of the distal stent end into kinks and tortuosities of the ICA should be avoided, especially when a Wallstent is selected. These anatomies cannot be eliminated but are displaced distally by the stiff stent and therefore are only exaggerated. Generally, nitinol

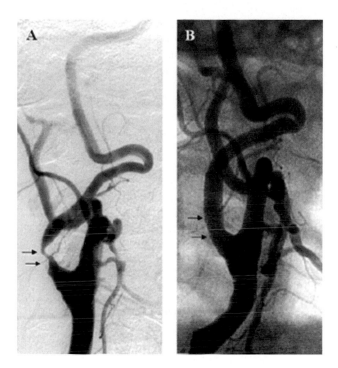

FIGURE 10-11. Stenting of the ostial left common carotid artery (CCA) using balloon-expandable stent. **A**: Prestenting angiograms. **B**: Poststenting angiograms with no residual stenosis.

stents are less rigid and conform better to the curve of the vessel without straightening the ICA as much as the Wallstent does (Fig. 10-11). A number of nitinol stents that are compatible with 0.014-inch guide wires and are loaded on 5-Fr and 6-Fr delivery catheters (in both over-the-wire and monorail systems) are currently in clinical trials.

Covering the origin of the ECA with the stent is not usually associated with adverse clinical consequences. Follow-up arteriograms have shown that, with rare exceptions, the ECA remained patent. However, should the ECA become significantly stenosed or occluded after the stent postdilatation, particularly if the patient is symptomatic (jaw and facial pain), which is very rare, this vessel can be approached through the stent mesh and is dilated using a coronary balloon. A 0.014-inch guide wire is used to enter the ECA, which is then dilated by a 2-mm or 4-mm–diameter balloon. The goal should be to establish normal thrombolysis in myocardial infarction (TIMI)-III flow in the ECA and not to completely obliterate the stenosis.

POSTDILATATION

The size of the postdilatation balloon is matched to the diameter of the ICA, and the dilatation is limited to the site of the stenosis within the stent (Fig. 10-3E). Typically, the self-expanding stent is postdilated with a 5-mm balloon, less commonly with a 5.5-mm balloon (Savvy, Cordis Inc., Miami, FL; Gazelle or Speedy Bypass, Boston Scientific Inc., Natick, MA), and almost never with a balloon that is more than or equal to 5.5 mm. The balloon is deflated very slowly. In heavily calcified lesions, a high-pressure balloon is used (e.g., Titan, Cordis Inc.). The stent postdilation is a critical step and requires careful attention. It is the time of the procedure when embolic neurological events are likely to develop.

To minimize the embolic risk during this step, we recommend: (a) using balloons that are no larger than 5.5 mm in diameter, (b) inflating the balloon to nominal pressures, (c) accepting a 10% to 20 % residual stenosis (Fig. 10-2B), (d) restricting it to a single postdilation that is limited to the lesion site (Fig. 10-3E), and (e) gradual deflation (over 30 to 45 seconds) and removal of the balloon.

Generally, it is safer to underdilate than to overdilate the self-expanding stent. Overdilatation with a high-pressure balloon may potentially squeeze the atherosclerotic material through the stent mesh, causing emboli. Minor residual stenosis following CAS is acceptable and does not cause any hemodynamic problems (Fig. 10-2B). In addition, the self-expanding stent has the tendency for late, progressive expansion, slowly reducing the residual stenosis. In some cases, continued flow via the stent struts into an ulcer crater is visualized at the end of the procedure (Fig. 10-2B). An attempt to obliterate this communication by using larger balloons or higher pressures should be avoided, as this communication usually seals off in the ensuing few days and is of no clinical consequence.

REMOVAL OF THE ANTI-EMBOLIZATION DEVICE

A. Distal Occlusion

Aspiration

Prior to the occlusion balloon deflation, a long beveled monorail aspiration catheter, the "export catheter,"is introduced over the wire into the ICA. The distal end of the aspiration catheter has a radio-opaque marker, and the catheter is advanced until this marker is just below the inflated occlusion balloon. Maintaining constant suction with a 20-cc or 30-cc syringe, the export catheter is slowly pulled back to the carotid bifurcation and then advanced forward to the occlusion balloon. This back-and-forth maneuver is repeated until approximately 50 to 60 cc of blood in total is aspirated. The goal is to aspirate the emboli-containing blood column proximal to the occlusion balloon, thereby preventing these emboli from traveling intracranially when the occlusion balloon is deflated.

Balloon Deflation

While the aspiration of blood is in progress, the assistant reassembles the end of the occlusion balloon deflation apparatus, the "microseal adaptor." As soon as aspiration is completed, the balloon is deflated, and the Anti-Embolization system is completely removed. The final angiograms are then acquired, and the balloon occlusion site within the ICA is carefully evaluated for possible dissections.

B. Filters

The filters are removed using dedicated retrieval catheter. The entire filter (e.g., AccuNet, NeuroShield) or part of the filter (Angioguard) is withdrawn into the retrieval catheter, which is then securely removed as one unit. Prior to filter retrieval, blood flow through the filter should be angiographically ascertained. In very rare occasions, the filter can be clogged by a large amount of embolic debris, and the flow through the ICA is interrupted. In this case, the technique of the export aspiration catheter should be used (see distal balloon occlusion Anti-Embolization technique).

C. Proximal Occlusion

Following postdilatation, both the ECA and the CCA balloons are deflated, and the system is removed from the artery.

FINAL ANGIOGRAPHIC ASSESSMENT

Lesion Site and Cervical Internal Carotid Artery

Following stent postdilation, final angiograms are acquired in the same projection(s) that demonstrated the maximum severity of the lesion in both digital subtraction angiography (DSA) or regular cineangiogram format. Careful attention must be paid to the segment of the ICA that contained the Anti-Embolization device. It is not unusual to encounter spasm in this segment, particularly if the ICA is tortuous. Guide-wire removal and partial retrieval of the guiding sheath to the proximal CCA will assist in relieving the spasm, as it relaxes the artery and helps the operator get a better assessment of the stented segment. A small dose of intraarterial nitroglycerin is rarely needed. It is important to note that as a consequence of stent-induced activation of the carotid baroreceptors, the patient might be relatively hypotensive and may not tolerate the nitroglycerin. Stent-related distal edge dissections are very rare and when present are short and for the most part inconsequential. Occasionally, such dissections may need treatment, and an additional stent is then placed. On rare occasions, linear dissections may result from the use of the occlusion balloon. These were more common with the first-generation devices when the balloon could only be inflated to two sizes (5.5 mm and 6 mm) and was frequently oversized to the ICA. The recently introduced second-generation device (GuardWire-plus) offers a wide range of sizes (3 to 6 mm in 0.5-mm increments), and the balloon can be more accurately matched to the size of the distal vessel, reducing the risk of these dissections. In any event, these small linear dissections usually do not compromise blood flow and very rarely require additional stents.

Intracranial Vasculature

We routinely acquire intracranial angiograms after the stenting procedure is completed. A comparison with the preinterventional angiograms is then made to assess the possibility of "silent embolization" and demonstrate improvement in the intracranial flow. Some operators reserve it for those patients who experience intraprocedural neurological events. Almost all the current carotid stent investigational protocols call for repeat intracranial views, which are acquired in the same projections as the baseline views.

GUIDING SHEATH REMOVAL AND ACCESS SITE HEMOSTASIS

The shuttle sheath is pulled back over a wire into the iliac artery and is exchanged for a short sheath of appropriate size (usually 7Fr, rarely 8Fr), which is removed in 3 to 4 hours when the activated clotting time (ACT) is less than or equal to 150 seconds. In our practice, access site hemostasis is achieved at the end of the procedure using a vascular closure device. This vascular sealing approach is particularly valuable for those patients who are proposed to be discharged on the same day (17).

CONCLUSIONS AND FUTURE DIRECTIONS

With today's equipment and techniques, stenting mortality and morbidity from stroke-related complications (all strokes, TIA, and death) are in the range of 2% to 3%, equivalent to or lower than comparable patient populations treated with CEA (1–11). Rigorous follow-up studies have confirmed the low restenosis rates after CAS and the low incidence of late cerebrovascular events (1,20). In both percutaneous stenting and endarterectomy, embolic stroke events can occur. In each technique, the incidence of ischemic or embolic stroke depends on the meticulous procedural techniques and the operator expertise, which is markedly dependent on the volume of cases performed. The availability of Anti-Embolization devices is expected to further reduce the risk for cerebral emboli and enhance future results of this treatment. There is also an ongoing improvement of the equipment available for carotid stenting. Lower-profile stent, monorail delivery systems, better guiding sheaths, and specially designed guide wires and balloons are now being introduced. It is likely that a variety of different stent designs will be required for optimal treatment of variable carotid bifurcation anatomy. Technical problems, attributed to the inadequacy of currently available devices, are increasingly rare.

REFERENCES

1. Roubin GS, New G, Iyer SS, et al. Immediate and late clinical outcomes of carotid artery stenting in patients with symptomatic and asymptomatic carotid artery stenosis: a 5-year prospective analysis. *Circulation* 2001;103:532–537.
2. Mathias K. Stent placement in arteriosclerotic disease of the internal carotid artery. *J Interv Cardiol* 1997;10:469–477.
3. Diethrich EB, Ndiaye M, Reid DB. Stenting in the carotid artery: initial experience in 110 patients. *J Endovasc Surg* 1996;3:42–62.
4. Theron JG, Payelle GG, Coskun O, et al. Carotid artery stenosis: treatment with protected balloon angioplasty and stent placement. *Radiology* 1996;201:627–636.
5. Shawl F, Kadro W, Domanski MJ, et al. Safety and efficacy of elective carotid artery stenting in high-risk patients. *J Am Coll Cardiol* 2000;35:1721–1728.
6. Wholey MH, Al-Mubarak N, Wholey MH. Updated review of the global carotid artery stent registry. *Catheter Cardiovasc Interv* 2003;60:259–266.
7. Ohki T, Feith FJ. Carotid artery stenting: utility of cerebral protection devices. *J Invasive Cardiol* 2001;13:47–55.
8. Henry M, Amor M, Klonaris C, et al. Angioplasty and stenting of the extracranial carotid arteries. *Tex Heart Inst J* 2000;27:150–158.
9. Reimers B, Corvaja N, Moshiri S, et al. Cerebral protection with filter devices during carotid artery stenting. *Circulation* 2001;104:12–15.
10. Parodi JC, Mura RL, Ferreira LM, et al. Initial evaluation of carotid angioplasty and stenting with three different cerebral protection devices. *J Vasc Surg* 2000;32:1127–1136.
11. Al-Mubarak N, Colombo A, Gaines PA, et al. Multicenter evaluation of carotid artery stenting with a filter protection system. *J Am Coll Cardiol* 2002;39:841–846.
12. Mathur A, Roubin GS, Iyer SS, et al. Predictors of stroke complicating carotid artery stenting. *Circulation* 1998;97:1239–1245.
13. Yadav JS, Roubin GS, Iyer S, et al. Elective stenting of the extracranial carotid arteries. *Circulation* 1997;95:376–381.
14. Ohki T, Marin ML, Lyon RT, et al. Ex vivo human carotid artery bifurcation stenting: correlation of lesion characteristics with embolic potential. *J Vasc Surg* 1998;27:463–471.
15. Al-Mubarak N, Roubin GS, Vitek JJ, et al. Effect of the distal-balloon protection system on microembolization during carotid stenting. *Circulation* 2001;104:1999–2002.
16. Gomez CR, Roubin GS, Dean LS, et al. Neurological monitoring during carotid artery stenting: the duck squeezing test. *J Endovasc Surg* 1999;6:332–336.

17. Al-Mubarak N, Roubin GS, Vitek JJ, et al. Procedural safety and short-term outcome of ambulatory carotid stenting. *Stroke* 2001;32:2305–2309.
18. Al-Mubarak N, Vitek JJ, Iyer S, et al. Embolization via collateral circulation during carotid stenting with the distal balloon protection system. *J Endovasc Ther* 2001;8:354–357.
19. Mathur A, Dorros G, Iyer SS, et al. Palmaz stent compression in patients following carotid artery stenting. *Cathet Cardiovasc Diagn* 1997;41:137–140.
20. Endovascular versus surgical treatment in patients with carotid stenosis in the Carotid and Vertebral Artery Transluminal Angioplasty Study (CAVATAS): a randomized trial. *Lancet* 2001;357:1729–1737.

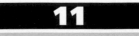

THE DIRECT CERVICAL CAROTID ARTERY APPROACH

EDWARD B. DIETHRICH

In the last several decades, the field of vascular surgery has been revolutionized by endovascular techniques that allow percutaneous vascular intervention. Advances in biomaterials and product design have given us a variety of low-profile equipment, hydrophilic catheter coatings, and improved balloon and stent designs. As these technological advancements have occurred, new and expanded applications and procedures have also appeared on the horizon. Carotid artery stenting (CAS) is currently a procedure that is receiving considerable worldwide attention. Although there is still a great deal of controversy regarding carotid stent procedures, success with the intervention has been described in a number of reports in the last 10 years (1–33). At the Arizona Heart Institute, we placed our first carotid stent in 1993 in a patient who presented with recurrent disease 5 years after a carotid endarterectomy (CEA). Following a successful intervention in her case, we went on to treat a total of 110 patients and published the first peer-reviewed report on stenting in the carotid artery in 1996 (4). The combined rate of stroke, transient ischemic attack (TIA), and death in that series totaled 10.6%—a rate we considered excessively high. Nevertheless, we and other investigators all over the world continued to study the technology, making procedural and device improvements and reducing complications. In the United States, we received Food and Drug Administration (FDA) Investigational Device Exemptions (IDEs) for the procedure, and our work is still governed by these protocols, as no stent has yet been approved for use in the carotid arteries.

The carotid stent procedure has evolved considerably over the years. Although the majority of stenting procedures can be performed using the retrograde femoral artery approach, in some cases, the arch vessels have severe angulations (Fig. 11-1), which may make retrograde femoral delivery of a stent virtually impossible. Other access routes, such as brachial (34) and radial (35) approaches, have been tried with successful results. We have found that, in many cases, a direct cervical carotid artery approach is the best solution. The results of our initial experience with balloon expandable stents deployed following a "mini" exposure technique we developed for direct carotid access were generally excellent. Long-term patency without intimal hyperplasia encouraged us to continue using these types of stents at the outset. However, the majority of our current stenting protocols now call for self-expanding stents. In this chapter, we review the direct carotid approach in detail, describing the procedure and illustrating the steps involved.

THE DIRECT CAROTID APPROACH
Patient Evaluation

One of the first steps in evaluating a patient for any carotid procedure is proper imaging. Noninvasive assessment with duplex imaging of the arch, vertebral, and extracranial arteries

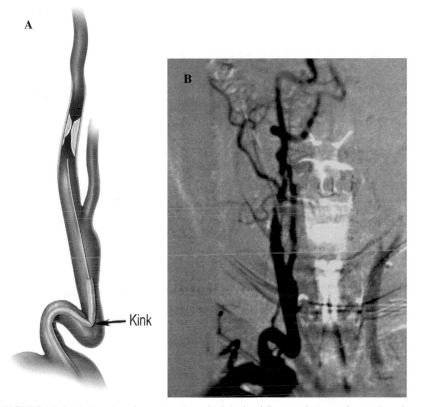

FIGURE 11-1. A: Drawing demonstrating a kink in the delivery catheter at the aortic arch. **B**: Angiogram showing marked tortuosity of the artery that prevents delivery of the stent to the desired location.

is completed, and computed tomography (CT) examination of the brain is often performed as well, particularly if the protocol mandates it. Duplex imaging of the arch vessels is sometimes technically difficult. Using several imaging modalities helps ensure adequate imaging and often assists the clinician in identifying patients who may be at high risk for a perioperative cerebrovascular accident during a stenting procedure. Brain scans and magnetic resonance angiography (MRA) are also used to evaluate patients based on history and current symptoms. Angiographic studies are required in all of the current protocols for CAS with embolic protection systems, and the images obtained via angiography are more accurate than those seen with MRA because the latter often contains artifacts and provides less definitive resolution of the lesion and arterial tree. In centers with state-of-the-art MRA equipment, images may be more accurate. At present, European centers are more likely to have these advanced MRA capabilities, as they have been working with the technology for many years.

At the Arizona Heart Institute, we treat both symptomatic and asymptomatic patients using endovascular procedures and have performed more than 500 carotid endovascular procedures. Approximately three-fourths of our cases have been in asymptomatic patients with high-grade lesions and assorted cardiac and peripheral vascular diseases that required intervention. Documented progression of disease is also a valid indication, even in patients who are asymptomatic. A separate category of patients seems to be on the rise: those who have previously undergone CEA and have developed restenosis. Likewise, patients with a contralateral occlusion and ipsilateral high-grade stenosis are ideal endovascular candidates because brain ischemia is reduced considerably by the relatively short occlusion time required for the stenting procedure.

Although there are many who support the use of CAS only in those deemed to be at high risk for endarterectomy, we prefer to evaluate patients on the basis of anatomy and plaque composition. Overall, we have defined four specific subgroups of patients in whom we believe the endovascular approach is either comparable or even superior to the classic endarterectomy procedure: (a) patients with high internal carotid artery lesions that are difficult to access via endarterectomy—mandibular subluxation is not a viable option given current availability of stent procedures, (b) patients who have undergone radiation to the cervical carotid area and/or a radical node dissection, (c) patients who have previously undergone one or more CEA procedures—especially because patients in this group and in group 2 (above) have higher rates of cranial nerve damage with endarterectomy, and (d) patients with combined or sequential lesions, which may require endarterectomy and angioplasty (Fig. 11-2). With improvements in embolic protection device design, there is no question that, over time, even some of the more complex bifurcation lesions will be successfully treated. Early results indicate CAS with Anti-Embolization protection is technically feasible and safe with generally favorable outcomes (36,37).

Medications

Aspirin and clopidogrel are administered before stenting. The former is continued indefinitely and the latter for a period of 30 days following the procedure. Although these two agents have been associated with a reduction in ischemic events in patients receiving carotid

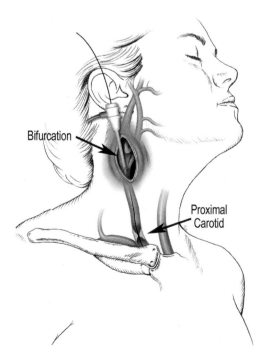

Bifurcation

Proximal Carotid

FIGURE 11-2. Drawing illustrating sequential lesions that are amenable to carotid artery stenting performed in concert with an endarterectomy.

artery stents (38), the use of the platelet glycoprotein IIb/IIIa receptor inhibitor, abciximab, has been less encouraging (39,40).

Anesthesia

The entire procedure may be performed under local anesthesia, and this allows the patient to respond to oral commands and helps the interventionist to monitor any neurologic changes. Occasionally, in the direct access technique we describe, general anesthesia is indicated for patient comfort and cooperation.

Access

At present, when anatomy precludes a retrograde femoral approach, we advocate exposing a short segment of the common carotid artery just above the clavicle on the side of the intended stent deployment (Fig. 11-3). This is the same location we used in our first series in 110 patients, employing a percutaneous "direct stick" into the common carotid artery (Fig. 11-4). Unfortunately, complications associated with this method included bleeding, hematoma formation, and stent deformity due to compression during sheath removal.

Stenting Procedure

The common carotid artery is dissected free from the carotid sheath and held with a heavy silk or vessel loop (Fig. 11-5). From this point on, the procedure is identical to a percutaneous retrograde approach. The only difference is the length of the sheaths, wires, and balloons—these are sometimes reduced considerably, which makes the procedure more conven-

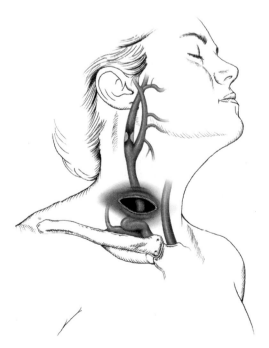

FIGURE 11-3. Drawing showing the site of the incision just above the clavicle for exposure of the common carotid artery. This approach can be used for either right- or left-sided angioplasty and stent deployment.

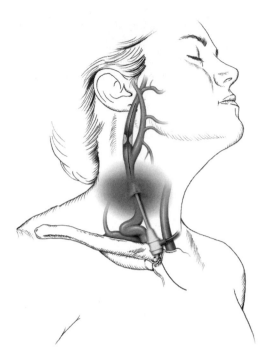

FIGURE 11-4. Drawing of our original technique for percutaneous entry into the common carotid artery. This approach was abandoned because of an excessive rate of complications associated with it.

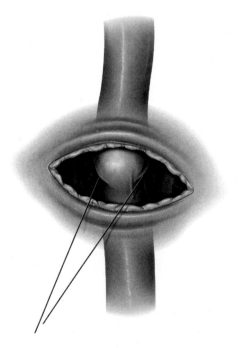

FIGURE 11-5. The common carotid artery is exposed for a 2 to 3 cm distance and is elevated with a heavy silk or vessel loop.

ient. However, with the advent of embolic protection devices, this "shortening" is not possible in every protocol.

An 18-gauge, $2\frac{3}{8}$-inch single-wall entry needle (Cook, Inc., Bloomington, IN) is used for the puncture, and the artery is gently retracted for better entry (Fig. 11-6). An angled hydrophilic guide wire, such as the Glidewire (Medi-tech/Boston Scientific, Watertown, MA), is passed cephalad for about 5 cm in order to avoid crossing the lesion or entering the internal carotid artery. A small contrast injection is made through the needle prior to introduction of the wire to identify the carotid bifurcation and the origin of the external carotid artery. Obviously, crossing the internal carotid artery is not advisable and may promote embolic complications, and, therefore, the wire is placed across the external carotid artery. The use of a dilator to expand the puncture site expedites sheath placement, which is followed by insertion of a 6F or 7F, 6-cm–long sheath (Cordis, Warren, NJ), depending on the size requirement for the proposed stent (Fig. 11-7). Intravenous heparin sodium (approximately 5,000 units) is given to maintain the activated coagulation time (ACT) above 250 seconds throughout the procedure, and sheaths and catheters are irrigated with a heparinized saline solution (10,000 units of heparin to 1,000 cc normal saline). A bolus of contrast is injected to identify the carotid bifurcation in preparation for the stenting procedure. If anterior-posterior and lateral cerebral angiograms have not been performed as part of the preoperative evaluation, these are obtained to establish the baseline anatomy.

The fluoroscopic unit is positioned in a manner that exposes both bifurcation vessels, eliminating a vessel overlap with the internal carotid artery. This is usually a steep oblique, or even a lateral projection (Figs. 11-8, 11-9). Once the correct fluoroscopic position is selected, the C-arm is fixed and not moved again so that road mapping will record the exact stent placement. Because the majority of carotid stenting procedures are performed according to protocols that use some form of cerebral embolic protection, the next step in the procedure depends upon which device is used.

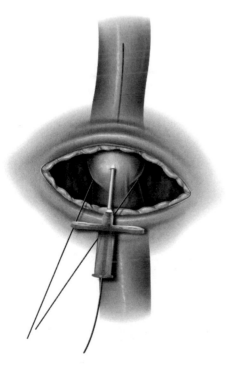

FIGURE 11-6. The common carotid artery is elevated gently and punctured with an 18-gauge needle, and an angled Glidewire is passed approximately 5 cm cephalad.

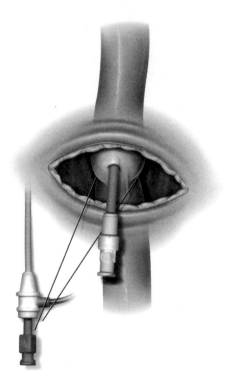

FIGURE 11-7. A dilator is introduced over the wire to expand the puncture site; this is followed by insertion of a short sheath of the desired French size.

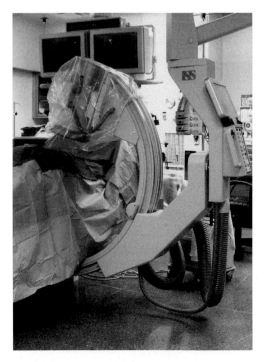

FIGURE 11-8. Photograph of the C-arm in a steep, oblique position for unobstructed visualization of the entire internal carotid artery.

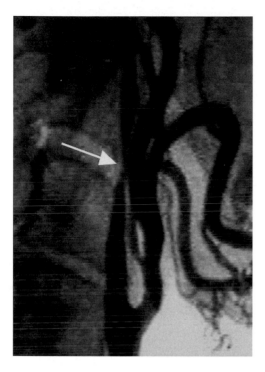

FIGURE 11-9. Angiogram obtained from the C-arm as positioned in Fig. 11-8.

Angiographic visualization is used to judge the length and diameter of the lesion before any predilation. In severely stenotic lesions, predilation is frequently necessary before stent deployment, and some protocols require balloon dilation. Balloon diameter is usually one or two sizes smaller than the stent delivery balloon, but never larger than 4 mm in diameter.

The diameter and length of the lesion are assessed to determine the most appropriate stent but, again, there is little room for creativity given that only one type of stent is specified by each protocol. This may change in the pivotal phase of the Carotid Revascularization with Endarterectomy and Stenting Systems (CARESS) Trial. The most common balloon dilation catheter size is a 4 mm $\times$ 2 mm balloon followed by stent delivery on the same size or next larger-sized balloon. None of the current protocols features the rigid, balloon-expandable Palmaz stent (Cordis, Warren, NJ), which was our original selection. The flexible, self-expanding stents, such as the Wallstent (Boston Scientific, Natick, MA), are common now. There are no stents currently approved for use in the carotid and, although several companies are considering new prototype designs for use in this location, commercialization depends on the results of clinical trials.

The guide wire is withdrawn from the external carotid artery and substituted with the wire that will be used for ballooning and stent delivery. Most protocols that specify protection devices (Fig. 11-10) also dictate the type of wire used to incorporate them. If that is not the case, we prefer to use an 0.018-inch Roadrunner wire (Cook, Inc., Bloomington, IN) to pass across the lesion into the internal carotid artery. One milligram of atropine is administered to prevent bradycardia and hypotension during balloon expansion. The balloon is centered across the lesion using the road mapping image for guidance, and a short burst of contrast is injected to reveal its final position. Approximately 8 to 10 atmospheres of pressure are used for balloon expansion. If bradycardia occurs, the balloon is deflated immediately. Following dilation of the vessel, the balloon is withdrawn and replaced with the stent specified

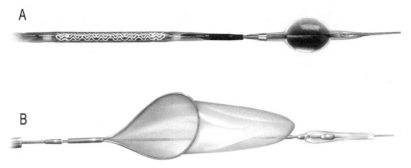

FIGURE 11-10. **A**: Photographs of PercuSurge balloon protection system and **(B)** the EPI filter protection system. These are just two of the current protection systems being evaluated.

by the protocol. Once the stent has been positioned correctly, it is deployed with the protection device in place (Fig. 11-11).

Contrast is injected following stent deployment to confirm patency and assess proper positioning. Inadequate stent expansion contributes to complications such as stent occlusion and thrombus formation. Therefore, most protocols call for a "gentle" balloon dilation following stent deployment in order to ensure good apposition between the stent and the artery wall. This is a change in technique from the earliest days of carotid stenting when we believed the stent required high-pressure balloon dilation. The results achieved with that technique were not satisfactory, and it is now clear that lower pressure dilation centered at the maximum stenosis level is all that is required. A perfect cosmetic result is not required for an excellent clinical outcome. Real-time intravascular ultrasound can be used to confirm proper stent deployment (41) if there is any serious concern about the result (Fig. 11-12). A cerebral angiogram is also performed at the conclusion of stent deployment for comparison with the prestent image to confirm the absence of cerebral embolization. In some cases where emboli are visualized, neurorescue techniques, such as thrombolytic infusion, are required, depending on the patient's condition. Periprocedural neurocomplications have been markedly reduced in stenting procedures now that most centers use low-profile systems and protection devices. In addition, we are much more knowledgeable about proper patient selection for these procedures.

Once the procedure is complete, a 5-0 suture is placed around the sheath, tightened as the sheath is withdrawn, and the incision is closed (Fig. 11-13). The majority of cases are performed under local anesthesia, but if a general anesthetic was used, the patient is awakened in the endovascular suite so that neurological function can be assessed. The patient is then transferred to the ICU and, in the first hour after transfer, we perform a duplex scan of the treatment site.

DISCUSSION

Although the Carotid and Vertebral Transluminal Angioplasty Study (CAVATAS) trial investigators (42) compared endovascular treatment with conventional carotid surgery and concluded that endovascular treatment avoided minor complications and had similar major risks and effectiveness at prevention of stroke over 3 years, there are still conflicting opinions regarding how to best use endovascular technologies to prevent TIAs and stroke. More

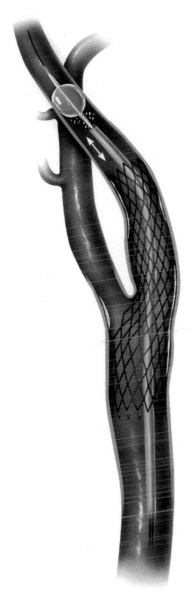

FIGURE 11-11. Drawing of inflated PercuSurge protection balloon and deployment of a Wallstent. This is an example of a procedure being followed in the Phase I Carotid Revascularization with Endarterectomy and Stenting Systems (CARESS) Trial.

recently, we have embarked upon further study of carotid procedures in the CARESS trial (43), which includes both symptomatic and asymptomatic patients. The CARESS trial is being conducted by the International Society of Endovascular Specialists (ISES), and Phase 1 enrollment was completed in December 2002—the pivotal study of approximately 2,500 patients was expected to begin in 2003. This important society-sponsored study will answer questions about carotid stenting in common practice, regardless of patient risk factors, symptomatology, or morbidity. The protocol enables the investigator to overcome access problems encountered in patients with difficult aortic arch anatomy because it allows use of the direct exposure technique described in this paper. Our results with this approach are identical to those achieved in less tortuous vessels using a retrograde femoral approach; use of the direct

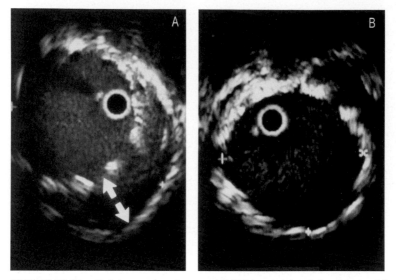

FIGURE 11-12.   A: Intravascular ultrasound (IVUS) image taken following carotid stent deployment that shows incomplete stent/artery wall contact. **B**: Repeat IVUS after a second balloon dilation that demonstrates a perfect result.

approach expands the pool of eligible candidates considerably because the exposure is made just above the clavicle, beyond vessel tortuosity. Even in patients who have previously had a CEA or radical node dissection, exposure is usually fairly straightforward because the incision site is generally caudal to scar tissue or a previous incision.

Carotid stenting is an evolving technology, and there is no doubt that there are many patients who will benefit from an endovascular approach. The direct carotid approach described here makes endovascular surgery possible in almost any patient. The only drawback of the method is that it demands surgical skills that some interventionists may not be trained

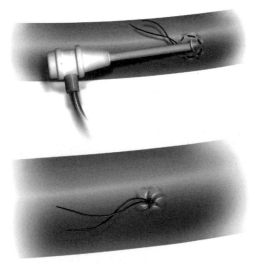

FIGURE 11-13. A 5-0 suture placed around the sheath provides hemostasis, and then the sheath is removed.

in. In these cases, cooperative efforts that involve a team approach to the procedure may help overcome that particular barrier to improved patient care.

REFERENCES

1. Kachel R, Basche S, Heerklotz I, et al. Percutaneous transluminal angioplasty of supra-aortic arteries, especially the internal carotid artery. *Neuroradiology* 1991;33:191–194.
2. Kachel R. Results of balloon angioplasty in the carotid arteries. *J Endovasc Surg* 1996;3:22–30.
3. Theron J. Angioplastie carotidienne protegee et stents carotidiens. *J Mal Vasc* 1996;21(Suppl A): 113–122.
4. Diethrich EB, Ndiaye M, Reid DB. Stenting in the carotid artery: initial experience in 110 patients. *J Endovasc Surg* 1996;3:42–62.
5. Wholey MH, Wholey M, Jarmolowski CR, et al. Endovascular stents for carotid artery occlusive disease. *J Endovasc Surg* 1997;4:326–338.
6. Teitlebaum GP, Lefkowitz MA, Giannotta SL. Carotid angioplasty and stenting in high-risk patients. *Surg Neurol* 1998;50:300–311.
7. Wholey MH, Wholey M, Bergeron P, et al. Current global status of carotid artery stent placement. *Cathet Cardiovasc Diagn* 1998;44:1–6.
8. Jordan WD Jr, Voellinger DC, Doblar DD, et al. Microemboli detected by transcranial Doppler monitoring in patients during carotid angioplasty versus carotid endarterectomy. *Cardiovasc Surg* 1999; 7:33–38.
9. Jordan WD Jr, Schroeder PT, Fisher WS, et al. A comparison of angioplasty with stenting versus endarterectomy for the treatment of carotid artery stenosis. *Ann Vasc Surg* 1997;11:2–8.
10. Jordan WD Jr, Roye GD, Fisher WS 3rd, et al. A cost comparison of balloon angioplasty and stenting versus endarterectomy for the treatment of carotid artery stenosis. *J Vasc Surg* 1998;27:16–22.
11. National Stroke Association. Current status of carotid stenting. *Stroke Clin Update* 1999;IX:1–4.
12. Al-Mubarak N, Roubin GS, Liu MW, et al. Early results of percutaneous intervention for severe coexisting carotid and coronary artery disease. *Am J Cardiol* 1999;84:600–602.
13. Mericle RA, Kim SH, Lanzino G, et al. Carotid artery angioplasty and use of stents in high-risk patients with contralateral occlusions. *J Neurosurg* 1999;90:1031–1036.
14. Chastain HD 2nd, Gomez CR, Iyer S, et al. Influence of age upon complications of carotid artery stenting. *J Endovasc Surg* 1999;3:217–222.
15. Lanzino G, Mericle RA, Lopes DK, et al. Percutaneous transluminal angioplasty and stent placement for recurrent carotid artery stenosis. *J Neurosurg* 1999;90:688–694.
16. Brown MM. Vascular Surgical Society of Great Britain and Ireland: Results of the carotid and vertebral artery transluminal angioplasty study. *Br J Surg* 1999;86:710–711.
17. Wholey MH, Wholey M, Mathias K, et al. Global experience in cervical artery stent placement. *Cathet Cardiovasc Interv* 2000;50:160–167.
18. New G, Roubin GS, Iyer SS, et al. Safety, efficacy, and durability of carotid artery stenting for restenosis following carotid endarterectomy: a multicenter study. *J Endovasc Ther* 2000;7:345–352.
19. Vitek JJ, Roubin GS, Al-Mubarak N, et al. Carotid artery stenting: technical considerations. *Am J Neuroradiol* 2000;21:1736–1743.
20. Malek AM, Higashida RT, Phatouros CC, et al. Stent angioplasty for cervical carotid artery stenosis in high-risk symptomatic NASCET-ineligible patients. *Stroke* 2000;31:3029–3033.
21. Cremonesi A, Castriota F, Manetti R, et al. Endovascular treatment of carotid atherosclerotic disease: early and late outcome in a non-selected population. *Ital Heart J* 2000;1:801–809.
22. Roubin GS, New G, Iyer SS, et al. Immediate and late clinical outcomes of carotid artery stenting in patients with symptomatic and asymptomatic carotid artery stenosis: a 5-year prospective analysis. *Circulation* 2001;103:532–537.
23. Chakhtoura EY, Hobson RW 2nd, Goldstein J, et al. In-stent restenosis after carotid angioplasty-stenting: incidence and management. *J Vasc Surg* 2001;33:220–225.
24. Dangas G, Laird JR Jr, Mehran R, et al. Carotid artery stenting in patients with high-risk anatomy for carotid endarterectomy. *J Endovasc Ther* 2001;8:39–43.
25. Brooks WH, McClure RR, Jones MR, et al. Carotid angioplasty and stenting versus carotid endarterectomy: randomized trial in a community hospital. *J Am Coll Cardiol* 2001;38:1589–1595.
26. Lepore MR Jr, Sternbergh WC 3rd, Salartash K, et al. Influence of NASCET/ACAS trial eligibility on outcome after carotid endarterectomy. *J Vasc Surg* 2001;34:581–586.

27. Al-Mubarak N, Roubin GS, Vitek JJ, et al. Procedural safety and short-term outcome of ambulatory carotid stenting. *Stroke* 2001;32:2305–2309.
28. Kirsch EC, Khangure MS, van Schie GP, et al. Carotid arterial stent placement: results and follow-up in 53 patients. *Radiology* 2001;220:737–744.
29. Ahmadi R, Schillinger M. Lang W, et al. Carotid artery stenting in older patients: is age a risk factor for poor outcome? *J Endovasc Ther* 2002;9:559–565.
30. AbuRahma AF, Bates MC, Wulu JT, et al. Early postsurgical carotid restenosis: redo surgery versus angioplasty and stenting. *J Endovasc Ther* 2002;9:566–572.
31. Drescher R, Mathias KD, Jaeger HJ, et al. Clinical results of carotid artery stenting with a nitinol self-expanding stent (SMART stent). *Eur Radiol* 2002;12:2451–2456.
32. Stankovic G, Liistro F, Moshiri S et al. Carotid artery stenting in the first 100 consecutive patients: results and follow-up. *Heart* 2002;88:381–386.
33. Ross CB, Naslund TC, Ranval TJ. Carotid stent-assisted angioplasty: the newest addition to the surgeons' armamentarium in the management of carotid occlusive disease. *Am Surg* 2002;68:967–975.
34. Al-Mubarak N, Vitek JJ, Iyer SS, et al. Carotid stenting with distal balloon protection via the transbrachial approach. *J Endovasc Ther* 2001;8:571–575.
35. Yoo BS, Lee SH, Kim JY, et al. A case of transradial carotid stenting. *Catheter Cardiovasc Interv* 2002;56:243–245.
36. Al-Mubarak N, Colombo A, Gaines PA, et al. Multicenter evaluation of carotid artery stenting with a filter protection system. *J Am Coll Cardiol* 2002;39:841–846.
37. Angelini A, Reimers B, Della Barbera M, et al. Cerebral protection during carotid artery stenting: collection and histopathologic analysis of embolized debris. *Stroke* 2002;33:456–461.
38. Bhatt DL, Kapadia SR, Bajzer CT, et al. Dual antiplatelet therapy with clopidogrel and aspirin after carotid artery stenting. *J Invasive Cardiol* 2001;13:767–771.
39. Hofmann R, Kerschner K, Steinwender C, et al. Abciximab bolus injection does not reduce cerebral ischemic complications of elective carotid artery stenting: a randomized study. *Stroke* 2002;33:725–727.
40. Qureshi AI, Suri MF, Ali Z, et al. Carotid angioplasty and stent placement: a prospective analysis of perioperative complications and impact of intravenously administered abciximab. *Neurosurgery* 2002;50:466–473.
41. Reid DB, Diethrich EB, Marx P, et al. Intravascular ultrasound assessment in carotid interventions. *J Endovasc Surg* 1996;3:203–210.
42. Brown MM. Vascular Surgical Society of Great Britain and Ireland: Results of the carotid and vertebral artery transluminal angioplasty study. *Br J Surg* 1999;86:710–711.
43. Roubin GS, Hobson RW, White R, et al. CREST and CARESS to evaluate carotid stenting: time to get to work! *J Endovasc Ther* 2001;8:107–110.

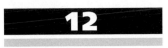

PROCEDURAL COMPLICATIONS

NADIM AL-MUBARAK
SRIRAM S. IYER
GARY S. ROUBIN
JIRI J. VITEK

The ability to treat obstructive carotid artery disease with stenting through a percutaneous arterial access without the need for general anesthesia has eliminated the various wound and anesthetic complications that were associated with the traditional treatment, carotid endarterectomy (CEA) (1,2). In order to accept the reported late freedom from stroke as an advantage of carotid artery stenting (CAS), the immediate procedural complications should be kept at a minimum (3). The developmental evolution and the technical learning curve of CAS have been associated with a variety of complications that were encountered at one time (Table 12-1) and have subsequently been avoided with improved patient selection, modifications in the technique, and the development of suitable equipment for this procedure (2). Today, major complications resulting in severe clinical sequelae are rare when carotid stenting is performed by experienced operators (1,2,4). In this chapter, we will detail our experience with a variety of complications that we have encountered mainly during the early learning curve and discuss methods necessary to avoid these complications and treat them should they arise.

VASCULAR ACCESS SITE COMPLICATIONS

Carotid stenting should be undertaken only within an endovascular program where the personnel are familiar with efficient and safe arterial sheath removal. Puncture site complications can be minimized by careful anterior wall puncture of the femoral artery and moderation of periprocedural anticoagulation. In our practice, if suitable, we routinely apply a vascular closure device at the end of the procedure to achieve immediate hemostasis. This allows early ambulation and discharge with the added benefit of counteracting the activated carotid sinus reflex and the occasionally observed postprocedural hypotension (5). If manual sheath removal technique is used, then the sheath should be removed by experienced personnel under additional local anesthesia 2 to 4 hours after the procedure is completed when the activated coagulation time (ACT) falls to less than or equal to 150 seconds. A good intravenous line, adequate hydration, and pretreatment with atropine are used to prevent or treat potential vasovagal hypotension associated with the sheath removal. Patients are usually kept on bed rest for 4 to 6 hours following the sheath removal.

TRANSIENT BRADYARRHYTHMIAS AND HYPOTENSION

Transient sinus bradycardia or asystole are relatively common physiological responses during balloon dilatation of the carotid bifurcation lesions, particularly during the stent postdilata-

TABLE 12-1. POTENTIAL COMPLICATIONS OF CAROTID ARTERY STENTING

Minor complications
  Puncture site complications
  Sustained hypotension
  Carotid artery spasm
  Compromise of the ECA origin
  Carotid artery dissection
  Minor embolic neurological events
  Carotid perforation (very rare)
  Contrast encephalopathy (very rare)
Major complications
  Major embolic stroke
  Cerebral hemorrhage
  Acute stent thrombosis (very rare)

ECA, external carotid artery.

tion (6). This phenomenon is seen more commonly with self-expanding stents, which exert sustained radial pressure on the carotid baroreceptors, and is less commonly observed following treatment of restenotic lesions after CEA where the receptors may have been denervated by the surgical dissection. During our initial experience, we routinely placed a temporary pacemaker prior to the stenting procedure. We have since abandoned this practice. These hemodynamic instabilities are effectively avoided by pretreatment with 1 mg of intravenous atropine. Asystole that is seen during balloon inflation in a minority of patients is always transient and resolves immediately following balloon deflation and very rarely requires intravenous atropine (1 mg). Large doses of atropine are avoided in the elderly patients, as this can result in confusion and make accurate neurological assessment more difficult.

SUSTAINED HYPOTENSION

Similar to CEA, sustained hypotension occurs infrequently in the immediate period following CAS. In our large experience, persistent hypotension was observed following 11% of the carotid stenting procedures lasting 2 to 24 hours and was not associated with any adverse clinical events in the hospital or during the 30-day follow-up period (6). Two other small series have reported adverse events related to this phenomenon (7,8). Age, transient hypotension during the balloon dilatation, and the use of self-expanding stents were identified as independent predictors of sustained hypotension following CAS (6,8). The degree of hypotension appears to be more pronounced in patients with heavily calcified lesions.

    The mechanism of sustained hypotension following CAS may be explained on the basis of the carotid sinus reflex arc. The baroreceptor nerve terminals located at the outer muscle layer of the carotid sinus respond to stretch and deformation of the arterial wall by transmitting impulses that inhibit the vasoconstrictor regions in the medulla oblongata, resulting in vasodilatation and subsequent hypotension (9). Additionally, bradycardia resulting from stimulation of the vagal regions in the medulla oblongata further contributes to the occurrence of hypotension (9). The balloon dilatation and the radial force of the self-expanding stent result in increased radial pressure within the carotid sinus, leading to inappropriate activation of the baroreceptors and subsequent development of sustained hypotension.

Plaque disruption may also enhance the arterial pressure transmission to the carotid sinus baroreceptors. With time, the stent conforms to the arterial wall and the baroreceptors adapt to the sustained stimulation, gradually terminating the hypotensive response.

Careful hemodynamic monitoring of all patients during the procedure and in the early hours following the intervention is crucial for early recognition and management, hence preventing adverse outcomes. It is important that other potential sources of hypotension in this clinical setting, such as bleeding from the vascular access site, volume depletion, and cardiac pathologies, be considered and carefully excluded. Generally, monitoring in the intensive care unit is not necessary, and a modest fall in blood pressure does not require any specific intervention. However, in patients with additional intracranial stenosis, contralateral internal carotid artery (ICA) occlusion, or significant vertebrobasilar disease, hypotension should be treated aggressively. Similarly, when patients develop periprocedural cerebral ischemia secondary to an embolic event, hypotension should be corrected expeditiously. Generally, this phenomenon responds well to intravenous hydration and/or small dose of intravenous vasopressors. Early ambulation following the procedure, which can be facilitated by the application of a vascular closure device, helps counteract the carotid sinus hypotensive effect. Sustained hypotension is less frequently observed in these patients (5).

CONTRAST ENCEPHALOPATHY

Contrast encephalopathy is very rare and is a transient syndrome that occurred in only one patient in our entire experience. An identical case has been reported by another group (10). In our case, the event occurred after a complicated and a prolonged procedure where a large volume of contrast medium was used. The patients developed profound neurological deficit related to the involved hemisphere with marked contrast enhancement "staining" in the basal ganglion and the cortex, but no radiographic brain abnormalities were noted on computed tomography (CT). There are usually no angiographic vascular abnormalities on intracranial angiography. Because the contrast medium does not pass through the blood–brain barrier, it has been suggested that this phenomenon is caused by a combination of fine particulate embolization and excessive local contrast injection (11,12). "Leaky capillaries" due to hyperperfusion have also been suggested as the underlying pathology (11,12). Patients typically recover fully within 24 hours without permanent neurological damage. It is important to clinically differentiate this phenomenon from a massive cerebral infarction or hyperperfusion syndrome.

CAROTID ARTERY SPASM AND PSEUDOSPASM

Spasm of the distal ICA is an infrequent angiographic occurrence that usually resolves spontaneously after the guide wire is removed from the vessel (Figs. 12-1–12-5). Theoretically, flow-limiting spasm could be a potential hazard in the presence of contralateral ICA occlusion or incomplete circle of Willis. However, this complication is very rare. We have not encountered any adverse events related to carotid artery spasm in our experience. Meticulous and gentle technique as well as the use of soft-tipped guide wires has minimized the frequency of carotid artery spasm. Intravascular administration of 100 to 200 μg of nitroglycerin through the guiding sheath facilitates a rapid resolution of the spasm (Fig. 12-3). External carotid artery (ECA) spasm occurring after removal of the stiff guide wire during the guiding sheath placement is benign and should be ignored.

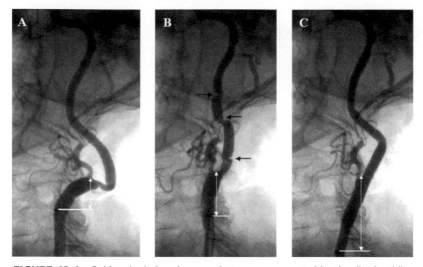

FIGURE 12-1. Guide wire-induced spasm that was exaggerated by the distal guiding sheath position. The vertical arrows display the distance between the guiding sheath tip and the carotid artery bifurcation. **A**: Preprocedural angiogram with moderate angulation of the proximal internal carotid artery (ICA). **B**: The ICA is straightened by the guide wire with multiple areas of spasms (*black arrows*). **C**: Resolution of the spasm after the guide wire was removed and the guiding sheath was withdrawn to a more proximal position.

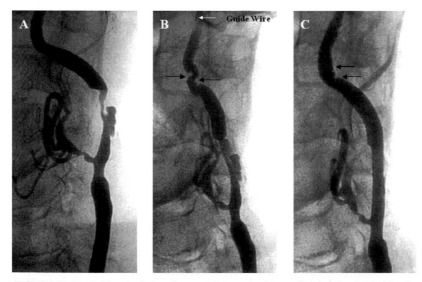

FIGURE 12-2. Guide wire-induced spasm that resolved immediately following guide wire removal. **A**: Preprocedural angiogram showing a long ulcerated lesion of the proximal internal carotid artery (ICA). **B**: Spasm (*black arrows*) of the distal ICA that occurred following guide wire (*white arrow*) placement. **C**: The spasm resolved following expeditious completion of the procedure and removal of the guide wire.

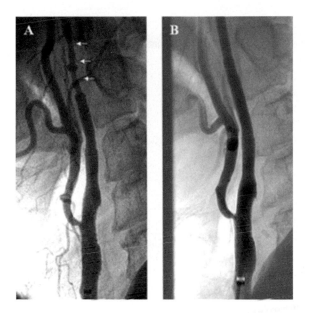

FIGURE 12-3. Intravascular filter-induced internal carotid artery (ICA) spasm. **A**: Spasm of the distal ICA (*arrows*) at the site of an Anti-Embolization filter. The spasm persisted despite filter removal, but resolved after intravascular nitroglycerin administration (**B**).

It is very important to distinguish spasm from carotid artery "kinks." In many patients, normal carotid anatomy includes redundant tortuous segments and even complete loops that can be seen in the distal common carotid artery (CCA) near the bifurcation or in the distal ICA below the siphon (Figs. 12-1, 12-4, 12-5). The distal ICA is very prone to spasm during interventional manipulation. The placement of stiff guide wire and the cephalad pressure placed on the CCA by the guiding sheath accentuates these loops and kinks, shifting

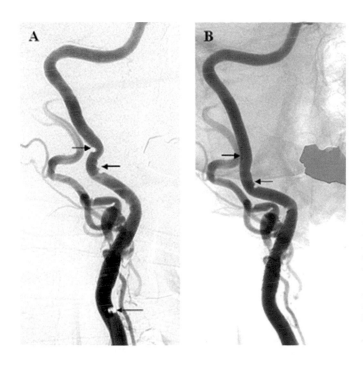

FIGURE 12-4. Sheath effect (pseudospasm). **A**: Pseudospasm (*top arrows*) of the distal internal carotid artery (ICA) that resulted from cephalad displacement of the ICA tortuosities by the distal position of the guiding sheath (*bottom arrow*) within the distal common carotid artery (CCA). **B**: The pseudospasm resolved following proximal withdrawal of the guiding sheath.

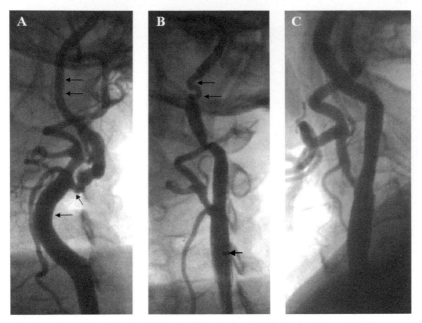

FIGURE 12-5. Combination of sheath effect and guide wire-induced spasm. **A**: Preprocedural angiogram displaying tortuosities of the common carotid artery (CCA) and internal carotid artery (ICA) as well as moderate angulation of the ICA origin (*arrows*). **B**: Spasm/pseudospasm is apparent within the distal cervical ICA (*thin arrows*) accentuated by the guide wire, a stiff stent, and the distal position of the guiding sheath, which is visible within the stent (*thick arrow*). **C**: Complete resolution of the spasm after guide wire removal and proximal repositioning of the guiding sheath, which is no longer visible.

them more cephalad. These kinks should be recognized but ignored, as they will resolve completely when the wire and sheath are removed. The operator *must not* be tempted to dilate or stent these kinks. It must be emphasized that severe kinks and tortuosities are contraindications to CAS.

A special situation arises when a tortuous ICA loop is located just distal to the carotid bifurcation. A "bend point" at this site could be the source of distal dissection after stent deployment or stent postdilatation. In these cases, the stent may unavoidably straighten the tortuous segment that is close to a lesion and create a new kink further distal (Figs. 12-1, 12-4, 12-5). This is particularly apparent when using a stiff stent that does not conform to the arterial tortuousities (Fig. 12-5). Occasionally, a kink may appear to produce a significant narrowing, and unless there is a reduced blood flow (which has not been observed by the authors), these angiographic findings should be ignored. Follow-up angiographic studies in our patients have confirmed that these anomalies are benign and are not associated with adverse outcomes (Fig. 12-6). Distal ICA kinks will often resolve when the guiding sheath is retracted to the proximal CCA. Special techniques to avoid dissections during stenting of these vessels are discussed below.

CAROTID DISSECTIONS

Carotid artery dissection is a rare but important complication of the CAS procedure. A number of factors predispose to the development of this complication including: (a) severe

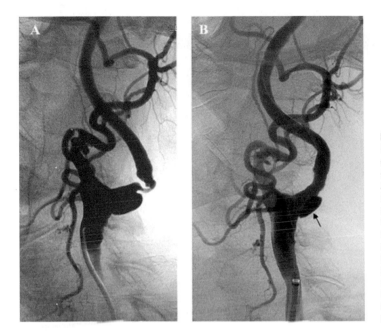

FIGURE 12-6. Stenting of a high-grade lesion that is located within a severe internal carotid artery (ICA) bend. **A**: Preprocedural angiogram. **B**: Final angiography. Equipment is carefully passed through the lesion over an extra-support guide wire, and a soft stent that conforms to the arterial bend is used. Aggressive postdilatation is generally avoided, and the residual cap observed outside the stent (*arrow*) is abandoned to avoid distal embolization.

"bends" or "kinks" of the ICA, (b) aggressive hardware (guide wires, balloon catheters, stents) manipulation within the ICA, (c) postdilatation of the distal stent edge within the ICA, and, less commonly, (d) aggressive manipulation of the guiding sheath tip, which is usually located in the CCA. Stenting of lesions that are adjacent to severe distal kinks or bends (Figs. 12-6, 12-7) can pose a technical challenge and predispose to the development of vascular dissections. In these cases, the dissections can occur by forcing a stiff peripheral balloon or a stiff-ended stent delivery system through the bend during an attempt to position the device within the lesion. The risk of dissection in these cases is increased by attempting to deliver these devices over a "soft" guide wire with poor support.

Generally, these dissections can be avoided by careful technique that considers the following technical maneuvers: (a) the lesion is crossed with a soft 0.014-inch coronary guide wire, and the tip is then advanced close to the siphon, (b) this wire is then exchanged over a coronary balloon (0.018-inch—compatible COBRA, SciMed Inc., Maple Grove, MN) to an extra-support 0.018-inch guide wire (Roadrunner, Cook Inc., Bloomington, IN), and (c) the stenosis is then dilated, and the stent is advanced to cover the lesion. It should be noted that most of the current stent systems are deliverable over a 0.014-inch guide wire, which obviates the need for this maneuver.

Spasms, pseudospasms, and distally displaced kinks should be recognized, and stenting of these side effects must be avoided (Figs. 12-1, 12-4, 12-5). An attempt to straighten the bend with the stent is strongly discouraged, as this will only displace the kinks more distally. Our practice is to use self-expanding stents that are at least 1 to 2 mm larger than the reference vessel diameter, and we avoid dilating the distal end of the stent. If stent edges need expansion, then dilatation is done carefully at low pressures to avoid edge dissection.

With the advent of Anti-Embolization devices, dissections have also occurred at the site of the protection device. These dissections are rare, in the majority are non-flow limiting, and do not require any intervention (Fig. 12-7). The risk of these dissections can be minimized by the careful application and sizing of the Anti-Embolization device. The final post-stenting angiography should include an angiographic assessment of the device placement site.

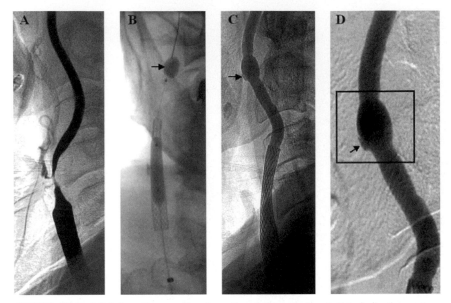

FIGURE 12-7. Mild dissection resulting from the distal occlusion Anti-Embolization system. **A**: Preprocedural angiogram displaying a high-grade stenosis of the proximal internal carotid artery (ICA). **B**: Stent postdilatation while the distal occlusion balloon is inflated (*arrow*). **C**: Final angiography showing an aneurysmal dilatation with a mild non–flow-limiting dissection of the distal ICA at the prior occlusion balloon site. **D**: A closer display of the aneurysmal dilatation and the dissection. No specific treatment was required. The patient remained asymptomatic with no neurological events.

Generally, dissections are treated by additional stenting prior to removal of the guiding sheath (Fig. 12-8). It is important to maintain the guide wire position until the final angiographic assessment is completed and the presence or absence of dissections is ascertained. Flexible self-expanding stents that conform to the arterial shape are preferred, particularly in the treatment of dissections that occur in the proximity to severe bends/kinks.

HYPERPERFUSION SYNDROME

Cerebral hyperperfusion syndrome was first described following carotid endarterectomy (CEA) with an incidence of 0.3% to 2.7% (13–15). Symptoms that include ipsilateral headaches, nausea, vomiting, focal seizures, and a variable degree of altered mental status are usually associated with markedly elevated blood pressure, and frequently precede the development of fatal intracranial hemorrhage. The syndrome typically occurs in patients with severe carotid stenosis and poor collateral circulation, particularly in those with complete occlusion of the contralateral ICA or patients with underdeveloped circle of Willis. The mechanism is related to long-standing hypoperfusion that results in impaired autoregulation of the microcirculation (13). In the presence of severe ipsilateral obstruction, cerebral blood flow is maintained at a normal level through marked arteriolar vasodilation. Following revascularization, the increased perfusion pressure overwhelms the ability of the dilated arterioles to constrict, resulting in the development of the clinical syndrome. Only a small number of the patients who develop this pathophysiology become symptomatic. In these patients, disruption of the endothelial cells may lead to bleeding into the surrounding brain tissue.

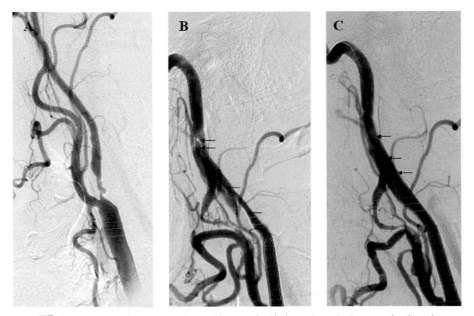

FIGURE 12-8. Severe distal internal carotid artery (ICA) dissection. **A**: Preprocedural angiogram showing a high-grade stenosis of the proximal ICA. **B**: Following ICA stenting with the distal occlusion Anti-Embolization device, a partially flow-limiting dissection *(arrows)* was notable on control angiography. **C**: The dissection was successfully stented and normal flow was restored *(arrows)*.

A syndrome identical to that observed following CEA has been described in patients undergoing CAS. In the authors' experience, this occurred in approximately 0.2% of the cases. The clinical presentation and outcomes are identical to those observed with the hyperperfusion syndrome following CEA (16–18). Several factors may contribute to its development during CAS. These include severe carotid artery stenosis with contralateral ICA occlusion, recanalization of a completely occluded carotid artery, and the concomitant bilateral carotid stenting during the same setting. Contrary to the surgical hyperperfusion syndrome where symptoms usually develop within few days following CEA, the endovascular hyperperfusion develops during the stenting procedure or during the immediate postprocedural period (16–18). This is likely related to the heparin administration and the use of antiplatelet agents, particularly intravenous glycoprotein (GP) IIB/IIIA antagonists. Based on the lack of evidence for a beneficial effect of the GP IIB/IIIA antagonists during CAS, we do not routinely administer these agents during carotid intervention. We have also abandoned the approach of concomitantly stenting both carotid arteries in patients with severe bilateral stenoses.

Current management of the hyperperfusion syndrome consists of identification of predisposed patients, careful monitoring, and meticulous control of the blood pressure, which appears to be the most important factor contributing to the adverse outcome (13). Therefore, it is important to control the blood pressure levels during the periprocedural period utilizing intravenous antihypertensive agents if necessary. Based on our anecdotal experience with the distal balloon protection, we recommend the expeditious utilization of intravenous Nipride infusion to reduce the blood pressure if still elevated after the final interventional stage and before the deflation of the protection balloon. Theoretically, the protection balloon may serve as a protective cushion that, if tolerated, may allow time for blood pressure control prior to exposing the microcirculation to the increased intracranial pressure following revascularization.

EXTERNAL CAROTID ARTERY COMPROMISE

The ECA is frequently involved by the atherosclerotic disease of the carotid artery bifurcation, and its origin can be compromised following stent placement and dilatation in the ICA (Figs. 12-7, 12-9). During CEA, the surgeons attempt to maintain patency of this vessel; however, many follow-up clinical and angiographic studies have shown that the ECA is frequently occluded and is well tolerated. Acute occlusion of the ECA is usually well tolerated owing to the well-developed collateral circulation for the ICA as well as the contralateral ECA. In the absence of a good collateral circulation, some patients may experience jaw muscle angina, but this usually resolves spontaneously over time. However, the ECA may in some patients provide an important path for collateral circulation to the brain via the ophthalmic artery and other collaterals. In these situations, its patency should be maintained, but not at the expense of excessive manipulation and increased risk for embolic complications or ICA compromise. The procedure for maintaining ECA patency is described in detail in the technical section. In general, it is not necessary to achieve a wide opening, but just to establish thrombolysis in myocardial infarction (TIMI)-III flow. In our experience, follow-up angiographic studies after CAS have frequently shown that even moderately compromised ECA origin at the end of the CAS procedure may spontaneously improve.

CAROTID ARTERY PERFORATION

Carotid artery perforation during CAS is an extremely rare event. In the authors' experience with over 1,500 stented carotid arteries, only one single case was observed. This perforation

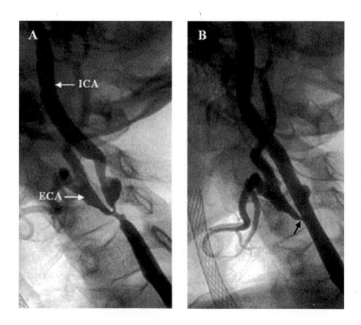

FIGURE 12-9. Compromise of the external carotid artery (ECA) origin following internal carotid artery (ICA) stenting. **A**: High-grade lesion that involves the carotid artery bifurcation. **B**: Angiography following stenting showing significant compromise of the origin of the ECA. Patient remained asymptomatic and without neurological events on follow-up.

occurred following aggressive balloon dilatation of the distal end of the stent using a 7-mm diameter balloon in a "misguided attempt" to optimize the luminal appearance of the stented segment and completely obliterate the residual stenosis. We now appreciate that residual luminal irregularities, or pockets of contrast in a residual ulceration external to the stent, are of no prognostic significance in terms of immediate or late results (Fig. 12-7). Our current approach is to conservatively size all balloons (most commonly 5.0 mm, and less commonly 5.5 mm) and expect that vessel perforation can be completely avoided.

ACUTE STENT THROMBOSIS

Acute stent thrombosis is a remarkably rare event after CAS. The low rate of stent thrombosis and the periprocedural embolic events are predicated upon correct and compulsive use of appropriate doses of adjunctive antiplatelet therapy (1,2). Basic and meticulous stenting techniques must be adhered to. These include: (a) stenting only in the presence of brisk flow without significant inflow or outflow obstruction; (b) stenting from an angiographically "smooth" proximal segment to an angiographically smooth distal segment; and (c) proper stent sizing and careful stent opposition to the arterial wall. The high-flow and low-resistance carotid circulation is the interventionist's friend, but good basic stenting techniques are essential to the complication-free results. Late in-stent thrombosis has been observed in two patients who were treated for radiation-induced obstructive carotid artery disease (Fig 12-10). It is now our practice to treat these patients with antiplatelet agents (clopidogrel) indefinitely.

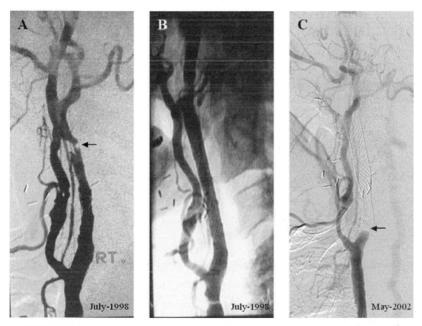

FIGURE 12-10. Late stent thrombosis in a patient that had a stent placed for radiation-induced obstructive disease of the distal internal carotid artery (ICA) that was inaccessible for conventional carotid endarterectomy (CEA). **A**: Presenting carotid angiogram displaying severe stenosis of the distal ICA (*arrow*). **B**: Poststenting angiogram. **C**: Follow-up angiogram approximately 4 years later showing complete occlusion of the stent (*arrow*). The patient was asymptomatic.

INTRACRANIAL HEMORRHAGE

Cerebral hemorrhage is a devastating and usually fatal complication (16–18). Fortunately, it is very rare and occurred in approximately 0.2% in our CAS experience in the setting of hyperperfusion syndrome. In these instances, cerebral hemorrhage was associated with a combination of excessive anticoagulation, poorly controlled hypertension, aggressive attempts at intracranial neurovascular rescue, presence of a vulnerable berry aneurysm, or CAS in the presence of a recent ischemic stroke (less than 3 weeks in duration). Therefore, anticoagulation should carefully be monitored with use of ACT measurements. Our practice is to use one single bolus of heparin at the beginning of the procedure (5000 units). Hypertension is treated with intravenous nitroglycerin or Nipride when necessary. During neurovascular rescue, extreme care is exercised in guide wire manipulation and the use of thrombolytics, particularly when the ACT levels are elevated and/or anti-GP IIB/IIIA agents are used.

If a cerebral hemorrhage is suspected, the procedure should be terminated. Anticoagulation should be reversed with protamine and an emergency CT scan performed. Operators should be familiar with the angiographic features of an intracranial "mass effect," which indicates cerebral hemorrhage (Fig. 12-11). Sudden loss of consciousness preceded by severe

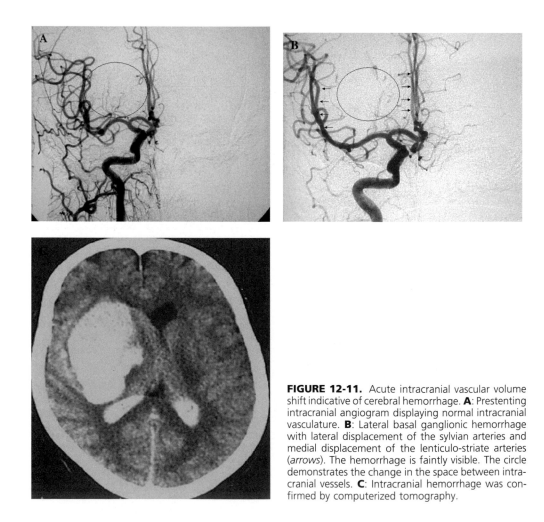

FIGURE 12-11. Acute intracranial vascular volume shift indicative of cerebral hemorrhage. **A**: Prestenting intracranial angiogram displaying normal intracranial vasculature. **B**: Lateral basal ganglionic hemorrhage with lateral displacement of the sylvian arteries and medial displacement of the lenticulo-striate arteries (*arrows*). The hemorrhage is faintly visible. The circle demonstrates the change in the space between intracranial vessels. **C**: Intracranial hemorrhage was confirmed by computerized tomography.

headaches in the absence of intracranial vessel occlusion should alert the operator to this devastating event. Fortunately, with careful and appropriate patient selection and strict attention to the above technical and anticoagulation issues, the risk of cerebral hemorrhage is very low.

DISTAL EMBOLIZATION

Symptomatic distal embolization is an important complication of carotid artery stenting (1,2). It is caused by the release of thrombotic, necrotic, or atherosclerotic material from the lesion during the intervention (19). Risk factor recognition, careful patient selection, and meticulous techniques can minimize this complication (Table 12-2). The availability of Anti-Embolization devices has shown promise to reduce this complication to a very rare event.

It is essential to monitor the patient's neurological status after every step of the procedure. Transient neurological changes should always prompt the operator to optimize the blood pressure and clarify the status of the intracranial vasculature. This is best done after expeditious completion of the procedure. If the change in neurological status is associated with slow flow from lesion recoil, guide wire spasm, or dissection, it is important to rapidly place the stent and remove the guide wire in order for the spasm to quickly resolve. Clearly, optimal treatment requires the operator to be proficient with the technique so this can be accomplished expeditiously. If a significant change in the neurological status does not resolve immediately, general patient care should be instituted with emphasis on maintaining normal blood pressure and intravenous volume expansion, stabilizing the patient's heart rate, and maintaining a viable airway with oxygen administration. The stenting procedure should be efficiently completed. If the patient becomes uncooperative, agitated, and especially if the airway is compromised, the assistance of an anesthesiologist should be utilized.

Intracranial angiography is performed in anteroposterior and lateral projections. If possible, angiography of the contralateral carotid artery and at least one vertebral artery should be performed to determine the status of anterior and posterior communicating arteries and leptomeningeal anastomoses. The angiograms are carefully examined to determine the site and extent of intracranial vessel embolism (Figs. 12-12, 12-13). Because of anatomical arrangements and flow pattern, the most likely sites of intracranial embolism are the distal ICA, and the middle cerebral artery with its branches. Large vessel occlusion is usually obvious (especially in lateral projection), but embolism in the smaller branches requires

TABLE 12-2. RISK FACTORS FOR EMBOLIZATION DURING CAS

Poor pretreatment with antiplatlet agents

Aggressive guide wire manipulation

Aggressive balloon dilatation prior to or after stent deployment

Forceful introduction of a high-profile stent across a heavily calcified tight lesion

Aggressive attempts to access a highly atherosclerotic, tortuous common carotid artery

CAS, carotid artery stenting.

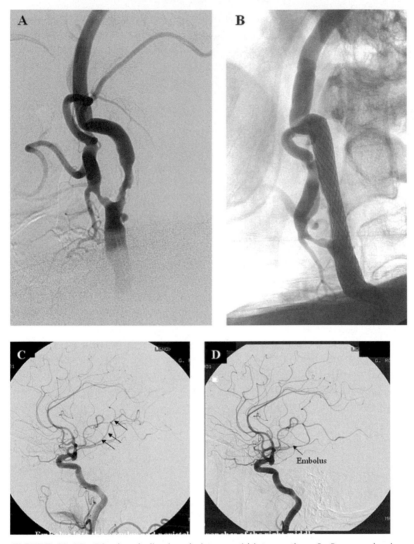

FIGURE 12-12. Distal embolization during carotid intervention. **A**: Preprocedural angiography with a high-grade internal carotid artery (ICA) stenosis. **B**: Final angiography after stenting. **C**: Lateral intracranial angiography prior to stenting of the ipsilateral ICA. The arrows point to the parietal branch of the parietal artery. **D**: The arrow points to the spot where the parietal artery is occluded by small embolus with no opacification of the distal segment of the vessel and an ensuing avascular zone. The proximal segment of the blocked parietal artery is still visible.

careful scrutiny (Figs. 12-12, 12-13). Acute occlusion of small branch vessels may be noted only in comparison to the preprocedural angiography (Figs. 12-12, 12-13). The availability of a good preprocedural intracranial angiogram is therefore essential in all patients undergoing carotid stenting. Appropriate steps are taken to recanalize the occluded vessel as soon as possible; "time is brain." If there is a neurological deficit and small branch occlusion, the "three Hs" (hydrate, heparinize, and higher blood pressure) are to be applied. It is important to remember that changes of neurological status can also ensue from intracerebral hemorrhage or hyperperfusion syndrome. If there are signs of localized expanding phenomenon on

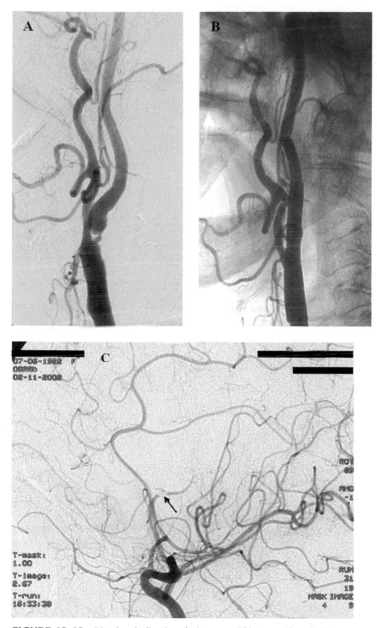

FIGURE 12-13. Distal embolization during carotid intervention: **A**: Preprocedural angiography with a high-grade internal carotid artery (ICA) stenosis. **B**: Final angiography after stenting. **C**: A visible embolus in the frontal branch of the ascending frontoparietal artery with an ensuing "avascular zone" and disruption of the frontal segment of the sylvian triangle.

angiography indicating intracerebral hemorrhage, heparin should be reversed and a brain CT scan performed (Fig. 12-11).

REFERENCES

1. Yadav JS, Roubin GS, Iyer S, et al. Elective stenting of the extracranial carotid arteries. *Circulation* 1997;95:376–381.
2. Roubin GS, New G, Iyer SS, et al. Immediate and late clinical outcomes of carotid artery stenting in symptomatic and asymptomatic carotid stenosis: a 5-year prospective analysis. *Circulation* 2001:103: 532–537.
3. Morey SS. AHA updates guidelines for carotid endarterectomy. *Am Fam Physician* 1998;58:1898, 1903–1904.
4. Wholey MH, Al-Mubarak N, Wholey MH. Updated review of the global carotid artery stent registry. *Catheter Cardiovasc Interv* 2003;60:259–266.
5. Al-Mubarak N, Roubin GS, Vitek JJ, et al. Procedural safety and short-term efficacy of ambulatory carotid stenting. *Stroke* 2001;32:2305–2309.
6. Al-Mubarak N, Liu MW, Dean LS, et al. Incidence and outcomes of prolonged hypotension following carotid artery stenting. *J Am Coll Cardiol* 1999;33:65A.
7. Dangas G, Laird JR Jr, Satler LF. Postprocedural hypotension after carotid artery stent placement: predictors and short- and long-term clinical outcomes. *Radiology* 2000;215:677–683.
8. Mendelsohn FO, Weissman NJ, Lederman RJ. et al. Acute hemodynamic changes during carotid artery stenting. *Am J Cardiol* 1998;82:1077–1081.
9. Berne RM, Levy MN. The peripheral circulation and its control. In: Berne RM, Levy MN, eds. *Cardiovascular physiology*, 6th ed. New York: Mosby, 1992:184–188.
10. Dangas G, Monsein LH, Laureno R, et al. Transient contrast encephalopathy after carotid artery stenting. *J Endovasc Ther.* 2001;8:111–113.
11. Torvik A, Walday P. Neurotoxicity of water-soluble contrast media. *Acta Radiol* 1995;399(Suppl): 221–229.
12. Caille JM, Allard M. Neurotoxicity of hydrosoluble iodine contrast media. *Invest Radiol* 1988;23(Suppl 1):5210–5212.
13. Naylor AR, Ruckley CV. The post-carotid endarterectomy hyperperfusion syndrome. *Eur J Endovasc Surg* 1995;9:365–367.
14. Sundt TM, Sharbrough FW, Piepgras DG, et al. Correlation of cerebral blood flow and electroencephalographic changes during carotid endarterectomy. *Mayo Clin Proc* 1981;56:533–543.
15. Breen JC, Caplan L, DeWitt LD, et al. Brain edema after carotid surgery. *Neurology* 1996;46:175–181.
16. McCabe DJH, Brown MM, Clifton A. Fatal cerebral reperfusion hemorrhage after carotid stenting. *Stroke* 1999;30:2483–2486.
17. Chamorro A, Vila N, Obach V, et al. A case of cerebral hemorrhage early after carotid stenting. *Stroke* 2000;31:792–793.
18. Al-Mubarak N, Roubin GS, Vitek JJ, et al. Subarachnoidal hemorrhage following carotid stenting with the distal-balloon protection system. *Catheter Cardiovasc Interv* 2001;54:521–523.
19. Ohki T, Marin ML, Lyon RT, et al. Ex vivo human carotid artery bifurcation stenting: correlation of lesion characteristics with embolic potential. *J Vasc Surg* 1998;27:463–471.

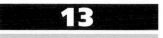

THE RISK OF EMBOLIZATION DURING CAROTID STENTING AND THE CONCEPT OF ANTI-EMBOLIZATION

TAKAO OHKI

Although good results regarding carotid artery stenting (CAS) have been reported by a number of investigators, concerns about its safety and efficacy have been raised, and its general role and comparative value to carotid endarterectomy (CEA) remains unclear (1–3). Among several issues related to CAS, the major concern has been the potential for CAS to produce embolic particles that may manifest as a neurological deficit. This chapter reviews the potential for CAS to produce emboli and presents a rationale for the use of Anti-Embolization devices during CAS.

EXPERIMENTAL AND CLINICAL EVIDENCE FOR EMBOLIZATION DURING CAROTID ARTERY STENTING

The main cause of perioperative neurological deficits following CAS is thought to be embolic particles released from the carotid plaque during the balloon dilatation and stent deployment (4). This hypothesis was further confirmed by our study, which analyzed the incidence of embolic events following CAS performed in an *ex vivo* model utilizing human carotid plaques. The plaques were collected from patients undergoing standard CEA procedures (5). This study demonstrated that embolic particles were consistently produced from all the plaques that were stented (Fig. 13-1).

These experimental observations have been further confirmed by clinical studies. The Carotid and Vertebral Artery Transluminal Angioplasty Study (CAVATAS) is a randomized prospective trial comparing the safety and efficacy of CEA with carotid angioplasty with and without stenting. A substudy of this trial that focused on the transcranial Doppler results showed that on average, balloon angioplasty produced four times more embolic signals, which represents embolic particles (including air) compared to CEA (202 ± 119 vs. 52 ± 64) (6). However, this difference was not translated into an overall difference in the stroke or death rates between the two arms (7). Another prospective randomized trial (the Leicester trial) also confirmed the fact that CAS generates significantly more embolic particles than CEA (8). This trial was aborted after enrolling only 17 patients because of the unacceptably high stroke/death rate following CAS (71%) compared to CEA (0%). Jordan et al. (9) have also confirmed these findings with regard to embolic events during the two treatment options.

More recently, Jaeger et al. (10) have reported on the incidence of silent embolic infarct

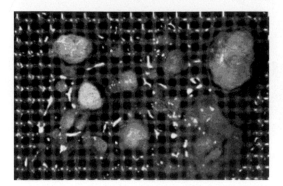

FIGURE 13-1. Macroscopic view of embolic particles generated following angioplasty and stenting. These particles consisted of atherosclerotic debris and calcified material. Filter size: 130 μm, original magnification ×40. (Reprinted from Ohki T, Marin ML, Lyon RT, et al. Human ex-vivo carotid artery bifurcation stenting: correlation of lesion characteristics with embolic potential. *J Vasc Surg* 1998;27:463–471, with permission.) (See also the color section following page 164 of this text.)

as detected by diffusion-weighted magnetic resonance imaging (DW-MRI) of the brain following CAS (10). DW-MRI of the brain was performed in 67 patients with 70 high-grade stenoses of the carotid artery before and 24 hours after stent implantation. During one procedure, symptomatic cerebral embolization occurred. DW-MRI showed new ipsilateral ischemic lesions after stent implantation in 20 patients (29%), including the symptomatic patient (Fig. 13-2). This study showed more convincing evidence for the occurrence of embolization during CAS.

These clinical and experimental observations led to the development of a number of Anti-Embolization devices that can capture these particles (11,12). Preliminary studies utilizing Anti-Embolization devices have confirmed the fact that significant amount of emboli are in fact released during CAS. Whitlow et al. (13) reported their initial results utilizing the distal occlusion balloon system (GuardWire Temporary Occlusion & Aspiration System, Medtronic AVA, Denvers, MA; formerly PercuSurge) to prevent embolization in 75 CAS procedures (13). Not surprisingly, visible particles consisting of fibrous plaque debris, lipid

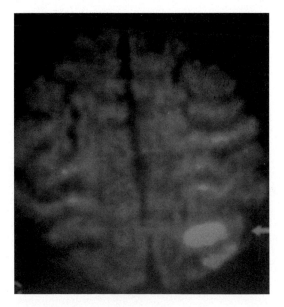

FIGURE 13-2. Postprocedural axial diffusion-weighted magnetic resonance imaging (DW-MRI) shows eight new ipsilateral lesions (15 to 20 mm) in the cortical territory of the middle cerebral artery (MCA) (*arrow*). (Reprinted from Jaeger HJ, Mathias KD, Hauth E, et al. Cerebral ischemia detected with diffusion-weighted MR imaging after stent implantation in the carotid artery *AJNR Am J Neuroradiol* 2002;23:200–207, with permission.)

or cholesterol vacuoles, and calcific plaque fragments were recovered from each case. The number of particles analyzed per patient ranged from 22 to 667, and the mean maximum diameter was 203 ± 256 μm (range 3.6 to 5262 μm).

CLINICAL SIGNIFICANCE OF EMBOLI

Despite the fact that there is growing evidence regarding the occurrence of embolization during CAS, the significance of such embolic particles and the need for cerebral protection device have been subjects of controversy. Although many believed that any embolization could not be good for the brain, some thought that unless the significance of emboli translated into clinical events such as stroke, its significance could not be determined and the need for Anti-Embolization devices remained questionable.

Although there is no level-1 evidence that supports the clinical effectiveness of Anti-Embolization devices, there is growing evidence that microembolization more often results in clinical sequelae (but not necessarily a stroke). For example, Fearn et al. (14) investigated the occurrence of cerebral embolization during cardiopulmonary bypass procedure with transcranial Doppler and evaluated its significance with careful neuropsychological tests (14). Cerebrovascular reactivity was measured in 70 patients before coronary operations in which nonpulsatile bypass was used. Throughout the operations, middle cerebral artery flow velocity and embolization were recorded by transcranial Doppler. Cognitive function was measured by a computerized battery of tests before the operation and 1 week, 2 months, and 6 months after surgery. More than 200 emboli were detected in 40 patients, mainly on aortic clamping and release, when bypass was initiated, and during defibrillation. Cognitive function deteriorated more in patients having cardiopulmonary bypass than in control patients having urological operations. The authors concluded that emboli were significantly associated with memory loss. Furthermore, Gaunt et al. (15) investigated the clinical significance of microembolization detected by transcranial Doppler ultrasonography by determining the quantity and character of emboli and correlating these with neurological and psychometric outcome, funduscopy, automated visual field testing, and computed tomographic brain scans in 100 consecutive patients undergoing CEA. Not surprisingly, embolization was detected in 92% of successfully monitored operations. More than 10 particulate emboli during initial carotid dissection correlated with a significant deterioration in postoperative cognitive function. Overall, 37% of patients undergoing CEA experienced deterioration in cognitive function. Although these studies were carried out in non–carotid-stenting procedures, it clearly shows that although embolization may not always result in a stroke, it has a significant negative effect on the brain.

Although the clinical benefit of recovering emboli from the brain has not been proven, the result of the Saphenous Vein Graft Angioplasty Free of Emboli Randomized (SAFER) trial is relevant (16). This trial randomized 550 patients with degenerated saphenous vein graft following coronary artery bypass grafting to either GuardWire-protected percutaneous transluminal coronary angioplasty (PTCA) or unprotected PTCA. The 30-day myocardial rate was 16.5% for the control arm, whereas it was reduced to 8.4% in the protected arm ($p < 0.001$). Based on this trial, the GuardWire received Food and Drug Administration (FDA) approval and is currently considered the standard of care for select patients undergoing PTCA for degenerated coronary saphenous vein grafts. If preventing emboli from reaching

TABLE 13-1. CAROTID STENTING WITH AND WITHOUT ANTI-EMBOLIZATION PROTECTION

	Total No. of Cases	S/D Rate Without Protection	S/D Rate With Protection
Henry et al. (17)	315	4.9%	2.2%
Roubin (18)	1276	6.9%	1.8%
Wholey et al. (19)	10693	5.3%	2.3%
Mathias (20)	406	3.0%	1.3%
German registry (21)	1353	2.5%	1.8%

S/D, stroke and death.

the heart is beneficial, one can speculate that it is also beneficial for the brain. Table 13-1 summarizes the stroke/death rate following carotid stenting with and without the use of Anti-Embolization devices (17–21). Although none of these studies was randomized, and although each study utilized historical control (unprotected CAS), it nonetheless shows the feasibility and safety of Anti-Embolization protection and, furthermore, provides some evidence that cerebral protection may be efficacious.

STRENGTH AND WEAKNESS OF VARIOUS APPROACHES

There are three different approaches to Anti-Embolization protection (Table 13-2) (12). The first approach is the use of a distal occlusion balloon to temporally occlude the outflow from the distal internal carotid artery (ICA). The second method is the use of a filtration device placed distal to the lesion. The third approach is to occlude the inflow to the brain by using a proximal occlusion balloon in the common carotid artery (CCA). Details of each approach are discussed in the chapters to follow.

Each approach is unique and possesses inherent advantages as well as disadvantages. The advantages of the distal occlusion balloon (GuardWire) include: (a) lower crossing

TABLE 13-2. VARIOUS APPROACHES TO AND DEVICES FOR CEREBRAL PROTECTION (12)

1) Distal occlusion
   Theron balloon
   Guardwire (GuardWire, Medtronic AVA, Denvers, MA)
2) Distal filter
   NeuroShield (MedNova, Inc., Galway, Ireland)
   Filterwire (Embolic Protection Inc, San Carlos, CA)
   Angioguard (Cordis, Warren, NJ)
   AccuNet (Guidant, Indianapolis, IN)
   Carotid Trap (Microvena, White Bear Lake, MN)
   E-Trap (Metamorphic Surgical Devices, Pittsburgh, PA)
   Bate floating filter (ArteriA, San Francisco, CA)
   Captura (Boston Scientific Corp., Natick, MA)
   SCION filter (SCION, Miami, FL)
3) Proximal occlusion
   Parodi Anti-Embolization Catheter (ArteriA, San Francisco, CA)
   Moma (Inventech, Italy)

profile and flexibility (compared to filtration devices), and (b) complete protection of the distal ICA. The disadvantages include: (a) interruption of flow during the protection (although tolerated by most patients), (b) somewhat cumbersome procedure (need to aspirate the particles, and also the need to keep the wire extremely stable during catheter exchange), (c) inability to perform angiogram during balloon protection, (d) difficulties in crossing tight and/or tortuous lesions, (e) potential for particles to embolize to the brain via the patent external carotid artery (ECA), and (f) potential to cause spasm and dissection in the distal ICA.

The strengths of the distal filters in general include: (a) preservation of flow, (b) ability to perform angiogram during the procedure, and (c) intuitiveness. The weaknesses are: (a) possibility of missing small particles, (b) larger crossing profile (in general), (c) difficulties in crossing tight and/or tortuous lesions, (d) somewhat cumbersome procedure (need to keep the wire extremely stable during catheter exchange), (e) potential to cause spasm and dissection in the distal ICA, and (f) potential for the filter to thrombose.

The advantages of the proximal occlusion system [Parodi Anti-Embolization catheter (PAEC); ArteriA, San Francisco, CA] are (a) ability to obtain complete protection prior to manipulating the lesion, (b) capture particles of all sizes, (c) ability to treat tight and/or tortuous lesions because one does not have to pass a relatively bulky and stiff system through the artery, and (d) ability to use guide wire of choice. The disadvantages include: (a) interruption of flow during protection, (b) potential to cause dissection or spasm in the ECA or CCA, and (c) requiring larger puncture site hole in the groin.

CYCLOSPORINE AND CEREBRAL PROTECTION DEVICES

There are several lesion characteristics that predict a successful outcome following endovascular interventions. These factors include: (a) focal rather than diffuse lesions, (b) stenotic lesions rather than complete occlusions, (c) large diameter vessels rather than smaller vessels, and (d) good runoff rather than poor runoff (22). Almost all carotid lesions completely fulfill all of these favorable factors. Therefore, with the exception of the risks associated with embolization, carotid artery stenoses may be ideal lesions for endovascular therapy. In fact, encouraging midterm patency and stroke prevention rates have been reported (7,23).

Liver transplantation also underwent a long period of scrutiny owing to the dismal early results, despite the fact that sophisticated surgical techniques were already developed in these early days. Cyclosporine was introduced as an adjunct in 1979, and it single-handedly made liver transplantation the best therapy for certain end-stage liver diseases (24). Until then, liver transplantation was considered an experimental procedure, much like carotid bifurcation angioplasty and stenting (CBAS) is today.

Anti-Embolization devices may play a similar or even greater role in CBAS. It is the final element that is needed in the maturation and the popularization of this new endovascular treatment. CEA is the most commonly performed major vascular operation in the United States, where 150,000 cases are performed annually. Three hundred thousand operations are performed worldwide. Moreover, it is estimated that 2 million U.S. citizens fulfill the Asymptomatic Carotid Atherosclerosis Study (ACAS) inclusion criteria, yet many are not treated. This signature operation for vascular surgeons may indeed be replaced with CBAS, and some form of Anti-Embolization device may play a key role in the transition of how patients with carotid stenosis are treated. However, many believe that such a transition must be based on randomized, prospective comparative trials, and such trials have been proposed and initiated [Carotid Revascularization Endarterectomy Versus Stenting Trial (CREST), stenting and angioplasty with protection in patients at high risk for endarterectomy study (SAPPHIRE)] (25,26).

For those who are currently not performing CBAS, it may be ethical and reasonable to wait until these promising devices become available. For those who are performing CBAS, it would seem reasonable to aggressively move to some form of brain protection.

SUMMARY

Based on these experimental and clinical observations, it is clear that CAS carries a significant risk for embolic events. Although we do not know with certainty the clinical significance of these embolic particles, there is growing evidence that suggests that emboli cause neurological damage. The early results of ongoing clinical trials evaluating the safety and efficacy of CAS in conjunction with protection devices are very promising, and the use of protection devices during CAS is considered mandatory by many experts in this field.

REFERENCES

1. Callahan TJ, Spyker D, Sapirstein W. Concern about safety of carotid angioplasty. *Stroke* 1996:27: 2144–2145.
2. Bettmann MA, Katzen BT, Whisnant J, et al. Carotid stenting and angioplasty: a statement for healthcare professionals from the Councils on Cardiovascular Radiology, Stroke, Cardio-Thoracic and Vascular Surgery, Epidemiology and Prevention, and Clinical Cardiology, American Heart Association. *Stroke* 1998;29:336–338.
3. Dorros G. Stent-supported carotid angioplasty. *Circulation* 1998;98:927–930.
4. DeMonte F, Peerless SJ, Rankin RN. Carotid transluminal angioplasty with evidence of distal embolization. *J Neurosurg* 1989;70:138–141.
5. Ohki T, Marin ML, Lyon RT, et al. Human ex-vivo carotid artery bifurcation stenting: Correlation of lesion characteristics with embolic potential. *J Vasc Surg* 1998;27:463–471.
6. Crawley F, Clifton A, Buckenham T, et al. Comparison of hemodynamic cerebral ischemia and microembolic signals detected during carotid endarterectomy and carotid angioplasty. *Stroke* 1997;28: 2460–2464.
7. Endovascular versus surgical treatment in patients with carotid stenosis in the Carotid and Vertebral Artery Transluminal Angioplasty Study (CAVATAS): a randomised trial. *Lancet* 2001;357:1729–1737.
8. Naylor AR, Bolia A, Abbott RJ, et al. Randomized study of carotid angioplasty and stenting versus carotid endarterectomy: a stopped trial. *J Vasc Surg* 1998;28:326–334.
9. Jordan WD Jr, Voellinger DC, Doblar DD, et al. Microemboli detected by transcranial Doppler monitoring in patients during carotid angioplasty versus carotid endarterectomy. *Cardiovasc Surg* 1999; 7:33–38.
10. Jaeger HJ, Mathias KD, Hauth E, et al. Cerebral ischemia detected with diffusion-weighted MR imaging after stent implantation in the carotid artery. *AJNR Am J Neuroradiol* 2002;23:200–207.
11. Theron J, Courtheoux P, Alachkar F, et al. New triple coaxial catheter system for carotid angioplasty with cerebral protection. *AJNR Am J Neuroradiol* 1990;11:869–874.
12. Ohki T, Veith FJ. Carotid artery stenting: utility of cerebral protection devices. *J Invasive Cardiol* 2001;13:47–55.
13. Whitlow PL, Lylyk P, Londero H, et al. Carotid artery stenting protected with an emboli containment system. *Stroke* 2002;33:1308–1314.
14. Fearn SJ, Pole R, Wesnes K, et al. Cerebral injury during cardiopulmonary bypass: emboli impair memory. *J Thorac Cardiovasc Surg* 2001;121:1150–1160.
15. Gaunt ME, Martin PJ, Smith JL, et al. Clinical relevance of intraoperative embolization detected by transcranial Doppler ultrasonography during carotid endarterectomy: a prospective study of 100 patients. *Br J Surg* 1994;81:1435–1439.
16. Baim DS, Wahr D, George B, et al. Randomized trial of a distal embolic protection device during

percutaneous intervention of saphenous vein aorto-coronary bypass grafts. *Circulation* 2002;105: 1285–1290.

17. Henry M, Amor M, Henry I. Carotid stenting with cerebral protection: first clinical experience using the PercuSurge GuardWire system. *J Endovasc Surg* 1999;6:321–331.
18. Roubin GS. Current status of carotid stenting. Presented at: TransCatheter Cardiovascular Therapeutics (TCT); September 2002; Washington, D.C.
19. Wholey M, Al-Mubarak N, Wholey MB, et al. Update on the global carotid stenting registry. Presented at: TransCatheter Cardiovascular Therapeutics (TCT); September 2002; Washington, D.C.
20. Mathias K. Diffusion weighted MRI analysis of carotid stenting. Presented at: 15th International Symposium on Endovascular Intervention (ISET); January 2003; Miami, Florida.
21. Mathias K. Results of the German Quality Assurance Program on CAS in 2,637 patients. Presented at: 15th International Symposium on Endovascular Intervention (ISET); January 2003; Miami, Florida.
22. Pentecost MJ, Criqui MH, Dorros G, et al. Guidelines for peripheral percutaneous transluminal angioplasty of the abdominal aorta and lower extremity vessels. A statement for health professionals from a special writing group of the Councils on Cardiovascular Radiology, Arteriosclerosis, Cardio-Thoracic and Vascular Surgery, Clinical Cardiology, and Epidemiology and Prevention, the American Heart Association. *Circulation* 1994;89:511–531.
23. Roubin GS, New G, Iyer SS, et al. Immediate and late clinical outcomes of carotid artery stenting in patients with symptomatic and asymptomatic carotid artery stenosis: a 5-year prospective analysis. *Circulation* 2001;103:532–537.
24. Clane RYl. Cyclosporine A initially as the only immunosuppressant in 34 patients of cadaveric organs. *Lancet* 1979;2:1033–1036.
25. Hobson RW 2nd. Status of carotid angioplasty and stenting trials. *J Vasc Surg* 1998;27:791.
26. Yadav J. Early results of the SAPPHIRE trial. Presented at: American Heart Association; November 2002; Chicago, Illinois.

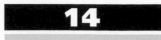

MICROEMBOLIZATION DURING CAROTID ARTERY STENTING

NADIM AL-MUBARAK

Despite advanced stenting techniques, clinical neurological events may complicate carotid artery stenting (CAS) procedures (1-3). Obstructive carotid artery lesions are known to contain friable thrombotic and atherosclerotic components that can embolize during the carotid intervention and are responsible for the majority of these neurological complications (4,5). Efforts are ongoing to optimize the outcome of this treatment: first, by identifying clinical and/or angiographic factors that predispose to these events, hence optimizing the patient selection for the procedure, and second, by developing strategies, so-called "Anti-Embolization devices," that capture the released embolic matter before it reaches the brain, minimizing the risk for embolic events (4). Detection and quantification of the embolic material during the procedure and the immediate postprocedural period could improve the patient selection for this treatment and facilitate the refinement of the Anti-Embolization strategies.

Live *in vivo* detection of microemboli passing through the cerebral circulation can be achieved using transcranial Doppler (TCD) (6–8). This technique is highly sensitive, specific, and provides a very good quantitative tool that detects microembolization during a variety of clinical settings. Microemboli produce very characteristic Doppler signals (microembolic signals, or MES) that are very specific when strict Doppler recognition criteria are applied (Fig. 14-1) (6). Although Doppler-detected microemboli are microscopic in size and clinically silent, their ability to predict embolic neurological events has been demonstrated in a number of clinical settings, such as during carotid endarterectomy (CEA), atrial fibrillation, and coronary artery bypass surgery (7). This chapter describes the TCD application for monitoring microembolization during CAS and discusses the clinical implications of the currently available data.

TRANSCRANIAL DOPPLER TECHNIQUE

The acoustic properties of the embolic material differ dramatically from the blood. Microemboli reflect the ultrasound waves much more strongly than the surrounding blood (9). This increased "reflectivity" results in a dramatic increase in the intensity of the signals received by the TCD probe. Using a 2-MH Doppler probe and pulsed-Doppler mode, the proximal segment of the ipsilateral middle cerebral artery (MCA) is sampled through the temporal bone window (Fig. 14-2). After obtaining an optimal Doppler signal, the probe is held in position for the entire procedure using a special holding device. The data are stored on a hard disk. MESs have distinct Doppler characteristics and audible acoustic components. These signals may occur at any time in the cardiac cycle, are usually transient, lasting for

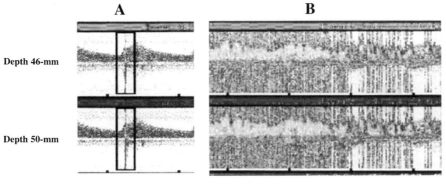

Depth 46-mm

Depth 50-mm

Microembolic Signal (MES)   Microembolic Shower

FIGURE 14-1. Microembolic Eq signals: The picture shows (**A**) an example of microembolic signals (MES) and (**B**) microembolic shower using a dual-channel transcranial Doppler (TCD) system at two different sample depths (46 mm and 50 mm). (See also the color section following page 164 of this text.)

10 to 100 milliseconds, and may be seen in clusters (Fig. 14-1A) (9). The audible component is described as a chirp, snap, or moaning sound. High concentration of microemboli does not usually produce discrete signals; rather, it increases the overall intensity of the Doppler spectral display, called the "embolic shower" (Fig. 14-1B). Strict guidelines for the identification of MESs have been published by an international expert committee (9). MES counts are usually expressed in mean values ± standard deviation (SD). For statistical purposes,

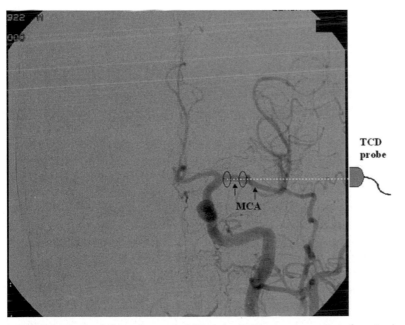

TCD
probe

MCA

FIGURE 14-2. Dual-channel transcranial Doppler (TCD) setup: Insonation of proximal horizontal segment of the middle cerebral artery (MCA; *arrows*) is achieved through the temporal bone window using two simultaneous pulsed-Doppler samples.

most investigators count 1 second of microembolic shower as 10 MES. Currently available dual-channel Doppler systems allow simultaneous sampling of two different sites within the MCA (Figs. 14-1, 14-2). Demonstrating the same MES at the two sites with a time gap increases the specificity of the signals, as it is strong evidence for its embolic nature. Using the currently available Doppler equipment, it is not possible to reliably distinguish air from solid material, nor it is possible to accurately estimate the size of the microembolus. Generally, solid microemboli have an intensity of more than 10 decibels above the background Doppler signal. Air bubbles produce more intense signals, of more than or equal to 60 decibels above the background signal (9).

TRANSCRANIAL DOPPLER-DETECTED MICROEMBOLIZATION DURING CAROTID ARTERY STENTING

Clinically silent microembolizations are frequently observed during percutaneous carotid interventions (6–8). Similar to CEA, several investigators have demonstrated that all patients undergoing CAS without Anti-Embolization protection have Doppler evidence of microembolization (6–8,10). However, the clinical significance of this phenomenon remains unclear, as the brain appears to have a remarkable tolerance for microembolization. In a substudy of a randomized trial that compared CEA to CAS [The Carotid and Vertebral Artery Transluminal Angioplasty Study (CAVATAS)], Crawley et al. (11) compared the microembolic loads and the neuropsychological sequelae among two groups of patients, 20 undergoing CAS and 26 undergoing CEA. Despite a significantly higher incidence of microemboli during carotid angioplasty (most of which was performed without stenting), similar decline in neuropsychological performance was observed between the two groups (11).

Although in many clinical conditions increased frequency of the Doppler-detected microemboli correlate well with an increased risk for adverse embolic neurological events, such a correlation during CAS has not yet been established (6,12). The ability of MESs to predict relevant embolic clinical endpoints during or immediately after CAS, when established, could have an important clinical implication. MESs serving as a surrogate marker of the clinical embolic risk in the assessment of the various Anti-Embolization strategies would facilitate its refinement. The higher frequency of MES observed during this procedure compared with the embolic clinical events would allow such an assessment in a small number of patients. The definition of the microembolic load during the various procedural stages could facilitate the development of protection strategies that specifically target the stages with increased microemboli release. The effect of Anti-Embolization devices on the microembolic load during these stages can be determined and provides important feedback on the performance of these strategies and their ability to minimize the clinical embolic risk. Further, defining the microembolic load associated with the various lesion types or clinical conditions would improve the patient selection and the patients' suitability for the procedure.

The use of the Doppler-detected microemboli as a surrogate marker of the clinical embolic risk during CAS may be limited by the inability of the current technology to distinguish gas from solid MESs (9). MESs recorded during carotid angiography may indicate microbubbles that are generally thought to be less hazardous than solids (13). During carotid intervention, microbubbles can be introduced into the circulation with the contrast injections or equipment. To minimize this uncertainty, most investigators exclude all the MES detected during the contrast injections from their analysis (8,14). Despite these potential limitations,

TCD studies have provided an important insight into the microembolization phenomenon during CAS with and without Anti-Embolization protection.

MICROEMBOLIC PROFILE DURING CAROTID ARTERY STENTING

The microembolic profile, i.e., the extent of microembolization during the various stages of the carotid stenting procedure, has been defined using continuous TCD monitoring during CAS (Fig. 14-3) (8). MESs are detected throughout the carotid stenting procedure performed without Anti-Embolization protection, with three critical phases being responsible for the majority of released microemboli (Fig. 14-3) (8). These stages include: (a) stent deployment, (b) lesion predilation, and (c) stent postdilatation, with the highest MES counts observed during the stent deployment phase, which is typically characterized by microembolic showers. All of these three phases are feasibly protectable and are currently being targeted by the various Anti-Embolization strategies. The guiding sheath and guide wire placements were associated with a relatively small microembolic load (Fig. 14-3). Notable are the increased MES counts observed during the stent deployment phase, which contradicts the general belief that stent deployment is associated with a low risk of embolization due to its scaffolding effect, which "supposedly" traps potential embolic matter against the arterial wall. The increased release of microemboli during the stenting phase could be explained by the sheer forces of the self-expanding stent, which is usually oversized to the ICA. A second theoretical possibility is the release of the air trapped within the stent sheath in the form of microbubbles.

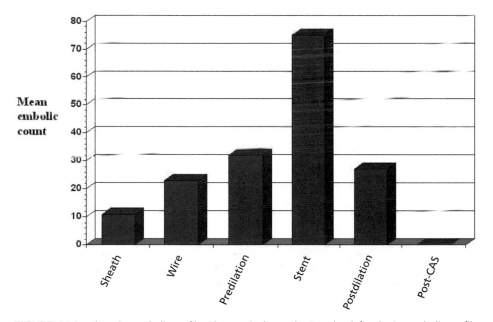

FIGURE 14-3. The microembolic profile: The graph shows the Doppler-defined microembolic profile during the different stages of carotid artery stenting (CAS) performed without Anti-Embolization devices. Microembolic signals (MES) are observed throughout the procedure including sheath placement, wire manipulation, predilatation, stent deployment, and postdilatation. Stent deployment and balloon dilatations account for to the highest MES counts. No MES were recorded during the immediate 15 minutes postprocedure.

Importantly, microemboli during the immediate postprocedural period have been very scarce. The Lenox Hill TCD analysis has shown that no microemboli were detected during the immediate 15 minutes following the completion of the procedure (8). Ohki et al. have demonstrated that carotid stents are not a source of microemboli during the late follow-up (5). These findings support the clinical observation that the majority of the neurological events occur during the procedure and that Anti-Embolization devices are rightfully targeting the critical phases of embolization during CAS. Mechanical Anti-Embolization systems with the exception of the Parodi Anti-Embolization device are designed to capture embolic particles following the passage of the guide wire through the lesion and until the end of the stent postdilatation (4). Emboli generated during sheath placement, wire manipulation, or following the removal of the protection devices are not captured. However, the microembolic profile suggests that these unprotected phases are associated with a relatively lower risk of embolization.

ASSESSMENT OF ANTI-EMBOLIZATION DEVICES

These devices are currently introduced into the carotid stenting procedure in order to prevent any embolic matter released during the intervention from reaching the brain, hence minimizing the risk of embolic neurological events. Similar to other endovascular devices, subsequent refinement after the initial phase of clinical testing is always necessary in order to optimize its application and efficacy. TCD monitoring during CAS procedures using these devices may facilitate its development and further refinement.

The most widely studied Anti-Embolization system is the distal occlusion protection (GuardWire, Medtronic AVA, Denvers, MA) (15). A low-pressure balloon is mounted at the end of a guide wire that is used to cross the lesion and deliver interventional equipment. By occluding the distal carotid artery with a balloon, embolic material released during the intervention is contained within the proximal blood column, which is aspirated at the end of the procedure prior to the protection balloon deflation. Although the preliminary clinical results are encouraging, embolic events have been observed in a minority of patients despite the application of this strategy (15). Several TCD studies have clearly demonstrated the ability of this strategy to reduce microembolization to the brain during carotid intervention and provided insight into the potential mechanisms of failures to provide full protection (8,14). In a series of 79 patients undergoing CAS (39 with no Anti-Embolization devices and 36 with the distal-balloon occlusion system), the use of the distal-balloon protection during CAS was associated with significantly lower total MES counts than those procedures performed without distal protection (Fig. 14-4, Table 14-1) (8). There was no significant difference in the microembolic load during sheath placement or guide wire manipulation between the two groups. However, the distal-balloon Anti-Embolization system was associated with significantly lower microembolization during the predilatation, stent deployment, and postdilatation, the three critical stages that are protected with this strategy (Fig. 14-5). The majority of MES recorded during the distal balloon system application occurred during sheath placement and wire manipulation, to a lesser extent during the distal balloon deflation (Fig. 14-4, Table 14-1). These findings support the validity of the Anti-Embolization protection concept and may translate into a reduction of the larger and clinically more important emboli, hence reducing the clinical embolic risk during CAS.

Several factors could have contributed to the MES that were still detectable during CAS with this Anti-Embolization system. These include emboli that could have been trapped within the space between the arterial wall and the occlusion balloon, "the dead zone," and

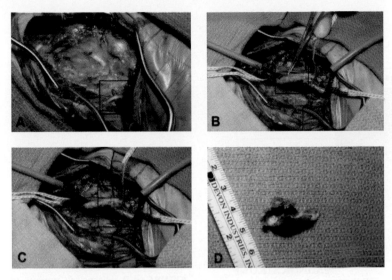

FIGURE 1-1. Carotid endarterectomy technique. **A:** Superficial dissection: patient's head on the right side of the figure, left carotid intervention. Detail: greater auricular nerve. **B:** Deeper plane: The jugular vein has been retracted, the facial vein ligated. Exposure of common carotid artery. Detail: ansa hypoglossi. **C:** Detail: The bifurcation of the common carotid artery has been exposed; the internal carotid artery lays in the lower part of the picture (initially runs lateral to the external carotid artery). **D:** Removed atherosclerotic plaque. Photographs courtesy of Mitesh Shah, MD, Section of Neurological Surgery, Indiana University School of Medicine, Indianapolis, Indiana.

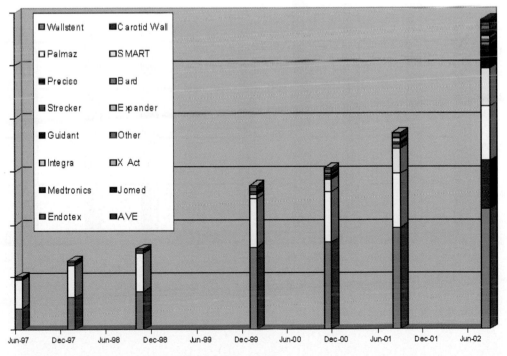

FIGURE 4-1. Historical review: stents placed by center.

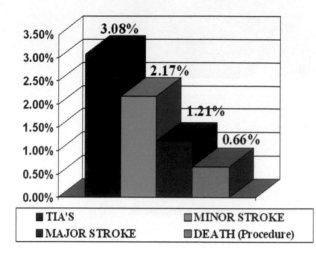

FIGURE 4-2. Historical review of stent complications.

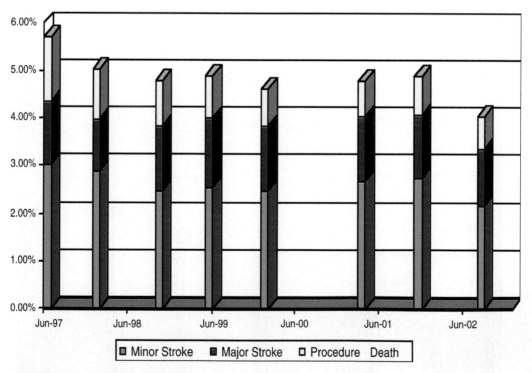

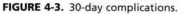

FIGURE 4-3. 30-day complications.

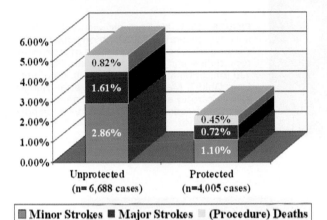

FIGURE 4-4. Complications with and without cerebral protection.

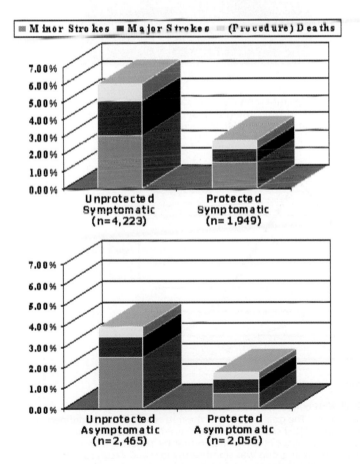

FIGURE 4-5. Complications with and without protection: symptomatic and asymptomatic patient populations.

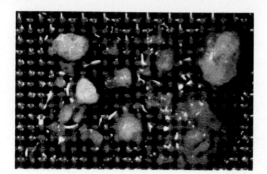

FIGURE 13-1. Macroscopic view of embolic particles generated following angioplasty and stenting. These particles consisted of atherosclerotic debris and calcified material. Filter size: 130 μm, original magnification x40. (Reprinted from Ohki T, Marin ML, Lyon RT, et al. Human ex-vivo carotid artery bifurcation stenting: correlation of lesion characteristics with embolic potential. *J Vasc Surg* 1998;27:463–471, with permission.)

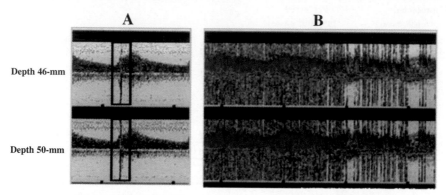

FIGURE 14-1. Microembolic signals: The picture shows **(A)** an example of a microembolic signals (MES) and **(B)** microembolic shower using a dual-channel transcranial Doppler (TCD) system at two different sample depths (46 mm and 50 mm).

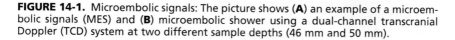
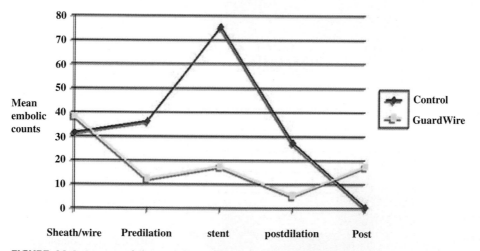

FIGURE 14-4. Impact of the occlusion balloon Anti-Embolization system on microembolization during carotid artery stenting (CAS): The graph compares the microembolic loads [defined as the mean total microembolic signal (MES) counts] in two groups during various stages of CAS. The occlusion balloon system was associated with significantly reduced MES counts. Microembolization in the occlusion balloon group was significantly low and occurred mainly during sheath placement, guide wire manipulation, and to a much lesser extent during the interventional stages. Some MESs were recorded during the occlusion balloon deflation.

STENT RELEASE

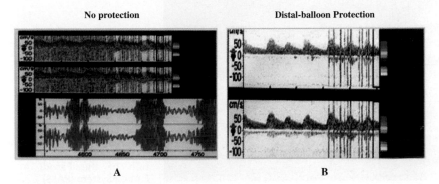

FIGURE 14-5. Microembolization during stent deployment with and without Anti-Embolization: Doppler display of microembolic signals (MES) recorded during the stent deployment phase during carotid artery stenting (CAS) with (**A**) *no* Anti-Embolization device (in this case showing microembolic shower) and (**B**) the occlusion balloon Anti-Embolization system where only few MESs were observed.

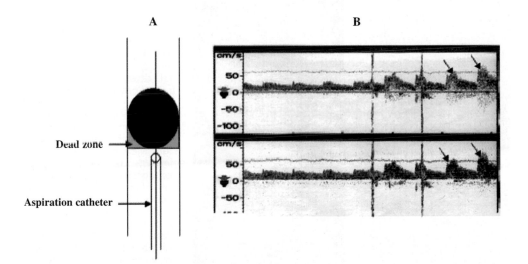

FIGURE 14-6. A: The "dead zone" of the occlusion balloon Anti-Embolization device. Embolic matter may be trapped between the occlusion balloon and the arterial wall, making it difficult to be accessed and removed by the aspiration catheter. **B:** The trapped debris may embolize during the occlusion balloon deflation as this picture shows. MESs are recorded during the occlusion balloon deflation. Note the improvement in the Doppler flow as the balloon deflates (*arrows*).

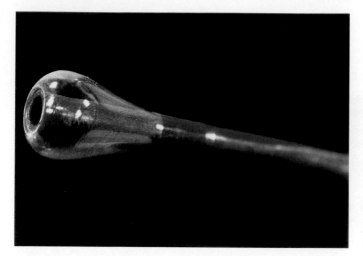

FIGURE 17-4. Picture of the distal balloon occlusion portion of the Parodi Anti-Emboli System (PAES).

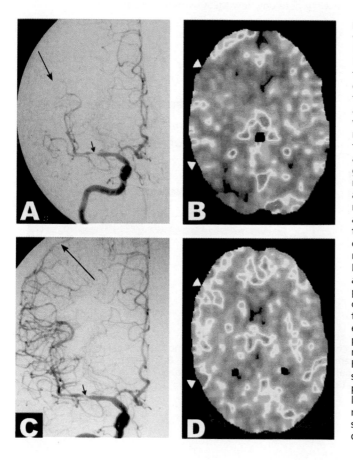

FIGURE 21-2. A 72-year-old woman with left upper extremity weakness, numbness, and intermittent limb shaking due to symptomatic right middle cerebral artery (MCA) stenosis failing medical therapy with aspirin, clopidogrel, and intravenous heparin. **A:** Right internal carotid arteriography in frontal projection during arterial phase demonstrates high-grade, focal stenosis of the right M1 segment (*short arrow*) and delayed filling of distal right MCA branch vessels (*long arrows*). **B:** Xenon computed tomography (CT) brain scan confirms asymmetric and reduced perfusion of the right MCA distribution (*white arrows*). **C:** Following angioplasty using a 1.5-mm-diameter coronary balloon (*short arrow*), the vessel diameter is only modestly increased although distal perfusion has increased markedly (*long arrows*). **D:** Repeat xenon CT perfusion study 24 hours following angioplasty demonstrates dramatically increased perfusion of the right MCA territory due to the small increase in cross-sectional diameter of the stenosis.

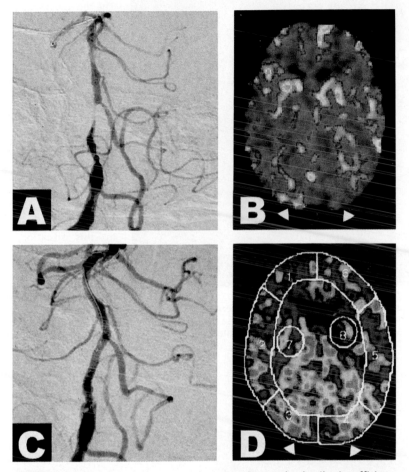

FIGURE 21-3. A 49-year-old man with crescendo vertebrobasilar insufficiency failing medical therapy with aspirin, clopidogrel, and intravenous heparin. **A**: Complete cerebral arteriography demonstrated high-grade focal stenosis of the intracranial right vertebral artery. The left vertebral artery was previously occluded, and there was no significant contribution to the posterior cerebral circulation by circle of Willis collaterals. **B**: Xenon computed tomography (CT) perfusion brain scan reveals diminished cortical perfusion in the posterior circulation (*white arrows*). **C**: Revascularization was performed under general anesthesia using a 2.5 x 9-mm metallic stent, which resulted in complete resolution of symptoms. **D**: Xenon CT perfusion scan within 24 hours of the procedure demonstrates hyperperfusion (increase in perfusion greater than 100%) in the posterior circulation (*white arrows*). This was managed by strict blood pressure control in the neurological intensive care unit until resolution. The patient recovered without complication.

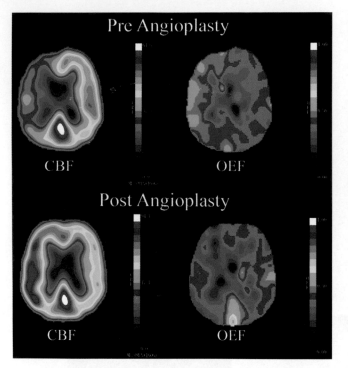

Pre Angioplasty

CBF   OEF

Post Angioplasty

CBF   OEF

FIGURE 21-4. Quantitative positron-emission tomography (PET) images of cerebral blood flow (CBF, *left*) and oxygen extraction fraction (OEF, *right*). The top row of images (immediately before angioplasty) shows the reduction of CBF and compensatory increase in OEF in the right hemisphere distal to the stenosis. There are two basic compensatory responses of the cerebrovasculature to reduced perfusion pressure—autoregulatory vasodilation and increased oxygen extraction (134). These serve to maintain normal oxygen metabolism and neuronal function. When perfusion pressure drops below a critical level, the capacity for autoregulatory vasodilation is exceeded, and CBF will fall passively as a function of pressure. In this situation, OEF can increase from a baseline of 30% to a maximum of 80%. This phenomenon has been called "misery perfusion." (135) The presence of increased OEF has been proven to be a powerful and independent predictor of subsequent stroke in patients with atherosclerotic occlusive cerebrovascular disease (34,39,136). The lower row of images acquired 36 hours after angioplasty shows the improvement in CBF and OEF. PET images courtesy of Colin P. Derdeyn, MD.

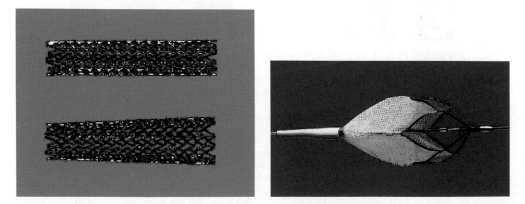

FIGURE 22-1. Carotid stent (AccuLink, Guidant Co., Indianapolis, IN) and Anti-Embolic device (AccuNet, Guidant Co.) being used by the Carotid Revascularization Endarterectomy Versus Stent Trial (CREST) investigators for performing CAS. **A:** AccuLink stents are made of self-expanding nitinol and are available in two configurations: straight (*above*) and tapered (*below*), each in several diameters and lengths. **B:** The AccuNet Anti-Embolic device is made of polyurethane and is available in several diameters.

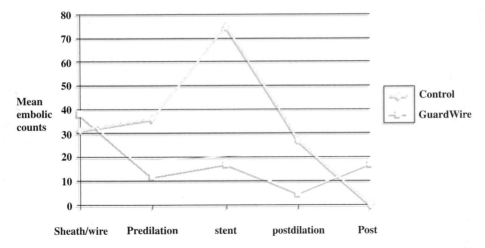

FIGURE 14-4. Impact of the occlusion balloon Anti-Embolization system on microembolization during carotid artery stenting (CAS): The graph compares the microembolic loads [defined as the mean total microembolic signal (MES) counts] in two groups during various stages of CAS. The occlusion balloon system was associated with significantly reduced MES counts. Microembolization in the occlusion balloon group was significantly low and occurred mainly during sheath placement, guide wire manipulation, and to a much lesser extent during the interventional stages. Some MESs were recorded during the occlusion balloon deflation. (See also the color section following page 164 of this text.)

therefore were inaccessible for removal by the aspiration catheter (Fig. 14-6A). These emboli could have accounted for the MES observed during the distal-balloon deflation (Fig. 14-6B), a non-occlusive protection balloon (Fig. 14-7), and embolization via collateral circulation through the external carotid artery (Fig. 14-8) (16). Some operators have applied the "saline flushing maneuver" into the ICA prior to the occlusion balloon deflation, thereby diverting potential embolic material to the ECA, which is generally thought to be of reduced risk for clinical emboli. However, this maneuver could promote embolization into the ipsilateral hemisphere through a well-developed collateral circulation (16).

TCD application during CAS has provided significant procedural feedback that improved the application of the distal-balloon Anti-Embolization system. To summarize a few important technical points: it is very important to achieve a complete occlusion with the

TABLE 14-1. MES COUNTS: CAS WITH DISTAL-BALLOON ANTI-EMBOLIZATION DEVICE VERSUS CONTROL

	Control Group	Distal Balloon Group	*p* Value
Sheath placement	11 ± 7	16 ± 24	NS
Wire manipulation	23 ± 22	22 ± 33	NS
Predilatation	32 ± 36	12 ± 31	0.001
Stent deployment	75 ± 57	17 ± 22	0.004
Postdilatation	27 ± 25	5 ± 9	0.002
Distal-balloon deflation	NA	17 ± 21	NA
Post CAS (up to 15 min)	0	0	0
Total	164 ± 108	68 ± 83	0.002

MES, microembolic signals; CAS, carotid artery stenting; NA, not applicable; NS, not significant.

STENT RELEASE

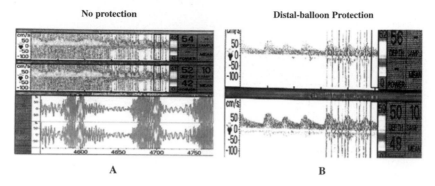

A

B

FIGURE 14-5. Microembolization during stent deployment with and without Anti-Embolization: Doppler display of microembolic signals (MESs) recorded during the stent deployment phase during carotid artery stenting (CAS) with (**A**) *no* Anti-Embolization device (in this case showing microembolic shower) and (**B**) the occlusion balloon Anti-Embolization system where only few MESs were observed. (See also the color section following page 164 of this text.)

balloon and to maintain this occlusion throughout the procedure and until the end. It is also critical to maintain the stability of the distal balloon position during the various catheter exchanges. An initially occlusive balloon may become nonocclusive if moved into a proximal segment of a tapering ICA (Fig. 14-7). This can be achieved by inflating the balloon to 6 mm, as possible, instead of 5.5 mm, taking care not to injure a small caliber carotid artery. It is also important to maximize the efficacy of aspiration by reaching as distal as possible with the aspiration catheter, keeping it just below the distal balloon for a few seconds, as there are possibly trapped emboli in this area.

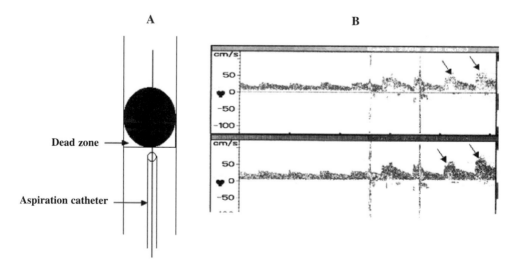

FIGURE 14-6. A: The "dead zone" of the occlusion balloon Anti-Embolization device. Embolic matter may be trapped between the occlusion balloon and the arterial wall, making it difficult to be accessed and removed by the aspiration catheter. **B**: The trapped debris may embolize during the occlusion balloon deflation as this picture shows. MESs are recorded during the occlusion balloon deflation. Note the improvement in the Doppler flow as the balloon deflates (*arrows*). (See also the color section following page 164 of this text.)

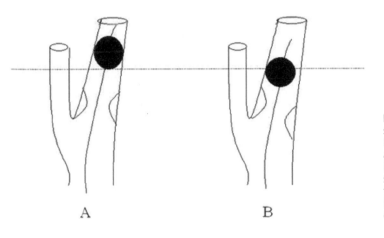

FIGURE 14-7. An initially stable and occlusion balloon (**A**) becomes unstable and nonocclusive (**B**) after it moved into a proximal segment of the tapering internal carotid artery during balloon/stent catheter exchanges.

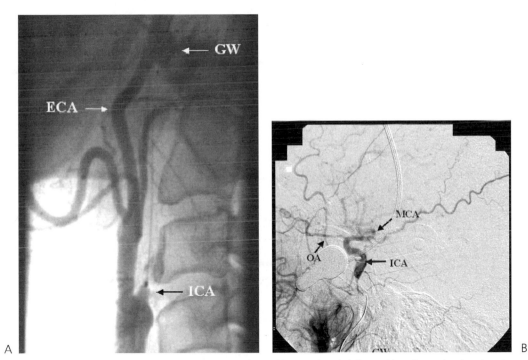

FIGURE 14-8. Microembolization via the external carotid artery (ECA): (**A**) carotid angiography showing the distal internal carotid artery (ICA) occluded by the GuardWire balloon (GW). The blood flow through the ECA is maintained. Despite the complete ICA occlusion, microembolic signals (MESs) were still recordable within the middle cerebral artery (MCA). This observation prompted ipsilateral intracranial angiography (**B**) during the distal ICA occlusion (inflated GW balloon visible at the bottom of the picture). Despite the ICA occlusion, the intracranial ICA and the MCA were filling from the ECA via a well-developed ophthalmic artery (OA). The patient remained asymptomatic and had no neurological events.

TRANSCRANIAL DOPPLER DURING NONOCCLUSIVE ANTI-EMBOLIZATION SYSTEMS

Data on microembolization assessment with other Anti-Embolization systems during CAS are limited. Parodi et al. (17) reported that a large number of MESs were recorded throughout CAS performed with a filter Anti-Embolization system. However, no quantification of this phenomenon was provided. This is consistent with our limited unpublished observation of significant TCD-documented microembolization throughout the stenting procedure performed with filter Anti-Embolization. However, one has to be careful drawing any conclusions based on this observation, as a negative clinical impact of microembolization has not yet been established in the carotid stenting setting. Additionally, although microemboli may still pass through the filter pores, large emboli with potential clinical relevance are very likely to be trapped by the filter system. Hence, a correlation between microembolization and embolic neurological events, particularly in this setting, must be uniquely established.

Similarly, unpublished experience from Lenox Hill suggested that MESs were scarce during the critical stages of CAS performed with the Parodi Anti-Embolization device. Few MESs are observed during the final stage of balloon deflation. However, no data are available on the extent of microembolization and the impact of these devices on overall embolic load during CAS.

REFERENCES

1. Roubin GS, New G, Iyer SS, et al. Immediate and late clinical outcomes of carotid artery stenting in symptomatic and asymptomatic carotid stenosis: a 5-year prospective analysis. *Circulation* 2001:103: 532–537.
2. Wholey MH, Wholey M, Mathias K, et al. Global experience in cervical carotid artery stent placement. *Catheter Cardiovasc Interv* 2000;50:160–167.
3. Shawl F, Kadro W, Domanski MJ, et al. Safety and efficacy of elective carotid artery stenting in high-risk patients. *J Am Coll Cardiol* 2000;35:1721–1728.
4. Ohki T, Veith F. Carotid stenting with and without protection devices: should protection be used in all patients? *Sem Vasc Surg* 2000;13:144–152.
5. Ohki T, Marin ML, Lyon RT, et al. Ex vivo human carotid artery bifurcation stenting: correlation of lesion characteristics with embolic potential. *J Vasc Surg* 1998;27:463–471.
6. Markus HS, Monitoring embolism in real time. *Circulation* 2000;102:826–828.
7. Markus HS, Clifton A, Buckenham T, et al. Carotid angioplasty: detection of embolic signals during and after the procedure. *Stroke* 1994;25:2403–2406.
8. Al-Mubarak N, Roubin GS, Vitek JJ, et al. Effect of the distal-balloon protection system on microembolization during carotid stenting. *Circulation* 2001;104:1999–2002.
9. Ringelstein EB, Droste DW, Babikian VL, et al. Consensus of microembolus detection by TCD: international consensus group on microemblus detection. *Stroke* 1998;29:725–729.
10. Gaunt ME, Martin PJ, Smith JL, et al. Clinical relevance of intraoperative embolization detected by transcranial Doppler ultrasonography during carotid endarterectomy: a prospective study of 100 patients. *Br J Surg* 1994;81:1435–1439.
11. Crawley F, Stygall J, Lunn S, et al. Comparison of microembolism detected by transcranial Doppler and neuropsychological sequelae of carotid surgery and percutaneous transluminal angioplasty. *Stroke* 2000;31:1329–1334.
12. Ackerstaff RG, Moons KG, Van de Vlasakker CJ. Association of intraoperative transcranial Doppler monitoring variables with stroke from carotid endarterectomy. *Stroke* 2000;31:1817–1823.
13. Markus HS, Loh A, Isreal D. Microscopic air embolism during cerebral angiography and strategies for its avoidance. *Lancet* 1993;341:784–787.
14. Whitlow PL, Katzan IL, Dagirmanjian A, et al. Embolization during protected versus unprotected carotid stenting. *Circulation* 2000;102:II–475(abst).

15. Henry M, Amor M, Knonaris C. et al. Angioplasty and stenting of extracranial carotid arteries. *Tex Heart Inst J* 2000;27:150–158.
16. Al-Mubarak N, Vitek JJ, Iyer S, et al. Embolization via collateral circulation during carotid stenting with the distal balloon protection system. *J Endovasc Ther* 2001;8:354–357.
17. Parodi JC, Mura RL, Ferreira LM, et al. Initial evaluation of carotid angioplasty and stenting with three different cerebral protection devices. *J Vasc Surg* 2000;32:1127–1136.

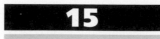

15

CAROTID ARTERY STENTING WITH THE DISTAL OCCLUSION ANTI-EMBOLIZATION SYSTEM

MICHEL HENRY
ANTONIOS POLYDOROU
ISABELLE HENRY
MICHÈLE HUGEL

Despite meticulous techniques and the advanced experience, embolic stroke represents a major drawback of the carotid stenting procedure (CAS). The majority of the neurological complications are due to the intracerebral embolism of plaque fragments or thrombus during different procedural steps. Anti-Embolization devices have been developed to reduce the incidence of embolic events during CAS (29–32). We have prospectively examined the outcome of CAS under cerebral protection using the distal occlusion balloon protection (GuardWire System, PercuSurge–Medtronic, Minneapolis, MN) to assess whether this therapy is comparable to historical controls of both carotid endarterectomy and CAS without Anti-Embolization.

Between February 1998 and February 2002, 238 patients (264 carotid stenoses) met the inclusion criteria and underwent CAS under protection using the GuardWire Anti-Embolization system. Patients were eligible for treatment if they had more than or equal to 70% diameter stenosis of the internal carotid artery (ICA) evaluated by angiography according to the North American Symptomatic Carotid Endarterectomy Trial (NASCET) criteria (2). We excluded the following patients from the treatment: multiple stenoses in the ICA, intracranial pathology, presence of angiographically visible thrombus, gastrointestinal bleeding in the last 6 months, and hemorrhagic disorders.

All patients should receive aspirin 75 to 300 mg per day indefinitely and ticlopidine 250 to 500 mg per day or clopidogrel 75 mg per day for at least 2 days and preferably 1 week before the procedure and for 1 month after it. Unfractionated heparin (5000 IU intravenously) and atropine (1 mg intravenously) are routinely administered just after the introducer sheath is placed. Patients were usually discharged the day after the procedure.

All patients underwent neurological examination, a duplex scan, and a computed tomography (CT) scan the day after CAS, a neurological examination and a duplex scan at 30 days and every 6 months thereafter, and an angiogram at 6 months. Any change in the neurological status after CAS required repeated CT brain scan. In our evaluation of the GuardWire system, we used the following endpoints:

The primary clinical end points included any major/minor stroke, death, or myocardial infarction (MI) within the first 30 days postprocedure. The periprocedural complications were defined as any major/minor stroke, death, or MI occurring in the early 48 hours. The secondary clinical end points were the need of new intervention, angioplasty, or endarterectomy at 6 months.

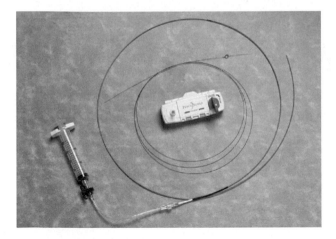

FIGURE 15-1. PercuSurge Guard-Wire system.

Angiographic endpoints were: angiographic success rate, defined as achieving a less than or equal to 30% residual stenosis, and angiographic restenosis, defined as a reduction of the arterial lumen diameter by more than or equal to 50%. The procedural success was defined as a reduction in the stenosis to less than or equal to 30% and absence of any neurological complication, MI, or death.

A total of 264 carotid angioplasties were attempted in 238 consecutive patients (190 males, 48 females, mean age 71.2 ± 9.4 years, range 40–91 years). Twenty-six patients had bilateral procedures. Ninety-five stenoses were asymptomatic (36%), and 169 were symptomatic (64%). A total of 224 lesions were atherosclerotic, 30 were restenoses (postsurgical: 27, postangioplasty: 3), and 8 were postradiation stenoses. One lesion was an inflammatory arteritis and another one a posttraumatic aneurysm. The mean percentage of stenosis was 82.3 ± 9.2 % (70–99). Mean lesion length was 14.4 ± 6.3 mm (5–50) and the mean arterial diameter was 5.0 ± 1.3 mm (4–7.1); 118 lesions (45%) were calcified, and 188 were ulcerated (72%).

DESCRIPTION OF THE GUARDWIRE SYSTEM

The device consists of three main components (see Figs. 15-1–15-3):

1. The GuardWire temporary occlusion catheter: a 0.014-inch or 0.018-inch wire con-

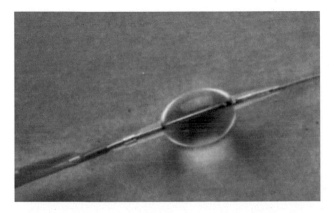

FIGURE 15-2. Export aspiration catheter mounted on a GuardWire temporary occlusion catheter.

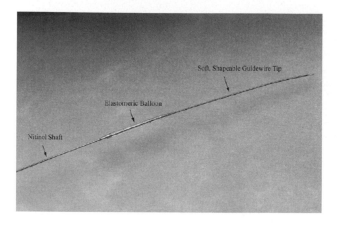

FIGURE 15-3. The PercuSurge GuardWire.

structed of a hollow nitinol hypotube incorporating into its distal segment an inflatable compliant balloon that is capable of occluding the ICA outflow. The balloon diameter (3 to 6 mm) is chosen depending on the artery diameter. The GuardWire is available in 2 lengths, 190 cm and 300 cm, and the wire accommodates monorail and over-the-wire delivery systems for dilatation and stenting. The terminal 3.5-cm segment of the wire can be shaped as needed to facilitate lesion-crossing maneuvers, much like coronary wires.

2. A Microseal that is incorporated at the proximal end of the wire, allowing inflation and deflation of the distal protection balloon (PB), utilizing a Microseal adapter. The Microseal keeps the electrometric balloon inflated while allowing catheter exchange at the proximal end, similar to commonly used guide wires.

3. The aspiration catheter placed over the GuardWire to aspirate generated debris. It may also be used to flush the ICA.

TECHNIQUES

Figures 15-4 through 15-7 offer a visual summarization of the procedure techniques. A 7F multipurpose guide catheter or a 6F long guiding sheath (depending on the stent type) is initially placed into the common carotid artery (CCA) via the femoral approach. The GuardWire is then gently advanced through the guide catheter, the lesion is crossed, and the marker of the protection balloon placed 2 or 3 cm beyond it. The Microseal adapter is then attached and the protection balloon slowly inflated with a fixed volume of dilute contrast, occluding the ICA and deriving vessel outflow towards the external carotid artery (ECA). It is important to verify by injection of contrast that the blood flow is totally interrupted in the ICA in order to ensure adequate antiembolization during the procedure. If the ICAs are large in diameter, it is advisable to place the protection balloon high in the ICA at the base of the skull, where the ICA is smaller and the stability of the balloon is achieved. Upon detaching the Microseal adapter, the occlusion balloon remains inflated. Predilatation of the lesion or direct stenting are then performed under protection. Any generated debris is removed from the ICA using aspiration alone or aspiration and flushing techniques.

Two protection techniques have been used:

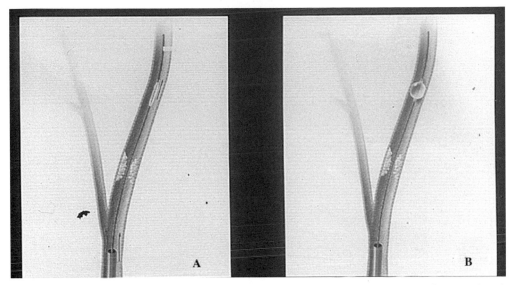

FIGURE 15-4. PercuSurge GuardWire system: procedure description. **(A)** The lesion is crossed with GuardWire. **(B)** The GuardWire balloon is inflated.

Technique 1: The occlusion balloon remains inflated during the whole procedure, and the aspiration is performed once after stent placement and postdilatation.

Technique 2: The occlusion balloon is deflated between predilatation and stent placement to restore the cerebral flow. Aspiration is performed after each of these two stages.

The technique used depends on patient tolerance to the occlusion, the cerebral collateral circulation, the status of the contralateral artery, the duration of the procedure, and the technical problems encountered. In both scenarios, the aspiration catheter is advanced over

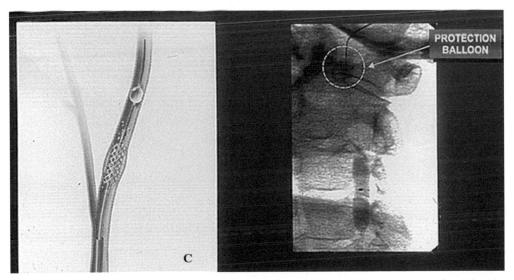

FIGURE 15-5. PercuSurge GuardWire system: procedure description. **(C)** Intervention is performed under protection. *(right)* GuardWire is used as a standard guide wire.

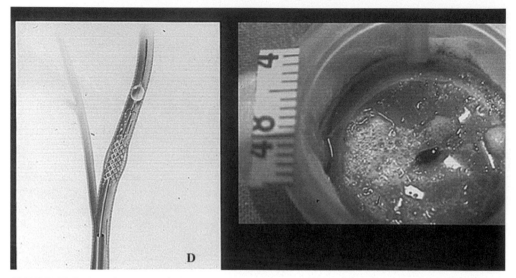

FIGURE 15-6. PercuSurge GuardWire system: procedure description. **(D)** Export catheter removes emboli and thrombus *(right)*.

the wire into the dilated area, with a 20-cc syringe connected to it to aspirate debris. A minimum of two aspirations are performed successively. Additionally, in our initial 40 cases, a flushing of the treated area was performed using saline injections through the guide catheter to drive the particles towards the ECA. The injection was performed with an injection pump at a rate of 2 mL per second for 10 seconds. Two flushes may be performed: the first with the guiding catheter positioned at the carotid bifurcation, and the second with the catheter

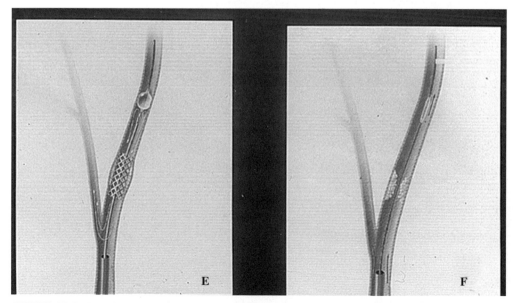

FIGURE 15-7. PercuSurge GuardWire system: procedure description. **(E)** Flushing saline to external carotid artery. **(F)** The GuardWire balloon is deflated.

near the protection balloon. If only a single flush is possible, it is advisable to position the guiding catheter tip close to the occlusion balloon. Finally, the Microseal adapter is reattached to the GuardWire, and the occlusion balloon is deflated, allowing normal flow to be restored. If the angiographic result is satisfactory, the device is removed.

TECHNIQUES OF CEREBRAL PROTECTION

- A total of 216 lesions were treated using the continuous occlusion technique. Mean occlusion time (seconds): 375 ± 182 (range 141–1480).
- A total of 46 lesions were treated by the second staged technique. Mean dilation occlusion time (seconds): 320 ± 150 (range 109–765), mean stent implantation occlusion time (seconds): 300 ± 140 (range 120–720).
- Mean occlusion time for all lesions (in seconds) was 410 ± 220 (120–1480).

IMMEDIATE TECHNICAL SUCCESS

Technical success (Figs. 15-8, 15-9) was achieved in 262 out of 264 (99.2%). There were two failures to cross the lesion with the GuardWire system because of very tight calcified stenoses and excessive tortuosities of the CCA and ICA. The procedures were successfully completed without cerebral protection. In one patient, after completion of the procedure, deflation of the occlusion balloon using the Microseal adapter was impossible, owing to a kink in the Microseal junction. This problem was managed by cutting the hypotube section of the GuardWire distally to the Microseal area, using scissors, and the balloon was then immediately deflated.

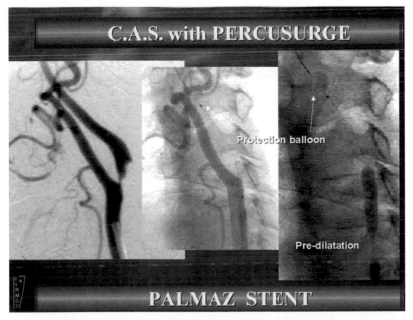

FIGURE 15-8. Tight left internal carotid artery stenosis. Carotid angioplasty and stenting under protection with PercuSurge (implantation of Palmaz stent).

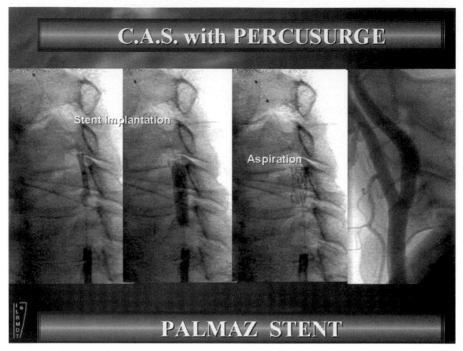

FIGURE 15-9. Tight left internal carotid artery stenosis. Carotid angioplasty and stenting under protection with PercuSurge (implantation of Palmaz stent).

Mild degrees of spasm have been seen at the location of the occlusion balloon in 10 patients, but without significant flow reduction. We have never seen severe spasm or a dissection of the arterial wall. All lesions were treated with endoprostheses except three postangioplasty restenoses. We implanted 128 Palmaz stents (P204: 73, P154: 53, Corinthian: 2), 36 Wallstent stents, 101 nitinol self-expandable stents, and 1 Jostent covered stent to treat the aneurysm. The nitinol and Wallstent stents covered the bifurcation without jeopardizing the flow in the ECA. All stents were well deployed.

TOLERANCE TO OCCLUSION BALLOON

The occlusion during protection balloon inflation was well tolerated in 251 out of 262 cases (95.8%), out of which 62 had a significant contralateral ICA disease (stenosis or occlusion). Two types of intolerance were observed:

1. Complete intolerance occurred in two patients (0.8%) immediately after inflation of the occlusion balloon:

   - One patient with total occlusion of the contralateral ICA who developed loss of consciousness and seizures. The patient totally recovered after rapid balloon deflation. CAS was successfully completed without Anti-Embolization.
   - One with poor collateral circulation from the circle of Willis who developed rapid loss of consciousness, but the procedure could be completed under protection. The patient immediately recovered after the occlusion balloon deflation.

2. Partial transient intolerance (occurred in nine patients: 3.4%) beginning approximately 2 minutes after flow interruption with transient symptoms such as agitation, brief loss of consciousness, or transient neurological deficit. The procedure was completed under protection. All patients had rapid and complete recovery while the protection balloon was still inflated. Seven of them had hypotensive response to dilatation with bradycardia, which could have promoted this intolerance. Ten patients developed a spasm of the ICA above the dilated area at the location of the protection balloon, which rapidly responded to vasodilator therapy.

COLLECTED DEBRIS

Aspiration of the debris was performed in all patients. The aspirated blood samples were collected in filters (with a pore size of 40 μm) and analyzed using optic and electron microscopic techniques. Visible debris was extracted from all patients [mean diameter: 250 μm (range 56–2652), mean number per procedure: 74 (range 7–145)]. Different types of particles were found: atheromatous plaques, cholesterol crystals, calcified crystals, necrotic cores, fibrin, recent and old thrombi, platelets, macrophage foam cells, lipoid masses, and acellular material. Figure 15-10 shows the images of the debris at electronic microscope and Figure 15-11 the distribution of particles for two patients.

1. Five neurological complications occurred (1.9%), including:

 (a) Four periprocedural complications (1.5%):

 ■ One amaurosis fugax in a symptomatic patient having a tight ulcerated right ICA stenosis after a Wallstent acute thrombosis during the procedure.

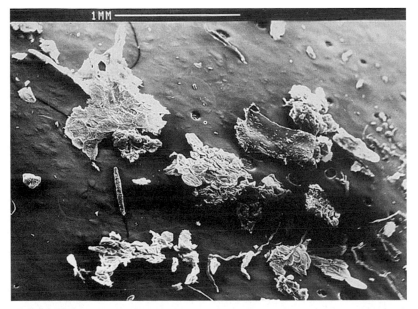

FIGURE 15-10. Debris retrieved with aspiration catheter. Electronic microscope examination.

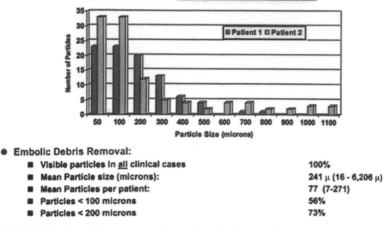

- ● Embolic Debris Removal:
  - ■ Visible particles in <u>all</u> clinical cases   100%
  - ■ Mean Particle size (microns):   241 μ (16 - 6,206 μ)
  - ■ Mean Particles per patient: 77 (7-271)
  - ■ Particles < 100 microns   56%
  - ■ Particles < 200 microns   73%

FIGURE 15-11. Distribution of debris retrieved with aspiration catheter in two patients.

The thrombosis was seen on the angiogram after occlusion balloon deflation. The balloon was quickly reinflated and abciximab injected (bolus of 0.25 mg per kg intravenously and 10 μg per mg continuous infusion for 12 hours thereafter). Thromboaspiration and flushing through the guide catheter were performed 10 minutes later and the protection balloon finally deflated. The final angiogram showed no residual thrombus inside the stent. Nevertheless, the patient developed amaurosis, which was probably the consequence of an embolism from the ECA through an ECA–ophthalmic artery communication. Indeed, a communication between the ECA and the ophthalmic circulation was noted after careful angiographic inspection.

A total of three transient ischemic attacks (TIAs) occurred:

- ■ One TIA with transient hemiparesis after a procedure of CAS for a tight asymptomatic left ICA stenosis in a patient who had a prolonged occlusion time (19 minutes). No evidence of ischemia was detected on subsequent serial CT examinations.
- ■ Two TIAs with brachial monoparesis, without sign of ischemia on CT scan examination.

(b) One intracerebral hemorrhage with hemiplegia on the third day after a CAS procedure under abciximab (same protocol as previously described) in a patient having a symptomatic subocclusion of the right ICA. He partially recovered 2 months later.

2. Cardiac events (0.4%) :

- ■ One symptomatic patient died from cardiac failure 3 weeks after the CAS procedure. No MI occurred during the hospital period or in the 30 days after CAS.

3. The overall 30-day incidence of neurological complications and death was 2.5% (amaurosis: 0.8%, TIA: 1.3%, and death: 0.4%).
4. No episode of cranial nerve palsy occurred.

FOLLOW-UP

At a mean follow-up of 23 ± 12 months (range 1–46 months), four deaths occurred: one patient died from a major stroke located at the contralateral side of the previously treated

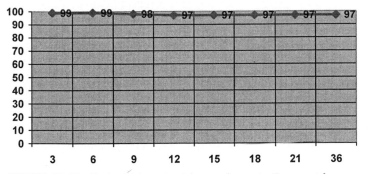

FIGURE 15-12. Kaplan-Meier actuarial curve demonstrating event-free survival (myocardial infarction, any stroke, death).

ICA at 6 months, two other patients died from myocardial infarction, and one patient died from cancer. No minor or major stroke occurred during the follow-up period. One asymptomatic restenosis was observed at 6 months and was treated successfully by balloon angioplasty. The event-free survival was 97% at 36 months (Fig. 15-12).

CLINICAL AND TECHNICAL IMPLICATIONS

The frequency of debris migration and distal embolism has been demonstrated by *ex vivo* human carotid stenting techniques (45) and confirmed by clinical studies (12,46–48). The number of embolic particles generated by percutaneous techniques seems to exceed that of endarterectomy (43,45,46). Although their clinical significance has not been documented yet (46,49), their presence could not have any beneficial effect on the brain. Furthermore, the minimum particle size capable of producing ischemic events has not been determined. Various patient and plaque characteristics have been suggested as predictors of debris generation and embolic events (36,45,50) to define high-risk groups for CAS procedures. In our study, debris was extracted from all patients, even in lesions that theoretically are thought to be at low risk for cerebral embolism (restenosis, echogenic plaques, concentric lesions), suggesting that the risk of embolization is independent of the nature of the plaques. Additionally, stent deployment does not provide sufficient protection against embolic plaque debris migration. In all series of CAS, embolic risk exists regardless of the implantation techniques and the stent characteristics. Manninen et al. (50) compared endovascular stent placement with percutaneous transluminal angioplasty (PTA) of carotid arteries in cadavers *in situ* and found no difference with respect to distal embolization.

Vitek et al. (51), in 1984, first reported a case of successful innominate artery angioplasty where the risk of cerebral embolization was reduced by temporary occlusion of the origin of the right CCA with a second balloon catheter. In the last decade, as a testimony to suboptimal results and the need for embolic risk elimination, several Anti-Embolization strategies during CAS have been proposed (52,53).

The GuardWire system was first tested in animals by Oesterle et al. (54), followed by clinical use (55) in 27 coronary interventions on saphenous vein grafts. It has been shown that the system was compatible with routine angioplasty procedures, capable of containing and retrieving atherosclerotic debris, and might aid in the prevention of distal embolization. The device has been proposed for cerebral protection during CAS. One of its advantages is that it behaves similar to the steerable coronary guide wires, allowing crossing of the stenosis easily and decreasing technical failures. We have encountered only two failures (0.8%) in crossing tight calcified stenoses in tortuous CCA and ICA. The Anti-Embolization device can be placed before stent placement in the majority of the cases. We do not recommend placement of the protection device after stent placement to avoid higher risk of embolism.

In case of failure of crossing the lesion, a predilatation can be done with a small coronary balloon before placing the protection balloon to facilitate the passage of the GuardWire. Additionally, the GuardWire provides sufficient support to advance the dilation balloon and the stent. The deflation time of the occlusion balloon is fast and lasts approximately 15 seconds.

LIMITATIONS OF THE TECHNIQUE

CAS with the distal occlusion Anti-Embolization is a feasible and safe procedure with very low 30-day neurological complication rates (1.9%). These results are favorable when compared with series using unprotected techniques (16,18,21,23,24,49,56,57) and historical surgical controls. Roubin (58) recently published favorable results from a single-center experience. In a series of 329 procedures performed under protection (232 with the GuardWire), the embolic events rate was 3%. Schlueter et al. (59) also showed the efficacy of this protection. In a series of 103 procedures, there were five (4.9%) periprocedural events, one minor stroke, and four TIAs, but there were only three TIAs (3%) among the 99 patients with successful deployment of the device. The major periprocedural neurological complications were encountered in two of these four failures of device deployment.

But cerebral protection cannot prevent all plaque debris embolization, and embolic events may still occur during all steps of the procedure. The occlusion balloon Anti-Embolization device offers protection against embolism only after the lesion has been crossed by the wire. This maneuver, as well the initial positioning of the guide catheter in the CCA, is also capable of releasing embolic material. Utilization of smaller tools and adaptation of coronary techniques may limit the risks and provide better outcomes.

Recently, Mathias and Jaeger conducted a very interesting study (48). They studied 70 CAS procedures without Anti-Embolization and 102 CAS with Anti-Embolization (GuardWire in 78%, AngioGuard filter in 22%) with transcranial Doppler monitoring (TCD) during the procedure and with magnetic resonance imaging (MRI) of the brain before and 24 hours after CAS. With TCD, the number of microembolic signals (MESs) for the patients was calculated during the different steps of carotid angioplasty (Table 15-1). Despite Anti-Embolization, emboli were registered, but the number of MESs was

TABLE 15-1. TRANSCRANIAL DOPPLER: NUMBER OF MES PER PATIENT DURING THE DIFFERENT STEPS OF CAROTID ANGIOPLASTY AND STENTING

	Unprotected	Protected
Probing of CCA	3	2
Introduction of long sheath	7	7
Passage of stenosis	9	3
Predilatation	78	9
Stent placement	89	8
In-stent dilatation	146	11

MES, microembolic signals; CCA, common carotid artery.

TABLE 15-2. MAGNETIC RESONANCE IMAGING AND CLINICAL OUTCOME

	Unprotected	Protected
New signal-intense lesions	28.5%	8.2%
TIAs	6.8%	3.2%
Minor stroke	2.2%	1.9%
Major stroke	1.3%	0%

TIA, transient ischemic attack.

much higher without protection, and the more critical step for brain embolism is predilatation, stent placement, and in-stent dilatation. With MRI, Mathias and Jaeger noticed that new signal intense lesions are more frequent with unprotected angioplasties (28.5% versus 8.2%) (Table 15-2).

Al Mubarak et al. (47) have recently published similar results with a greater number of emboli in the control group of patients treated without protection (Table 15-3). Using this Anti-Embolization strategy during CAS, the blood flow must be totally interrupted and diverted towards the ECA. Particles of all sizes are blocked in the ICA. The operator needs to be aware of potential problems during the application of this technique (Fig. 15-13):

1. The occlusion balloon may deflate or might become nonocclusive during the procedure, sometimes only during the systole or after dilatation of the stenosis (the diameter of the artery can increase owing to the improved flow). Some particles can still migrate to the brain. It is very important to ascertain a complete occlusion of the ICA using a contrast injection after inflation of the occlusion balloon and prior to the intervention. If difficulties in interrupting the flow within the ICA are encountered, it is better to place the balloon high in the ICA at the base of the skull.
2. Some particles could be too large for suction (very rare).
3. A shadow zone exists below the inflated balloon and some particles, trapped at this part, may be difficult or impossible to aspirate with the aspiration catheter. These particles may migrate to the brain when the balloon is deflated. In this case, saline flushing of this area with the aspiration catheter may be useful to clean up this shadow zone.
4. During ICA balloon occlusion, blood flow is diverted to the ECA with the potential for cerebral and retinal embolization through the large collateral (to midcerebral artery and vertebral artery). Collateral circulation exists between the ECA and ICA through the ophthalmic artery, ascending pharyngeal artery, internal maxillary artery, and between the ECA and vertebral artery through occipital and ascending pharyngeal arteries. So

TABLE 15-3. MEAN DENSITY VALUE

	Control 39 Cases	GuardWire 37 Cases	p Value
Sheath/wire	31 ± 24	38 ± 29	NS
Predilatation	33 ± 36	12 ± 31	0.001
Stent	75 ± 57	17 ± 22	0.004
Postdilatation	27 ± 26	5 ± 9	0.002
GuardWire deflation	NA	17 ± 21	
Total (mean $\pm$ SD)	164 ± 108	68 ± 83	0.002

NA, not applicable; NS, not significant.

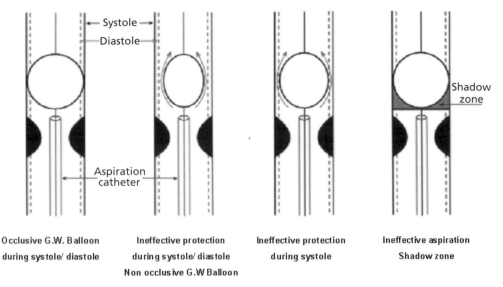

FIGURE 15-13. Carotid angioplasty and stenting under protection: risk of embolization with protection balloon.

this risk of brain embolism due to this collateral circulation must be well known, and it is important to have a good cerebral angiography prior to the procedure to identify this collateral circulation, and, in that case, a different protection strategy should be envisaged (filter or reversal flow). This complication has been well described recently by Al-Mubarak et al. (47).

Cerebral protection cannot prevent late embolic phenomenon. Approximately 30% of late TIAs occurred between 2 and 10 days after the procedure, and 30% of the minor strokes occurred 4 to 10 days after stent placement (24). These late TIAs and minor strokes may have been related to dislodged plaque and/or thrombus from between the stent struts or adjacent to the stent. These events represent a delayed embolic phenomenon described recently by Wholey et al. (24) in a series of 472 angioplasty procedures performed without protection and by Qureshi et al. (60). Mehran et al. (61) recently reported the results of the CAFE USA Trial, a prospective multicenter registry (seven centers). In this series of 212 procedures, the device was successfully placed in 97% of the cases, and only 3 (1.4%) intraprocedural strokes were described, showing the efficacy of the GuardWire. However, during the first 30 days, there were three deaths (1.4%), of which two were neurologic, 11 (5.2%) minor strokes, and 5 (2.4%) TIAs, but no major stroke. The mean time to neurologic event was 5.0 ± 1.2 hours, considerably delayed when compared with other experiences. We have never seen these late neurological complications in our series. We think that a meticulous aspiration with the aspiration catheter is an important technical point to eliminate the remaining particles after angioplasty and stenting and to avoid neurological complications. A strict monitoring of blood pressure and heart rate is also very important. Some patients are at higher risk: those of advanced age and patients with prior history of stroke, high grade stenosis, and echolucent plaques. The use of glycoprotein (GP) IIB/IIIA inhibitors (61) and final activated clotting time (ACT) are factors as well. The learning curve also plays an important role, as pointed out by Ahmadi et al. (62) in their series of 320 procedures. The 30-day complication rate was 15% for the first 80 procedures and only 5% for the others.

Cerebral protection also cannot prevent a brain hemorrhage, which can appear after the procedure and is encountered in most of the published series (23,24,60,63–65). Most of the time, it is a catastrophic event with a poor prognosis that can appear despite blood pressure control and can be due to cerebral hyperperfusion following successful angioplasty and stenting. This syndrome is thought to be a failure of normal cerebral autoregulation of blood flow secondary to long-standing decreased perfusion pressure (63). Several factors may favor this hyperperfusion syndrome: severe ipsilateral stenosis more than or equal to 90%, impaired collateral blood flow secondary to advanced occlusive disease in other extracranial cerebral vessels or an incomplete circle of Willis, perioperative hypertension, and the use of antiplatelet agents or other type of anticoagulation (24,63).

Fibrinolytic agents may favor a brain hemorrhage. Despite their marginal success (about 40% of the cases), they are the appropriate treatment in catastrophic events with angiographic evidence of occlusion (24), which are, in general, due to large plaque-like emboli. These plaques are not effectively dissolved by thrombolytic agents, which reinforces the need for distal protection devices during carotid stenting.

Some complications may also appear with these protection devices. A spasm may be seen at the site of the protection balloon, easily solved with antispasmodic drugs. A dissection of the ICA due to protection balloon with occlusion of the artery has been described by Castriota et al. (66). This complication should be very rare with the balloon being inflated at very low pressure.

TOLERANCE OF OCCLUSION

Before the procedure, complete angiographic assessment of the four supraaortic vessels is mandatory to determine the adequacy of the collateral flow supply through the circle of Willis, the vertebrobasilar artery, and contralateral carotid artery. Patients with congenital absence or acquired disease of these structures may not tolerate flow occlusion. This problem is similar but not identical to the surgical clamping during carotid endarterectomy because flow through the ECA is unaffected with an occlusion balloon. This vessel also provides collateral flow to both the anterior and posterior cerebral circulation, useful when the ICA is occluded but potentially harmful in cases in which flushing is used to clean the treated area. In this study, occlusion of the ICA was well tolerated in the majority of cases. We had 11 intolerances (4.2%) but only two complete major intolerances (rapid development of symptoms immediately after flow interruption), in which cerebral protection was not used to complete the procedure.

More commonly, a delayed intolerance of brief duration started while the procedure was well advanced, usually after stent deployment and before debris aspiration. In these cases, the procedure could be completed with aspiration and reestablishment of the cerebral flow, thus maintaining the benefits of the protection. We have to notice the small number of intolerance despite the fact that 48 patients had a significant contralateral ICA stenosis and 14 a contralateral ICA occlusion. Mehran et al. reported an intolerance rate of 8% (61).

FLUSHING

After aspiration, some debris could remain in the treated area. Flushing has been proposed to clean up this area. However, this technique may lead to ischemic complications in cases of collateral circulation, as previously described (76). A diagnostic angiography prior to

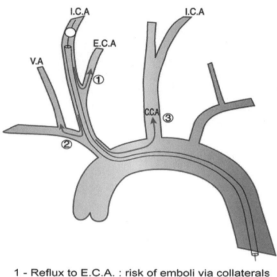

1 - Reflux to E.C.A. : risk of emboli via collaterals
2 - Risk of reflux to ipsilateral V.A.
3 - Risk of reflux to contralateral C.C.A.

FIGURE 15-14. Carotid angioplasty and stenting under protection with distal-balloon protection: risks during flushing.

treatment is mandatory for diagnosis of these particulars, which suggests ruling out the flushing step and restricting the debris removal to aspiration. In our series, one neurological complication (amaurosis) appeared after flushing. We abandoned the flushing maneuver after this occurrence. Flushing vigorously at high pressure during the cleaning procedures may lead to reflux to the origin of the CCA (more critical on the right side because the length of the CCA is usually shorter) and/or to the right vertebral artery with the risk of neurological deficit in this territory (Fig. 15-14). We now believe that a meticulous aspiration is sufficient to clean up the treated area in most of the cases. A flushing of the shadow zone could be discussed in some circumstances, particularly in patients with high risk of neurological complications.

PROCEDURAL CONSIDERATIONS AND LATE OUTCOME

The importance of pretreatment with aspirin and ticlopidine or clopidogrel, as well as its duration, in preventing complications seems critical but has not been proved. A randomized trial is needed to rigorously examine this issue. However, given the demonstrated importance of these agents in coronary stenting, such a trial seems unlikely to be undertaken. Abciximab has been proposed (71) as an adjunct therapy. Its potential benefit and indications remain to be evaluated. We think that this medication is indicated just in case of complications during the procedure.

In a select low surgical risk patient population randomized into NASCET and Asymptomatic Carotid Atherosclerosis Study (ACAS), relief of the carotid obstruction has been shown to reduce the risk of cerebrovascular events. Whether the relief of the obstruction in other patient groups with different baseline characteristics would have resulted in an identical treatment advantage is not known with certainty, nor is the relative effectiveness of CAS and CEA in preventing stroke and death in the high-risk patients. In the series by Shawl et al. (21), during the 19-month follow-up of patients there were very few neurological events, suggesting that the effectiveness of obstruction relief may well be reflected in long-term clinical benefit. In their series of 528 consecutive patients, Roubin et al. (23) described a 3-year freedom from ipsilateral or fatal stroke of 92 ± 1%, suggesting that carotid stenting may be comparable to surgery. The results of our CAS under cerebral protection series are similar and very promising (Fig. 15-12).

Randomized controlled trials of CEA versus CAS are now the next step in evaluating CAS. Until the results of these randomized trials are available, caution should be exercised in discarding CEA in patient groups in which it has been proven effective. One randomized trial, the Carotid and Vertebral Artery Transluminal Angioplasty Study (CAVATAS), which examined the role of angioplasty versus CEA, has been completed (27). This trial, although underpowered, suggested that balloon angioplasty without routine stenting has a similar safety profile to elective CEA. These data suggest that routine stent implantation will further improve the percutaneous management of carotid artery disease. Brooks et al. (28) also compared CAS and CEA in a randomized trial (104 symptomatic patients) and found that CAS is equivalent to surgery.

Other randomized trials that compare CEA and CAS, like the Carotid Revascularization Endarterectomy Trial (CREST), sponsored by the NIH, are planned (72). Unfortunately, the final results of CREST will not be available for at least 5 to 6 years. In the interim, there are sufficient published reports to support the use of CAS by experienced operators in patients known to be at high risk for CEA (16–18,20–25,49,56,57). Such procedures require an experienced team of neurologists and interventionists.

Patients at high risk for CEA include patients with carotid artery lesions above the C-2 or C-3 cervical vertebrae or at the ostium of the CCA and patients with cervical spine disease or fixation, previous radical neck dissection, fibromuscular dysplasia, previous cervical radiation, previous CEA, and the presence of important comorbid conditions, including unstable angina, recent MI, and severe congestive heart failure. In addition, there will be continuing evolution of new stents, dilation and postdilation strategies, and Anti-Embolization devices that will require evaluation (73).

CONCLUSION

CAS has been demonstrated as feasible and safe, even in high-risk patients with a complication rate comparable to that of patients in the ACAS and NASCET trials. CAS without Anti-Embolization is associated with a risk for brain embolism. The addition of the Anti-Embolization systems to CAS may reduce the associated embolic risk, expand the application to all cerebral angioplasty procedures, and might widen the scope of indications with complication rates that are comparable or even lower than those obtained with CEA, particularly in the high risk and elderly patients (74,75).

REFERENCES

1. *Heart and stroke facts: 1996 statistical supplement.* Dallas: American Heart Association, 1996.
2. Beneficial effect of carotid endarterectomy in symptomatic patients with high-grade carotid stenosis. North American Symptomatic Carotid Endarterectomy Trial collaborators. *N Engl J Med* 1991;325: 445–453.
3. MRC European Carotid Surgery Trial: Interim results for symptomatic patients with severe (70-90%) or with mild (0-29%) carotid stenosis. European Carotid Surgery Trialists' Collaborative Group. *Lancet* 1991;337:1235–1243.

4. Executive committee for the asymptomatic carotid atherosclerosis study: endarterectomy for asymptomatic carotid artery stenosis. *JAMA* 1995;273:1421–1428.

5. Graor RA, Hetzer NR. Management of coexistent carotid artery and coronary artery disease. *Stroke* 1988;23:19–23.

6. Newman DC, Hicks RG. Combined carotid and coronary artery surgery: a review of the literature. *Ann Thorac Sur* 1988;45:574–581.

7. Sundt TM, Jr, Meyer FB, Piepgras DG, et al. Risk factors and operative results. In: Meyer FB, ed. *Sundt's occlusive cerebrovascular disease*, 2nd ed. Philadelphia: W.B. Saunders, 1994:241–247.

8. Link MJ, Meyer FB, Cherry KJ, et al. Combined carotid and coronary revascularization. In: Meyer FB, ed. *Sundt's occlusive cerebrovascular disease*, 2nd ed. Philadelphia: W.B. Saunders, 1994:323–331.

9. Zierler RE, Brandyk DF, Thiele BL, et al. Carotid artery stenosis following endarterectomy. *Arch Surg* 1982;117:1408–1415.

10. Lusby RJ, Wylie EJ. Complications of carotid endarterectomy. *Surg Clin North Am* 1983;63: 1293–1301.

11. Winslow CM, Solomon DH, Chassin MR, et al. The appropriateness of carotid endarterectomy. *N Engl J Med* 1988;318:721–727.

12. Rothwell PM, Slattery J, Waslow CP. A systematic review of the risks of stroke or death due to endarterectomy for symptomatic carotid stenosis. *Stroke* 1996;27:260–265.

13. McCrory DC, Golstein LB, Samsa GP, et al. Predicting complications of carotid endarterectomy. *Stroke* 1993;24:1285–1291.

14. Gasecki AP, Eliasziw M, Ferguson GG, et al. Long-term prognosis and effect of endarterectomy in patients with symptomatic severe carotid stenosis and contralateral stenosis or occlusion: results from NASCET. North American Symptomatic Carotid Endarterectomy Trial (NASCET) Group. *J Neurosurg* 1995;83:778–782.

15. Das MB, Hertzer NR, Ratcliff J, et al. Recurrent carotid stenosis: a five year series of 65 operations. *Ann Surg* 1985;202:28–35.

16. Yadav JS, Roubin GS, Iyers SS, et al. Elective stenting of the extracranial carotid arteries. *Circulation* 1997;95:376–381.

17. Diethrich EB, Ndiaye M, Reid DB. Stenting in the carotid artery: initial experience in 110 patients. *J Endovasc Surg* 1996;3:42–46.

18. Roubin GS, Yadav S, Iyer SS, et al. Carotid stent-supported angioplasty: a neurovascular intervention to prevent stroke. *Am J Cardiol* 1996;78(Suppl 3A):8–12.

19. Henry M, Amor M, Masson I, et al. Angioplasty and stenting of the extracranial carotid arteries. *J Endovasc Surg* 1998;5:293–304.

20. Henry M, Amor M, Klonaris C, et al. Angioplasty and stenting of the extracranial carotid arteries. *Tex Heart Inst J* 2000;27:150–158.

21. Shawl F, Kadro W, Domanski MJ, et al. Safety and efficacy of elective carotid artery stenting in high-risk patients. *J Am Coll Cardiol* 2000;35:1721–1728.

22. Henry M, Amor M, Masson I, et al. Endovascular treatment of atherosclerotic stenosis of the internal carotid artery. *J Cardiovasc Surg* 1998;39(Suppl 1):141–150.

23. Roubin GS, New G, Iyer S, et al. Immediate and late clinical outcomes of carotid artery stenting in patients with symptomatic and asymptomatic carotid artery stenosis. *Circulation* 2001;103:532–537.

24. Wholey MH, Wholey MH, Tan WA, et al. Management of neurological complication of carotid artery stenting. *J Endovasc Ther* 2001;8:341–353.

25. Cremonesi A, Castriota F, Manetti R, et al. Endovascular treatment of carotid atherosclerotic disease: early and late outcome in a non selected population. *Ital Heart J* 2000;1:801–809.

26. Gupta A, Bhatia A, Ahuja A, et al. Carotid stenting in patients older than 65 years with inoperable carotid artery disease: a single-center experience. *Catheter Cardiovasc Interv* 2000;50:1–8.

27. Endovascular versus surgical treatment in patients with carotid stenosis in the Carotid and Vertebral Artery Transluminal Angioplasty Study (CAVATAS): a randomised trial. *Lancet* 2001;357:1729–1737.

28. Brooks WH, McClure RR, Jones MR. Carotid angioplasty and stenting versus carotid endarterectomy: randomized trial in a community hospital. *J Am Coll Cardiol* 2001;38:1589–1595.

29. Henry M, Amor M, Henry I, et al. Carotid stenting with cerebral protection: first clinical experience using the PercuSurge GuardWire system. *J Endovasc Surg* 1999;6:321–331.

30. Henry M, Henry I, Klonaris C, et al. Benefits of cerebral protection during carotid stenting with the PercuSurge GuardWire system: mid term results. *J Endovasc Ther* 2002;9:1–13.

31. Theron J, Payelle G, Coskun O, et al. Carotid artery stenosis: treatment with protected balloon angioplasty and stent placement. *Radiology* 1996;201:627–636.

32. Parodi JC, Lamura R, Ferreira LM, et al. Initial evaluation of carotid angioplasty and stenting with three different cerebral protection devices. *J Vasc Surg* 2000;32:1127–1136.

33. Orgogozo JM, Calpideo R, Anagnostou CN, et al. Mise au point d'un score neurologique pour l'évaluation clinique des infarctus sylviens. *Presse Med* 1983;12:3039–3044.

34. Biasi GM, Mingazzini PM, Baronio L, et al. Carotid plaque characterization using digital image processing and its potential in future studies of carotid endarterectomy and angioplasty. *J Endovasc Surg* 1998;5:240–246.

35. Biasi GM, Sampaolo A, Mingazzini P, et al. Computer analysis of ultrasonic plaque echolucency in identifying high risk carotid bifurcation lesions. *Eur J Vasc Endovasc Surg* 1999;17:476–479.

36. Biasi GM, Ferrari SA, Nicoläides AN, et al. The ICAROS Registry of carotid artery stenting. *J Endovasc Ther* 2001;8:46–53.

37. Benefit of carotid endarterectomy in patients with symptomatic moderate or severe stenosis. North American Symptomatic Carotid Endarterectomy Trial Collaborators. *N Engl J Med* 1998;339:1415–1425.

38. European Carotid Surgery Trialists Collaborative Group. Randomized trial of endarterectomy for recently symptomatic carotid stenosis: final results of the MRC European Carotid Study Trial (ECST). *Lancet* 1998;351:1379–1387.

39. Ouriel K, Hertzer NR, Beven EG, et al. Preprocedural risk stratification: identifying an appropriate population for carotid stenting. *J Vasc Surg* 2001;33:728–732.

40. Grotta J. Elective stenting of extracranial carotid arteries. *Circulation* 1997;95:303–305.

41. Bergeron P, Chambran P, Bianca S. Traitement endovasculaire des artères à destinée cérébrale: échecs et limites. *J Mal Vasc* 1996;21:123–131.

42. Bergeron P, Chambran P, Hartung O, et al. Cervical carotid artery stenosis: which technique, balloon angioplasty or surgery? *J Cardiovasc Surg* 1996;37(Suppl 15):73–75.

43. Gil Peralta A, Mayol A, Gonzalez M Jr, et al. Percutaneous transluminal angioplasty of the symptomatic atherosclerotic carotid arteries. Results, complications, and follow-up. *Stroke* 1996;27:2271–2273.

44. Wholey MH, Wholey M, Jarmolowsi CR, et al. Endovascular stents for carotid occlusive disease. *J Endovasc Surg* 1997;4:326–338.

45. Ohki T, Marin ML, Lyon RT, et al. Ex vivo human carotid artery bifurcation stenting: correlation of lesion characteristics with embolic potential. *J Vasc Surg* 1998;27:463–471.

46. Jordan WD, Voellinger DC, Doblar DD, t al. Microemboli detected by transcranial Doppler monitoring in patients during carotid angioplasty versus carotid endarterectomy. *Cardiovasc Surg* 1999;7:33–38.

47. Al-Mubarak N, Roubin GS, Vitek JJ, et al. Effect of the distal-balloon protection system on microembolization during carotid stenting. *Circulation* 2001;104:1999–2002.

48. Mathias K, Jaeger M. How much cerebral embolization occurs during CAS? Presented at: International Symposium on Endovascular Therapy; 2001; Miami, Florida:73–75.

49. Mathur A, Roubin GS, Iyer SS, et al. Predictors of stroke complicating carotid artery stenting. *Circulation* 1988;97:1239–1245.

50. Manninen HI, Rasanen HT, Vanninen RL, et al. Stent placement versus percutaneous transluminal angioplasty of human carotid arteries in cadavers in situ: distal embolization and findings at intravascular US, MR imaging and histopathologic analysis. *Radiology* 1999;212:483–492.

51. Vitek JJ, Raymon BC, Oh SJ. Innominate artery angioplasty. *AJNR Am J Neuroradiol* 1984;5:113–114.

52. Kachel R. Results of balloon angioplasty in the carotid arteries. *J Endovasc Surg* 1996;3:22–30.

53. Theron J. Angioplastie carotidienne protégée et stents carotidiens. *J Mal Vasc* 1996;21:113–122.

54. Oesterle SN, Hayase M, Baim DS, et al. An embolization containment device. *Catheter Cardiovasc Interv* 1999;47:243–250.

55. Webb JG, Carere RG, Virmani R, et al. Retrieval and analysis of particulate debris after saphenous vein graft intervention. *J Am Coll Cardiol* 1999;34:468–475.

56. Shawl FA, Efstratiou A, Hoff S, et al. Combined percutaneous carotid stenting and coronary angioplasty during acute ischemic neurologic and coronary syndromes. *Am J Cardiol* 1996;77:1109–1112.

57. Wholey MH, Al-Mubarak N, Wholey MH. Updated review of the global carotid artery stent registry. *Catheter Cardiovasc Interv* 2003;60:259–266.

58. Roubin GS. Carotid angioplasty and stenting under cerebral protection: the standard of care. Presented at: International Congress XV; February 11–14, 2002; Scottsdale, Arizona.

59. Schlueter M., Tuebler T, Haufe M, et al. Single-center experience with balloon protected carotid artery stenting in 98 patients. Presented at: American Heart Association Meeting; November 12, 2001; Anaheim, California.

60. Qureshi AI, Luft AR, Janardhan V, et al. Identification of patients at risk for periprocedural neurological deficits associated with carotid angioplasty and stenting. *Stroke* 2000;31:376–382.

61. Mehran R, Roubin GS, New G, et al. Neurologic events after carotid stenting with distal protection using an occlusion balloon: final results from the CAFE USA Trial. Presented at: American Heart Association Meeting; November 12, 2001; Anaheim, California.
62. Ahmadi R, Willfort A, Lang W, et al. Carotid artery stenting: effects of learning curve and intermediate-term morphological outcome. *J Endovasc Ther* 2001;8:539–546.
63. Meyers PM, Higashida RT, Phatouros CC, et al. Cerebral hyperperfusion syndrome after percutaneous transluminal stenting of the craniocervical arteries. *Neurosurgery* 2000;47:335–345.
64. McCabe DJ, Brown MM, Clifton A. Fatal cerebral reperfusion hemorrhage after carotid stenting. *Stroke* 1999;30:2483–2486.
65. Al-Mubarak N, Roubin GS, Vitek JJ et al. Subarachnoidal hemorrhage following carotid stenting with the distal balloon protection. *Catheter Cardiovasc Interv* 2001;54:521–523.
66. Castriota F, Cremonesi A, Manetti R, et al. Carotid angioplasty and stenting with and without cerebral protection: single-center experience in 275 consecutive patients. Presented at: International Congress XV; February 11–14, 2002; Scottsdale, Arizona.
67. Ohki T, Veith FJ. Carotid stenting with and without protection devices: should protection be useful in all patients? *Sem Vasc Surg* 2000;13:144–152.
68. Ohki T, Roubin GS, Veith FJ, et al. Efficacy of a filter device in the prevention of embolic events during carotid angioplasty and stenting. An ex vivo analysis. *J Vasc Surg* 1999;30:1034–1044.
69. Reimers B, Corvaja N, Moshiri S, et al. Cerebral protection with filter devices during carotid artery stenting. *Circulation* 2001;104:12–15.
70. Angelini A, Reimers B, Della Barbera M, et al. Embolized debris during carotid artery stenting with cerebral protection device: an histopathologic survey. Presented at: American Heart Association Meeting; November 13, 2001; Anaheim, California.
71. Bhatt DL, Kapadia SR, Yadav JS, et al. Update on clinical trials of antiplatelet therapy for cerebrovascular diseases. *Cerebrovasc Dis* 2000;10(Suppl 5):34–40.
72. Hobson RW 2nd, Brott T, Ferguson R, et al. CREST: carotid revascularization endarterectomy versus stent trial. *Cardiovasc Surg* 1997;5:457–458.
73. Hanley HG, Sheridan FM, Rivera E. Carotid stenting: a technology in evolution. *J La State Med Soc* 2000;152:235–238.
74. Reimers B, Castriota F, Corvaja N, et al. Carotid artery stent implantation with cerebral protection: a multicenter experience of 320 procedures. *J Am Coll Cardiol* 2002;39(Suppl A):30A.
75. Brennan C, Roubin GS, Iyer S, et al. Neuroprotection reduces the risk of peri-procedural major strokes and death in octogenarians. *J Am Coll Cardiol* 2002;39(Suppl A):66A.
76. Al-Mubarak N, Vitek JJ, Iyer S, et al. Embolization via collateral circulation during carotid stenting with the distal balloon protection system. *J Endovasc Ther* 2001;8:354–357.

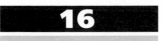

INTRAVASCULAR FILTER ANTI-EMBOLIZATION SYSTEMS

GORAN STANKOVIC
ANTONIO COLOMBO

In recent years, we have witnessed the rapid evolution of endovascular therapy for several vascular diseases where previously surgery was the only available treatment (1–6). As a result, interventional revascularization procedures of the brachiocephalic vasculature have been developed as an alternative to medical and surgical treatment (7–31).

However, there have been concerns regarding the safety of such interventions because of the associated risk of cerebral embolization (32–34). The observation of surgical specimens of the carotid bifurcation showed that at this location, the atherosclerotic plaque is often fragile, ulcerated, and hemorrhagic, implicating high risk for embolization (35). Not surprisingly, in many of the earlier trials, the perioperative stroke and death rates remained higher than those for carotid endarterectomy (CEA) (8,9,11–13,36). One randomized trial, comparing carotid angioplasty with CEA for symptomatic severe internal carotid artery (ICA) disease, was aborted after enrolling only 17 patients because of the unacceptably high stroke and death rates following angioplasty (71%) compared to CEA (0%) (37). It is, however, important to point out that those patients were treated by an interventionist with limited experience in carotid intervention, and the required antiplatelet therapy was inadequate by today's standards. Less discouraging are the results from the recently published Carotid And Vertebral Artery Transluminal Angioplasty Study (CAVATAS) (38), which randomized 504 patients with symptomatic carotid stenosis to either balloon angioplasty (bail-out stenting was performed in 26%) or CEA. CAVATAS demonstrated equal benefit for prevention of stroke and death in both groups at 30 days (incidence of any stroke lasting more than 7 days or death was 10%), which was sustained for 3 years. The authors of CAVATAS acknowledged that the results of balloon angioplasty would be out of date when their study was published, as carotid stenting has emerged in the past few years as the preferred method.

In 1998, one of the largest early series of carotid artery stenting (CAS) (from 24 worldwide centers, with 2048 patients) reported a technical success rate of 98.6% with a combined periprocedural stroke and death rate of 5.77% (this rate varied from 0% to 10% from the various centers) (15). Most of the procedures were performed without the benefits of Anti-Embolization protection. The authors concluded that periprocedural risks of CAS, although high, are generally acceptable and within the American Heart Association guidelines for CEA: risks less than 6% for patients with transient ischemic attacks (TIAs) and less than 7% for patients with symptomatic strokes (3). An updated survey has recently been published (23). The survey collected outcomes of CAS in a total of 12,392 carotid stenting procedures involving 11,243 patients. The combined all-stroke and procedure-related death rates were 3.98% (23). Marked increase in the utilization of Anti-Embolization protection was observed. The authors pointed out early evidence favoring Anti-Embolization protection during CAS.

During CAS, embolic particles may be released at any stage of the procedure: placement of the guiding catheter in the common carotid artery, which is most of the time atheromatous; crossing of the lesion with the guidewire and placement of the balloon across the stenosis; dilatation of the lesion; and stent implantation, particularly during its postdilatation (39,40). However, it is also important to note that distal embolizations after the intervention is completed are relatively rare, and transcranial Doppler monitoring and diffusion-weighted magnetic resonance imaging (MRI) have shown that many emboli are asymptomatic (34,41). Therefore, the clinical significance of the number of embolic particles created during revascularization procedure is not completely elucidated, although there is some evidence that patients with higher numbers of particles generated during the intervention would have a higher periinterventional stroke rate than patients among whom fewer particles are produced (29,32,41,42). During the last several years, Anti-Embolization devices have been developed for the prevention of distal embolization during the carotid intervention. The beneficial use of such devices seems to be supported by a growing number of publications reporting a markedly low rate of neurological events or death. Kastrup et al. (43) presented a systematic review of a single-center CAS study with (839 patients) and without Anti-Embolization devices (2357 patients) and concluded that protection devices appear to reduce thromboembolic complications during CAS. The combined stroke and death rate within 30 days was 1.8% in patients treated with cerebral protection devices compared with 5.5% in patients treated without cerebral protection devices ($p < 0.001$). This effect was mainly due to a decrease in the occurrence of minor strokes (3.7% without cerebral protection versus 0.5% with cerebral protection; $p < 0.001$) and major strokes (1.1% without cerebral protection versus 0.3% with cerebral protection; $p < 0.05$), whereas the death rate was nearly identical (approximately 0.8%; $p = 0.6$). Cremonesi et al. also recently reported their single-center experience with protected CAS in 442 patients (44). The percutaneous procedure was successful in 440 of 442 patients (99.5%). Predilatation was necessary in 37% of patients before the protection device was placed. No periprocedural death occurred with any embolic protection device. The in-hospital and 30-day combined all-stroke and death rate was 1.1%. The overall complication rate was 3.4%. Major adverse events included one major stroke (0.2%), four intracranial hemorrhages (0.9%), one carotid artery wall fissuration (0.2%), and one diffuse cardioembolism (0.2%). Minor adverse events included four minor strokes (0.9%) and four TIAs (0.9%). A low number of technical complications (total 0.9%), such as dissection of the ICA (0.7%) or trapped guide wire needing surgical approach (0.2%), were observed, and all these events were clinically well tolerated. Transient loss of consciousness, tremors, and fasciculation were present in 6 of 40 patients (15%) in whom occlusive protection devices were used. Mathias presented at Advanced Endovascular Therapies 2003 his own data on 691 patients with 793 arteries treated with CAS from 1999 till 2002, using various protection devices. The technical failure rate for all protection devices was 4.3%. At 30 days, the total death and stroke rate was 1.7% (minor stroke 0.8%, major stroke 0.4%, cerebral hemorrhage 0.2%, mortality 0.2%). TIAs occurred in 2.1% of patients. Mathias also presented data from a large German CAS registry on 2385 patients from 38 institutions (45). CAS was successful in 97.8% of patients. Cerebral protection devices were used in 873 patients. Neurological complications occurred in 10.5% of patients with protection: amaurosis fugax 0.6%, TIA less than 10 minutes 4.5%, TIA more than 10 minutes 2.6%, prolonged reversible ischemic neurological deficit (PRIND) (more than 24 hours in duration compared to TIA) 1.1%, minor stroke 0.9%, and major stroke 0.9%. When all successful CAS interventions are analyzed, the rate of minor/major stroke was 2.0% in patients with cerebral protection and 2.8% in patients without protection, a significant 30% reduction in the incidence. In the same period, the incidence of death and stroke was 2.4% in the German registry of more than 40,000 CEA procedures.

FILTER ANTI-EMBOLIZATION SYSTEMS

Anti-Embolization devices are classified in two major categories: (a) occlusion systems, distal and proximal (46–51), and (b) the filter-based devices. The occlusion systems have been discussed in the previous chapters. This chapter will discuss the technical application of the intravascular filter Anti-Embolization protection.

Recently, a variety of filter-based systems have been designed to capture and remove atheromatous debris released during percutaneous interventions in the carotid arteries. In contrast to the balloon-based protection system, filters can prevent embolic events without interrupting blood flow distally. Another important advantage of the filters is the ability to perform angiography during the procedure and therefore verify stent position prior to its final deployment. The main disadvantage of the filter systems is the pore-size dependence in their efficacy to capture released emboli with the possibility of missing particles that are smaller than the filter pores. Additionally, the relatively large crossing profiles may result in difficulties crossing very severe lesions or tortuous vessels, potentially causing spasm and dissection in the distal ICA (26).

All filters basically consist of three components: (a) a guide wire with a filter at its distal end, (b) delivery catheter, and (c) retrieval catheter. The basic technical application of these filters is identical in almost all systems. After preshaping the tip of the guide wire, the delivery catheter is introduced and gently advanced across the lesion such that the filter can be deployed at least 2 cm distal to the target lesion. The filter is deployed by withdrawal of the delivery catheter and its position verified by contrast injection. The same guide wire is then used to deliver balloon catheters and stents to the target lesion. Following treatment, the retrieval catheter is advanced towards the filter until the distal end of the catheter completely envelops the filter. Thereafter, the retrieval catheter with its content is withdrawn. Currently, there are several protection devices with different characteristics. An ideal protection device should combine several characteristics. First, the guide wire placement has to be performed easily, and the device needs to be flexible and deliverable. The protection device should have low profile for passage and for safe withdrawal through the stented segment. Most importantly, these devices need to be effective in capturing embolic matter without inducing obstruction of the distal flow. The goal of distal perfusion with optimal protection has not been yet accomplished, as incomplete capture and retrieval of debris cannot be excluded. The devices must not induce more complications than they prevent. They should not cause distal embolization during the crossing process of the target lesion and should be able to capture most of the particles. The specific features of the different filter devices that are currently available are demonstrated in Table 16-1.

THE ANGIOGUARD XP SYSTEM

The system consists of a filter, a deployment sheath, a capture sheath, one torque device, and one peel-away (Cordis, Warren, NJ). The filter is fixed on a 0.014-inch guide wire and is designed as a basket made of polyurethane (with the pore size of 100 μm) and eight nitinol struts (four of them have radiopaque markers) (Fig. 16-1). The length of the filter is 4.11 to 6.91 mm and is available in diameters from 4.0 to 8.0 mm (with 1 mm increases).

TABLE 16-1. FEATURES OF DIFFERENT PROTECTION DEVICES

Device	Pore Size (μm)	Crossing Profile (inches)	Capture Sheath Profile (inches)	Diameters Available (mm)
AngioGuard XP	100	0.042–0.052	0.066	4–8
MedNova III	120	0.048	0.096	4–6
MedNova IV	120	0.037	0.084	3–7
Boston Scientific Filter Wire	110	0.049	0.049	One size fits 3.5–5.5
Medtronic AVE	100	0.039	0.039	3.5–5.5
Guidant AccuNet	115	0.045–0.048	0.071	4.5–7.5
Microvena TRAP	200	0.037	0.066–0.078	2.5–7.5
ev3 Spider	80	0.038	0.054–0.063	3–7
PercuSurge	NA	0.028–0.036	0.042–0.070	3–6

NA, not applicable.

The crossing profile ranges from 3.2 French (for 4 mm filter diameter) to 3.9 French (for 8 mm filter diameter). The capture sheath has a crossing profile of 5F. The tip of the pod is very flexible in order to facilitate the passage through the implanted stent at the target lesion. A 6 French sheath or an 8F guiding catheter is used to deliver the filter. The delivery procedure is identical to the placement of the other filters. The main advantages of this system are longitudinal force, adequacy of basket volume, good visibility, and ease of use. As with most filter-based systems, the main disadvantage is difficulty in crossing tight or tortuous lesions, although this may be overcome by the upcoming improved generation.

THE MEDNOVA EMBOSHIELD PROTECTION SYSTEM

The MedNova EmboShield System (MedNova Ltd., Galway, Ireland) consists of an umbrella-like "floating basket" that in the early generation is mounted to the distal tip of the

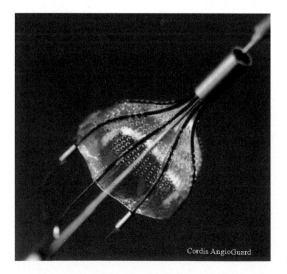

FIGURE 16-1. The AngioGuard XP System (Cordis Inc., Warren, NJ).

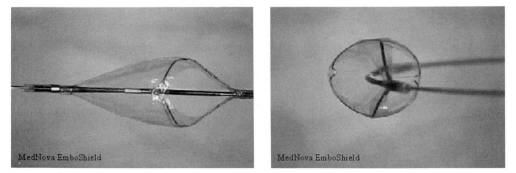

FIGURE 16-2. The MedNova NeuroShield System (MedNova Ltd., Galway, Ireland).

0.014-inch guide wire, and in the new generation is delivered to the desired segment after the lesion is crossed with a bare soft guide wire "over the wire." The filter is designed to conform well to vessel lumen and is made of polyurethane with a nonthrombotic hydrophilic coating, which has four proximal entry ports and multiple distal holes of 150 μm for the maintenance of distal perfusion (Fig. 16-2). The available filter sizes for Generation I and II are 4.0 to 6.0 mm (requires 4.5 French delivery catheters) and for Generation III 3.0 to 6.0 mm (requires 3 French delivery catheters). A monorail version has recently been developed. The filter contains a preshaped nitinol expansion system and is loaded into the delivery catheter. That system assists in filter deployment and apposition and improves fluoroscopic visualization. At the proximal end of the catheter, a strain relief collar is situated. The capture sheath has a filter retrieval pod at the distal end that facilitates expansion during the filter retrieval process. A 6 French guiding sheath or an 8F guiding catheter is required to advance this filter system. The wire tip is preshaped and loaded into the delivery catheter. The filter is then placed at least 2 cm distal to the lesion, and it is deployed by withdrawal of the delivery catheter. Importantly, independent wire movement is preserved. After the treatment, the retrieval catheter is advanced towards the filter until the distal retrieval pod fully envelops the filter. The filter with its content is then withdrawn. The main advantages of this system are: (a) the ability to cross the lesion with a bare guide wire prior to the filter delivery, improving the technical success even in the very severe and tortuous anatomy, (b) almost atraumatic passage of lesion allowed by the short and smooth transition from filter to nose cone, (c) complete withdrawal of filter into retrieval pod, and (d) the floating basket system, which allows wire reposition without filter movement, resulting in less distal vessel spasm.

THE FILTERWIRE EZ

The FilterWire EZ (Boston Scientific, Natick, MA) consists of a delivery catheter and a filter. The unique feature of the device is a modest off-center filter design attached to a guide wire (Fig. 16-3). This fact constitutes an improvement compared to the prior version, which was fully asymmetric. The "fish-mouth" filter opening design improves flexibility of this filter and allows a low crossing profile (3.5 French). The filter consists of polyurethane with distal pores of 80 μm in diameter. The system is manufactured in one size suitable for vessels of 3.5 to 5.5 mm in diameter and can be delivered through a 6 French guiding catheter. This adaptive property is due to a nitinol loop at the proximal end of the filter, which adapts to the vessel size during the expansion and provides complete circumferential

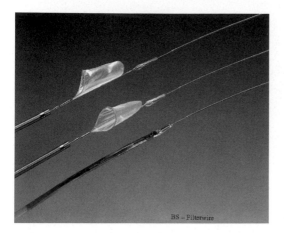

FIGURE 16-3. The Filter Wire EZ (Boston Scientific, Natick, MA).

contact with the arterial wall. Good flexibility enhances usage of this system in patients with severe disease and tortuous vessels. Other advantages of this device include the low crossing profile, the unimpeded entry of particles into the filter, and the ease of handling. The important characteristic is that this filter can be recaptured and retrieved using the standard peripheral balloon that is used for stent postdilatation. The delivery catheter (3.9F) is also used for retrieval of the filter. The main advantages of this system are ease of use, excellent visibility of nitinol loop, one-size-fits-all vessel sizes, and single deployment and capture catheter. The main disadvantages are: (a) limited range of vessel sizes in which device can be used, and (b) wire and sheath are side by side during crossing and tracking.

THE MICROVENA TRAP

The TRAP system (Microvena, White Bear Lake, MN) consists of a delivery and capture catheter and a filter. The 0.014-inch filter wire has a nitinol basket at its tip. The delivery catheter (3.5F) is delivered over an ordinary 0.014-inch guide wire. Thereafter, the guide wire is exchanged to the filter wire. This device has a low crossing profile (3.5F) and is designed as a nitinol wire woven basket on a 0.014-inch extra-support guide wire, with a polyurethane filter that allows normal blood flow to the distal vessel. The basket diameter varies between 2.5 and 7 mm. The advantages of the system are the low profile of the device, a retrieval mechanism that effectively prevents loss of captured particles, and the possibility to use the preferable guide wire. The main disadvantages are the crucial importance of precise system sizing and bulky retrieval catheter (6 French).

MEDTRONIC AVE CAROTID DISTAL PROTECTION DEVICE

The Medtronic AVE Carotid Distal Protection Device (DPD) (Medtronic, Santa Rosa, CA) is a self-expanding, braided nitinol filter with four proximal entry ports (approximately 80% of cross sectional area) and 100-μm distal pores. Large proximal ports and the tapered design allow emboli to enter the filter. The filter is available in a range of 3.5-mm to 6-mm diameters and is characterized by a low crossing profile (2.9 French) and 6 French guiding catheter

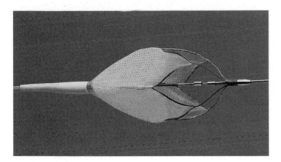

FIGURE 16-4. The AccuNet filter system (Guidant Co., Temecula, CA).

compatibility. The main disadvantages are average visibility of the filter and longer device length, which may preclude usage in distal lesions.

GUIDANT ACCUNET EMBOLIC PROTECTION SYSTEM

The AccuNet system (Guidant Co., Temecula, CA) consists of a filter, a delivery catheter, and a capture sheath. The filter uses a 0.014-inch ACS Hi-Torque Balance Heavyweight guide wire and is designed as a basket made of polyurethane (with the pore size of 120 μm) and six nitinol struts (Fig. 16-4). The system is available in diameters from 4.0 to 8.0 mm

THE SPIDER FILTER

The Spider filter (ev3, Plymouth, MN) is a nitinol filter design with a gold radiopaque proximal loop. The filter is structured on a delivery system over the wire system, which can be converted to a monorail system (Fig. 16-5).

IN VITRO AND CLINICAL EVALUATION OF FILTER DEVICES

Muller-Hulsbeck et al. (52) compared the effectiveness of five basic cerebral protection devices designed for carotid stenting in an *in vitro* bench-top model. Devices tested were:

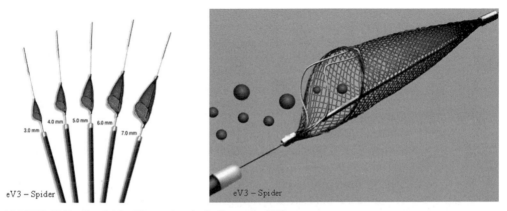

FIGURE 16-5. The Spider filter system (ev3, Plymouth, MN).

the AngioGuard, Filter Wire EX, TRAP, NeuroShield, and GuardWire Plus. For small, medium, and large particles, the lowest weight of emboli in the effluent of the ICA was obtained with the NeuroShield (0.28 mg, 0.18 mg, and 0.07 mg, respectively; $p<0.001$ compared to all other devices except the GuardWire for small particles only). The GuardWire had the highest embolization rate into the external carotid artery (ECA) for all particle sizes. Authors concluded that *in vitro*, none of the tested devices or modifications has the ability to prevent embolization completely, although the NeuroShield was the most effective for preventing particle embolization.

NONRANDOMIZED REGISTRIES OF FILTER ANTI-EMBOLIZATION

One of the first published clinical experiences of filter safety comes from a three-center registry by Reimers et al. (27) that included 84 patients with 86 lesions in the ICA (more than 70% diameter stenosis). Three different filter designs were used during carotid stenting: AngioGuard (n = 48), MedNova NeuroShield (n = 30), and Filter Wire EX filters (n = 8). The procedural success rate was 96.5%. In 53% of filters, macroscopic evidence of debris was found. Neurological complications during the first 30 days occurred in only one patient (1.2%). This patient suffered a minor stroke that resolved within 1 week. There were no major strokes. Two major adverse cardiac events (2.3%) occurred during the 30 days of follow-up. Al-Mubarak et al. (53) reported the results of CAS in 162 patients (164 lesions) using the MedNova NeuroShieldfilter device. Angiographic success was achieved in 162 of the procedures (99%), and filter placement was successful in 154 (94%) procedures. Carotid access was unsuccessful in two cases (1%) and filter placement in eight cases (5%).On an intention-to-treat basis, the overall combined 30-day rate of all-stroke and death was 2% (four events: two minor strokes and two deaths). This includes one minor stroke in a patient with failed filter placement and CAS completed without protection.The same type of filter device was also evaluated in a series of 50 consecutive patients (42 symptomatic) with internal carotid artery stenosis more than 70% (54). Procedural success was 100% for stenting and 98% for filter placement/retrieval. Nevertheless, at 30 days, the death and major disability from stroke rate was 4% (two patients). The AccuNet Distal Embolic Protection for Carotid Stenosis (ACCUNET) registry will evaluate procedural safety of the AccuNet embolic protection system in the ICA when used in conjunction with the AccuLink carotid stent system. Inclusion criteria are: discrete lesion in common carotid artery or ICA, stenosis more than or equal to 50% in symptomatic or more than or equal to 70% in asymptomatic patients, vessel diameter 4 to 9 mm, lesion length less than or equal to 32 mm, and 4 cm or more of straight segment in the distal ICA to allow device placement. Primary endpoints are: (a) acute device success and (b) composite of death, stroke, and myocardial infarction at 30 days. The AccuLink for Revascularization of Carotids in High Risk Patients (ARCHER) study will evaluate the safety and efficacy of the AccuLink carotid stent system in patients at high risk or unsuitable for CEA. Using similar inclusion criteria as the ACCUNET registry, a total of 513 patients were enrolled at 41 sites in North and South America. Clinical endpoints were composite of death, stroke, and myocardial infarction at 30 days and at 1 year. Preliminary 30-day results: AccuLink device success (successful stent placement and residual stenosis less than 50%) was achieved in 97.8% of patients and AccuNet success, defined as successful delivery/retrieval, was achieved in 92.7% of patients. Major adverse events at 30 days, defined as all-cause stroke, death, and myocardial infarction, are 7.8%. The ARCHER RX study started in May 2003 and utilizes Guidant's next-generation embolic protection device RX AccuNet and rapid exchange stent system RX AccuLink. By September

23, 2003, the study had enrolled 145 patients. Another trial comparing surgery versus carotid artery stentingwith cerebral protection is the Registry Study to Evaluate the NeuroShield Bare Wire Cerebral Protection System and XActStent in Patients at High Risk for CarotId Endarterectomy (SECURITY study). Between January 2002 and February 2003, 414 patients had been enrolled in this trial at 30 clinical sites. Inclusion criteria were patients at high risk for CEA based on comorbid and anatomical risk characteristics. Patients included in the study had to have symptomatic carotid stenosis *more than or equal to* 50% or asymptomatic carotid stenosis *more than or equal to* 80%, both measured by angiogram. The patients also had to have at least one other feature that would classify them as high risk. These criteria included: previous coronary artery bypass graft (CABG) with valve surgery within 30 days, unstable angina, EF less than 30%, need for dialysis because of renal failure, uncontrolled diabetes, restenosis after prior endarterectomy, or surgically inaccessible lesions. Overall stroke rate was 6.9% (minor stroke 4.6% and major stroke 2.3%), major stroke/ death 0.7%, other death 0.3%, and non-Q wave myocardial infarction 0.3%. The combined endpoint of myocardial infarction, any stroke, or death at 30 days was 7.2%.

RANDOMIZED CLINICAL TRIALS OF FILTER ANTI-EMBOLIZATION

Stenting and angioplasty with protection in patients at high risk for endarterectomy (SAPPHIRE) is a randomized multicenter trial comparing stenting with protection (Cordis PRECISE Nitinol Carotid Artery Stent with the AngioGuard XP distal protective device) to CEA in high-risk surgical patients with carotid artery disease. Inclusion criteria were: common carotid artery or ICA stenosis more than or equal to 50% in symptomatic or more than or equal to 80% in asymptomatic patients, vessel diameter 4 to 9 mm, and target lesion amenable to both CAS and CEA. Clinical endpoints are: (a) composite of major adverse events (MAE) comprising death, stroke, and myocardial infarction at 30 days, and (b) composite of 30-day MAE plus death and ipsilateral stroke between 30 days and 12 months. Twelve month results were presented by Yadav at TCT 2003. A total of 334 patients were randomized and 310 were treated (159 by CAS and 151 by CEA) at 29 participating centers. Owing to surgical refusal, 406 patients were enrolled in the stent registry, and owing to interventional refusal, 7 patients were enrolled in the surgical registry. The AngioGuard success (successful delivery and retrieval of the system) was achieved in 95.6% of the patients in the randomized stent population and 91.6% of the patients in the stent registry. Perioperative (30 days) stroke and death rates were 4.4% for CAS and 7.3% for CEA. The total major adverse event rate (death, any stroke, or myocardial infarction) for CEA was 12.6% and for CAS was 5.8%. Rates of myocardial infarction were 7.3% for CEA and 2.6% for CAS. At 12 months, the death rate was similar in CAS and CEA groups (6.9% versus 12.6%, $p = 0.12$), as well as the total stroke rate (5.7% versus 7.3%, $p = 0.65$), with a significantly lower rate of major ipsilateral stroke in CAS patients (0% versus 3.3%, $p = 0.03$). The incidence of myocardial infarctions (non-Q wave and Q wave) was also lower in CAS patients (2.5% versus 7.9%, $p = 0.04$). Cumulative incidence of major adverse events was also lower in CAS patients (11.9% versus 19.9%, $p = 0.048$). Authors concluded that stenting with emboli protection had superior 12-month event-free survival. In the Registry Stent patients, the incidence of major adverse events was 15.8% (death 10.1%, stroke 9.1%, and myocardial infarction 2.7%).

The AccuNet protection system will be utilized in the large (2,500 patients) multicenter Carotid Revascularization Endarterectomy Versus Stent Trial (CREST) (55,56). In the study, 2,500 patients will be randomized, giving researchers power to detect a greater than

1.2% per year absolute difference in primary end points. Eligible patients have had a TIA or nondisabling stroke in the past 180 days and have an ipsilateral carotid stenosis of more than or equal to 50% by angiography or more than or equal to 70% by ultrasound. Data from 441 patients enrolled in lead-in phases showed a 30-day stroke/death rate of 2% in asymptomatic and 5% in symptomatic patients.

CONCLUSION

Observational studies have provided evidence that percutaneous procedures in carotid arteries performed with Anti-Embolization protection are safe and effective compared to historical controls. Although there are still no published randomized trials supporting this statement, all registries evaluating distal protection devices demonstrated that in the majority of patients treated, debris was retrieved following stent implantation. However, there are several issues that remain to be addressed. In the following years, currently ongoing large clinical trials will provide a clear picture regarding the role of Anti-Embolization during percutaneous carotid interventions and answer the questions raised in this review.

REFERENCES

1. Beneficial effect of carotid endarterectomy in symptomatic patients with high-grade carotid stenosis. North American Symptomatic Carotid Endarterectomy Trial Collaborators. *N Engl J Med* 1991;325: 445–453.
2. Hobson RW 2nd, Weiss DG, Fields WS, et al. Efficacy of carotid endarterectomy for asymptomatic carotid stenosis. The Veterans Affairs Cooperative Study Group. *N Engl J Med* 1993;328:221–227.
3. Moore WS, Barnett HJ, Beebe HG, et al. Guidelines for carotid endarterectomy. A multidisciplinary consensus statement from the ad hoc committee, American Heart Association. *Stroke* 1995;26:188–201.
4. Endarterectomy for asymptomatic carotid artery stenosis. *JAMA* 1995;273:1421–1428.
5. Randomised trial of endarterectomy for recently symptomatic carotid stenosis: final results of the MRC European Carotid Surgery Trial (ECST). *Lancet* 1998;351:1379–1387.
6. Barnett HJM, Taylor DW, Eliasziw M, et al. The North American Symptomatic Carotid Endarterectomy Trial Collaborators. Benefit of carotid endarterectomy in patients with symptomatic moderate or severe stenosis. *N Engl J Med* 1998;339:1415–1425.
7. Bockenheimer SA, Mathias K. Percutaneous transluminal angioplasty in arteriosclerotic internal carotid artery stenosis. *AJNR Am J Neuroradiol* 1983;4:791–792.
8. Gil-Peralta A, Mayol A, Marcos JR, et al. Percutaneous transluminal angioplasty of the symptomatic atherosclerotic carotid arteries. Results, complications, and follow-up. *Stroke* 1996;27:2271–2273.
9. Diethrich EB, Ndiaye M, Reid DB. Stenting in the carotid artery: initial experience in 110 patients. *J Endovasc Surg* 1996;3:42–62.
10. Yadav JS, Roubin GS, King P, et al. Angioplasty and stenting for restenosis after carotid endarterectomy. Initial experience. *Stroke* 1996;27:2075–2079.
11. Theron JG, Payelle GG, Coskun O, et al. Carotid artery stenosis: treatment with protected balloon angioplasty and stent placement. *Radiology* 1996;201:627–636.
12. Wholey MH, Jarmolowski CR, Eles G, et al. Endovascular stents for carotid artery occlusive disease. *J Endovasc Surg* 1997;4:326–338.
13. Yadav JS, Roubin GS, Iyer S, et al. Elective stenting of the extracranial carotid arteries. *Circulation* 1997;95:376–381.
14. Henry M, Amor M, Masson I, et al. Angioplasty and stenting of the extracranial carotid arteries. *J Endovasc Surg* 1998;5:293–304.
15. Wholey MH, Wholey M, Bergeron P, et al. Current global status of carotid artery stent placement. *Cathet Cardiovasc Diagn* 1998;44:1–6.

16. Vitek J, Iyer S, Roubin G. Carotid stenting in 350 vessels: problems faced and solved. *J Invasive Cardiol* 1998;10:311–314.

17. Bergeron P, Becquemin JP, Jausseran JM, et al. Percutaneous stenting of the internal carotid artery: the European CAST I Study. Carotid Artery Stent Trial. *J Endovasc Surg* 1999;6:155–159.

18. Henry M, Amor M, Henry I, et al. Carotid stenting with cerebral protection: first clinical experience using the PercuSurge GuardWire system. *J Endovasc Surg* 1999;6:321–331.

19. Henry M, Amor M, Klonaris C, et al. Angioplasty and stenting of the extracranial carotid arteries. *Tex Heart Inst J* 2000;27:150–158.

20. Shawl F, Kadro W, Domanski MJ, et al. Safety and efficacy of elective carotid artery stenting in high-risk patients. *J Am Coll Cardiol* 2000;35:1721–1728.

21. Parodi JC, La Mura R, Ferreira LM, et al. Initial evaluation of carotid angioplasty and stenting with three different cerebral protection devices. *J Vasc Surg* 2000;32:1127–1136.

22. Ohki T, Veith FJ. Carotid stenting with and without protection devices: should protection be used in all patients? *Sem Vasc Surg* 2000;13:144–152.

23. Wholey MH, Al-Mubarak N, Wholey MH. Updated review of the global carotid artery stent registry. *Catheter Cardiovasc Interv* 2003;60:259–266.

24. Biasi GM, Ferrari SA, Nicolaides AN, et al. The ICAROS registry of carotid artery stenting. Imaging in Carotid Angioplasties and Risk of Stroke. *J Endovasc Ther* 2001;8:46–52.

25. Dangas G, Laird JR Jr, Mehran R, et al. Carotid artery stenting in patients with high-risk anatomy for carotid endarterectomy. *J Endovasc Ther* 2001;8:39–43.

26. Ohki T, Veith FJ. Carotid artery stenting: utility of cerebral protection devices. *J Invasive Cardiol* 2001;13:47–55.

27. Reimers B, Corvaja N, Moshiri S, et al. Cerebral protection with filter devices during carotid artery stenting. *Circulation* 2001;104:12–15.

28. Roubin GS, New G, Iyer SS, et al. Immediate and late clinical outcomes of carotid artery stenting in patients with symptomatic and asymptomatic carotid artery stenosis: a 5-year prospective analysis. *Circulation* 2001;103:532–537.

29. Tubler T, Schluter M, Dirsch O, et al. Balloon-protected carotid artery stenting: relationship of periprocedural neurological complications with the size of particulate debris. *Circulation* 2001;104:2791–2796.

30. Veith FJ, Amor M, Ohki T, et al. Current status of carotid bifurcation angioplasty and stenting based on a consensus of opinion leaders. *J Vasc Surg* 2001;33:S111–S116.

31. Angelini A, Reimers B, Della Barbera M, et al. Cerebral protection during carotid artery stenting: collection and histopathologic analysis of embolized debris. *Stroke* 2002;33:456–461.

32. Ohki T, Marin ML, Lyon RT, et al. Ex vivo human carotid artery bifurcation stenting: correlation of lesion characteristics with embolic potential. *J Vasc Surg* 1998;27:463–471.

33. Manninen HI, Rasanen HT, Vanninen RL, et al. Stent placement versus percutaneous transluminal angioplasty of human carotid arteries in cadavers in situ: distal embolization and findings at intravascular US, MR imaging and histopathologic analysis. *Radiology* 1999;212:483–492.

34. Jordan WD Jr, Voellinger DC, Doblar DD, et al. Microemboli detected by transcranial Doppler monitoring in patients during carotid angioplasty versus carotid endarterectomy. *Cardiovasc Surg* 1999;7:33–38.

35. Imparato AM, Riles TS, Gorstein F. The carotid bifurcation plaque: pathologic findings associated with cerebral ischemia. *Stroke* 1979;10:238–245.

36. Roubin GS, Yadav S, Iyer SS, et al. Carotid stent-supported angioplasty: a neurovascular intervention to prevent stroke. *Am J Cardiol* 1996;78:8–12.

37. Naylor AR, Bolia A, Abbott RJ, et al. Randomized study of carotid angioplasty and stenting versus carotid endarterectomy: a stopped trial. *J Vasc Surg* 1998;28:326–334.

38. Investigators C. Endovascular versus surgical treatment in patients with carotid stenosis in the Carotid and Vertebral Artery Transluminal Angioplasty Study (CAVATAS): a randomised trial. *Lancet* 2001; 357:1729–1737.

39. Ohki T, Roubin GS, Veith FJ, et al. Efficacy of a filter device in the prevention of embolic events during carotid angioplasty and stenting: an ex vivo analysis. *J Vasc Surg* 1999;30:1034–1044.

40. Martin JB, Pache JC, Treggiari-Venzi M, et al. Role of the distal balloon protection technique in the prevention of cerebral embolic events during carotid stent placement. *Stroke* 2001;32:479–484.

41. Jaeger HJ, Mathias KD, Drescher R, et al. Diffusion-weighted MR imaging after angioplasty or angioplasty plus stenting of arteries supplying the brain. *AJNR Am J Neuroradiol* 2001;22:1251–1259.

42. Burdette JH, Ricci PE, Petitti N, et al. Cerebral infarction: time course of signal intensity changes on diffusion-weighted MR images. *AJR Am J Roentgenol* 1998;171:791–795.

43. Kastrup A, Groschel K, Krapf H, et al. Early outcome of carotid angioplasty and stenting with and without cerebral protection devices: a systematic review of the literature. *Stroke* 2003;34:813–819.

44. Cremonesi A, Manetti R, Setacci F, et al. Protected carotid stenting: clinical advantages and complications of embolic protection devices in 442 consecutive patients. *Stroke* 2003;34:1936–1941.

45. Mathias K. Carotid artery stenting with and without cerebral protection: outcomes from a large single center experience and from the multicenter German registry. Presented at: Advanced Endovascular Therapies (AET) 2003; June 2003; New York, NY.

46. Theron J, Courtheoux P, Alachkar F, et al. New triple coaxial catheter system for carotid angioplasty with cerebral protection. *AJNR Am J Neuroradiol* 1990;11:869–874, 875–877.

47. Henry M, Henry I, Klonaris C, et al. Benefits of cerebral protection during carotid stenting with the PercuSurge GuardWire system: midterm results. *J Endovasc Ther* 2002;9:1–13.

48. Al-Mubarak N, Roubin GS, Vitek JJ, et al. Effect of the distal-balloon protection system on microembolization during carotid stenting. *Circulation* 2001;104:1999–2002.

49. Tubler T, Schluter M, Haufe M, et al. Protected carotid artery stenting: acute results and 30-day follow-up. *Eur Heart J* 2000;21:143(abst).

50. Whitlow P, Lylyk P, Londero H, et al. Protected carotid stenting with the PercuSurge guardwire: results from a multi speciality study group. *J Am Coll Cardiol* 2000;35:85(abst).

51. Roubin G, Mehran R, Diethrich E, et al. Carotid stent-supported angioplasty with distal neuroprotection using the GuardWire: 30-day results from the Carotid Angioplasty Free of Emboli (CAFÉ-USA) Trial. *J Am Coll Cardiol* 2001;37:1A–648A (abst).

52. Muller-Hulsbeck S, Jahnke T, Liess C, et al. Comparison of various cerebral protection devices used for carotid artery stent placement: an in vitro experiment. *J Vasc Interv Radiol* 2003;14:613–620.

53. Al-Mubarak N, Colombo A, Gaines PA, et al. Multicenter evaluation of carotid artery stenting with a filter protection system. *J Am Coll Cardiol* 2002;39:841–846.

54. Macdonald S, Venables GS, Cleveland TJ, et al. Protected carotid stenting: safety and efficacy of the MedNova NeuroShield filter. *J Vasc Surg* 2002;35:966–972.

55. Hobson RW 2nd, Brott T, Ferguson R, et al. CREST: carotid revascularization endarterectomy versus stent trial. *Cardiovasc Surg* 1997;5:457–458.

56. Roubin GS, Hobson RW 2nd, White R, et al. CREST and CARESS to evaluate carotid stenting: time to get to work! *J Endovasc Ther* 2001;8:107–110.

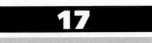

THE PROXIMAL BALLOON CATHETER: "THE PARODI ANTI-EMBOLI SYSTEM"

MARK C. BATES
JUAN CARLOS PARODI

Carotid artery stenting (CAS) seems to be a durable alternative to carotid endarterectomy (CEA), but ubiquitous acceptance of this new technology has been delayed by concerns regarding embolization (1–4). In fact, the literature is replete with cautionary statements regarding CAS, particularly in patients who are at low risk for CEA (5–8). The recent maturation of Anti-Embolization devices has renewed enthusiasm for this less-invasive technology. The Parodi Anti-Emboli System (PAES) is such a device and has many unique characteristics that separate it from all other cerebral protection systems. The PAES works based on the fundamental properties of gradient-driven passive flow reversal in the internal carotid artery (ICA) and is the only device that allows activation of protection prior to interaction with the target lesion.

The development of the flow reversal system described herein was in response to the preemptory challenge of designing a device that will provide cerebral protection during all stages of CAS and capture all embolic debris including particles less than 100 microns. Currently, there are no other devices that answer this challenge. The ability of the PAES to provide complete control of flow in the ICA may prove to be important as we begin seeking evidence based randomized data to confirm that CAS with adjuvant Anti-Embolization provides clinical equipoise to surgery. The following discussion will provide the reader with insight into the genesis of the idea for flow reversal as a means of cerebral protection during CAS. A brief review of technical considerations on use of the device and discussion of early clinical outcomes is also provided.

BACKGROUND

In the late 1980s, the team at the Instituto Cardiovascular de Buenos Aires, under the direction of Dr. Juan Parodi, was performing CEAs with transcranial Doppler (TCD) monitoring of the middle cerebral artery. During one such intervention, the team observed that middle cerebral artery flow reversal was frequently seen during passive back bleeding from the distal ICA (9). This led Dr. Parodi to begin developing transcatheter techniques that would utilize flow control as a means of achieving cerebral protection during CAS.

In the mid-1990s, proof of concept came in the way of early animal work by Tan et al. (10), who recorded ICA Doppler patterns with a flow wire during different transcatheter occlusive maneuvers. This porcine model confirmed that occlusion of the common carotid artery (CCA) caused retrograde collateral flow in the ipsilateral external carotid artery (ECA), thereby resulting in persistent antegrade flow into the ICA (Fig. 17-1). The importance of controlling flow in the ECA was also illustrated when persistent antegrade flow in the human ICA was noted after clamping the CCA during CEA (11). This explained why the early attempts by Kachel (12) and others to protect the brain with transcatheter occlusion of the CCA were unsuccessful in reducing the risk of stroke during CAS. The early Doppler flow wire animal studies also confirmed that ICA flow arrest could be initiated by occlusion of the CCA and ECA without interacting with the ICA. Also, continuous flow reversal could be initiated with the simple addition of an arterial venous communication allowing gradient driven passive flow reversal in the ICA (Fig. 17-2), eliminating the need for active aspiration using assisting devices or pumps.

Ohki et al. (13) then confirmed the ability of flow reversal using the PAES to retrieve radiopaque particles from the ICA in a canine model for CAS. Subsequent survival studies by Davies et al. (14) demonstrated that flow reversal is well tolerated in the pig model with no late ipsilateral hemispheric cerebral injury. The carotid arteries harvested in the survival study showed no evidence of late neointimal response or intimal disruption in the CCA or ECA from the balloon occlusive devices.

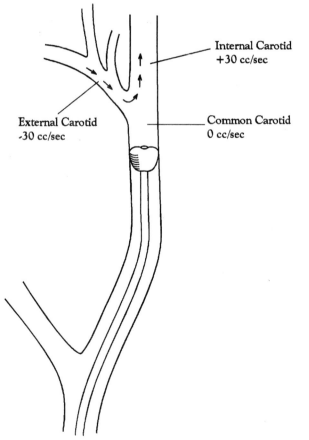

Internal Carotid
+30 cc/sec

External Carotid
-30 cc/sec

Common Carotid
0 cc/sec

FIGURE 17-1. Illustration of porcine Doppler flow patterns during transcatheter occlusion of the common carotid artery. Note the absolute value for the retrograde flow velocity is the same in the external carotid artery as the antegrade flow in the internal carotid artery.

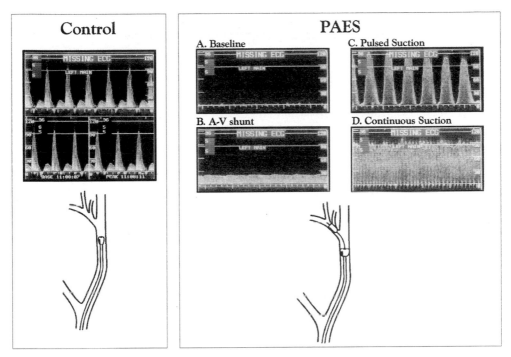

FIGURE 17-2. Illustration of Doppler flow patterns in the porcine internal carotid artery during different maneuvers with the Parodi Anti-Emboli System (PAES). The panel to the right demonstrates flow patterns before activation of the PAES. In the panel to the right, internal carotid artery (ICA) flow is recorded during different conditions; **(A)** Baseline − Doppler flow in the ICA during occlusion of the external carotid artery (ECA) and common carotid artery (CCA) with the system closed. **(B)** Same condition as **(A)** but after connecting the external arterial venous (AV) shunt; **(C)** and **(D)** are same as **(A)** but during active flow reversal with pulsed and continuous suction, respectively. Note: Control flow is recorded with the Doppler wire in the standard antegrade position so the Doppler pattern is measuring antegrade flow. The wire is retroflexed during the recordings on the right, thus recording retrograde flow.

DEVICE DESCRIPTION

The PAES is a closed system that allows ICA flow arrest, continuous passive ICA flow reversal, or augmented "active" ICA flow reversal, such that any particles that are released during angioplasty and stenting will pass retrograde through the catheter to be retrieved in the arterial venous conduit filter outside the body (Fig. 17-3). The three components of the device were specifically designed to allow retrograde laminar flow in the ICA and minimize margination of particles or collection of material that could subsequently embolize.

1. Parodi Anti-Emboli Catheter (PAEC): The first component of the system is the Parodi Anti-Emboli guide catheter. This is a 10 French guide catheter with a unique proprietary funnel shape balloon at the tip (Fig. 17-4). This atraumatic balloon allows occlusion of the CCA and flow reversal with minimal interruption in laminar flow. It also serves as the access port for the stent delivery system and other therapeutic devices.
2. Parodi External Balloon (PEB): The Parodi External Balloon is a soft, atraumatic, and oval balloon without hydrophilic coating mounted on a 0.019-inch guide wire. The distal, shapeable, floppy guide wire facilitates easy navigation into the ECA (Fig. 17-5).
3. Parodi Blood Return System (PBRS): The third component of the system is a conduit that connects the afferent arm of the PAEC flow reversal port to a venous sheath. This

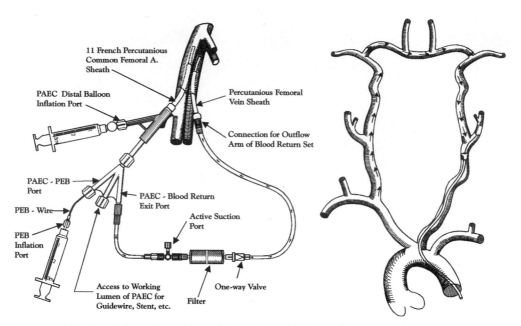

FIGURE 17-3.   Graphic illustration of the entire closed Parodi Anti-Emboli System. On the left are the workings of the proximal end of the Parodi Anti-Emboli Catheter (PAEC) and the Parodi Blood Return System (PBRS). On the right is an illustration of flow reversal in the internal carotid artery (ICA) and source of collateral support from the contralateral carotid system.

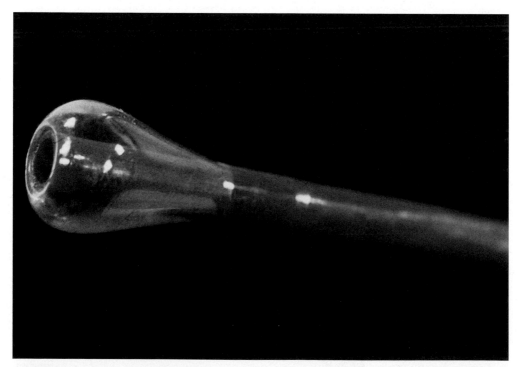

FIGURE 17-4.   Picture of the distal balloon occlusion portion of the Parodi Anti-Emboli System (PAES). (See also the color section following page 164 of this text.)

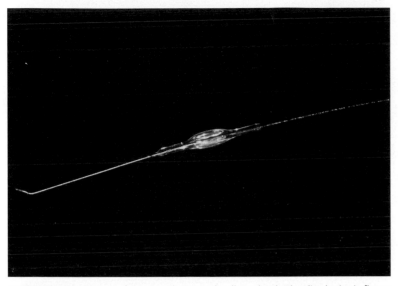

FIGURE 17-5. Picture of the Parodi External Balloon (PEB). The distal wire is floppy and shapeable. The wire proximal to the balloon is a 0.019-inch stainless steel hypotube.

conduit contains a 180-micron filter that collects particulate debris before the blood reenters the venous system. The filter may be important because as many as 27% of patients have a patent foramen ovale, and during Valsalva, paradoxical embolization could theoretically occur (Fig. 17-6) (15).

FLOW REVERSAL TECHNIQUE FOR ANTI-EMBOLIZATION

The unique mechanism of cerebral protection provided by this system generates a perceived complexity that is replaced by a sense of simplicity after experience with the device. The steps to the procedure are detailed below. In comparison to traditional carotid stenting with a distally deployed protection device, the only additional maneuvers are the introduction of the external carotid balloon and connection of the arterial venous (AV) blood return set. In addition, the PAES method eliminates the complicated step of navigating a device through the target lesion and then properly deploying it in the distal ICA. Once the PAES is deployed, the operator can perform contrast angiography and treat the vessel without concern that protection may be compromised.

The first step is the placement of the PAEC. This can be done using any of the accepted techniques for guide catheter placement in the carotid artery published elsewhere (16). The PEB is then placed through the dedicated proximal port of the PAEC and navigated under fluoroscopic guidance into the ECA. The third step is purging and attaching the PBRS to a 6 French venous sheath. The venous sheath can be placed in the ipsilateral or contralateral femoral vein.

After the device is positioned, the CCA is occluded with the PAEC, and the PEB is inflated in the ECA. Opening the PBRS stopcock initiates continuous flow reversal through the arterial venous shunt. The lesion is then crossed with a guide wire, and the stenting procedure is completed under continuous flow reversal. It is recommended that after the

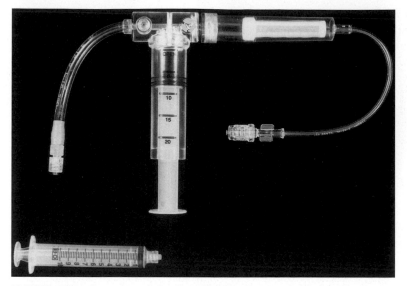

FIGURE 17-6. Illustration of the filter device in the Parodi Blood Return System (PBRS). The unique valve allows for one-way low resistance passive flow or active flow reversal by suction from an attached syringe.

stages of the procedure with the highest burden of particle release (balloon angioplasty and post stent dilatation) (17), 10 cc of blood be actively withdrawn with a syringe and reintroduced into the blood return set. After stent placement and postdilatation is completed, the PEB and PAEC are deflated while active suction is performed to retrieve any particles that may be contiguous to the balloon occlusion device. Final angiography is performed, and the system is removed.

PROCEDURE CAVEATS

Intolerance to flow reversal may be seen in patients with contralateral occlusion or an incomplete circle of Willis. In these patients, intermittent flow reversal can be used to complete the procedure. With the PAEC and PEB balloons remaining inflated in their carotids, some patients will have resolution of symptoms just with closure of the AV shunt. If the patient's intolerance persists after discontinuing passive flow reversal, then the CCA balloon can be quickly deflated to restore antegrade arterial flow. For the duration of the procedure, intermittent flow reversal can be used, reversing blood flow only during those times when the operator is interacting with the lesion. The ability to use intermittent complete occlusion and flow control is an advantage over the distal balloon occlusion devices that require completion of the stage of the procedure, including particle retrieval, before deflation of the distal balloon. Because all particles are continuously and completely cleared throughout the procedure with the PAES, one can quickly allow antegrade flow to occur and then use flow control with occlusion or passive flow reversal as needed during different steps of the procedure. Most patients with intolerance exhibit symptoms only after a few seconds to minutes of occlusion.

Caution should be exercised during active flow reversal. Rapid suction of large amounts of blood from this closed system could result in transient loss of consciousness and is not necessary for clearing the system. Alternatively, multiple blood withdrawals can be performed to completely clear the guide catheter prior to contrast injection and after the PAEC balloon is deflated because all blood is injected back into the venous system. Once the common carotid balloon is deflated, one can withdraw blood with impunity after confirmation of CCA flow by return of normal arterial pressure at the tip and fluoroscopic confirmation. One should generally withdraw at least 20 to 40 cc of blood, returning the blood back into the venous sheath via the blood return set filter, prior to any additional injection through the guide catheter. This ensures complete clearance of any particles that may be adherent to the guide catheter surface.

CLINICAL RESULTS

The PAES is currently approved for use in Europe, having received "Conformité Européen" (CE) mark in January 2001. There have been over 600 cases done worldwide with no reported embolic strokes. The controlled data and results are limited to four relatively small prospective trials.

The group at the Instituto Cardiovascular in Buenos Aries reported the first experience with the PAES in 100 high-risk patients in 2001 at the Society of Cardiovascular Interventional Radiology (SCVIR) (18). In this series, flow reversal was successfully initiated in all patients, and intolerance was noted in 8%. There were no embolic strokes. Two major complications resulted in the series: one case of hyperperfusion syndrome on day 5, which ended with an intracranial hemorrhage and death, and a second case of prolonged and severe hypotension from stretching the carotid sinus, which ended in a massive myocardial infarction (MI) and death.

Adami et al. (19) reported on the outcome of 30 patients in a seven-center Italian trial. This was with the first generation device, and access was not successful in two patients for flow reversal. One patient did not tolerate flow reversal, but the procedure was completed without incident, and there were no embolic strokes.

Sievert et al. (20) described similar results in 36 patients. There were no early embolic strokes, and one patient had a transient ischemic attack (TIA) several hours after the procedure. The PBRS filter captured debris in 34 of 36 patients, and average occlusion time was 15 ± 8 minutes. There were three groin hematomas, and two of these patients required thrombin injection for pseudoaneurysm.

A survey was sent to all sites outside the United States participating in clinical trials with the PAES. The results of the study have not been published but were presented at the Transcatheter Cardiovascular Therapeutics (TCT) meeting in Washington D.C. in 2002. These data were not controlled or randomized and are limited by the retrospective survey design. However, 302 patients were reported, and the procedure was technically successful in 97.7% of patients. Intolerance to flow reversal was noted in 22 out of 302 patients (6.7%). Procedural cerebral complications were limited to 2 out of 302 TIAs (0.7%) and three minor embolic strokes (0.99%). No major strokes were reported. Late minor stroke was 0.7%, major embolic stroke 0%, and hemorrhagic stroke 2 out of 302 (0.7%). The U.S. phase I clinical trial has been completed, but the results are pending at this time.

DISCUSSION

The PAES is unique and easy to distinguish from other Anti-Embolization systems. The PAES is the first "proximal" protection system to enter animal and human clinical trials and, unlike all other devices, provides the ability to activate cerebral protection prior to interaction with the lesion. This is an important advantage over distal protection devices because *ex vitro* studies suggest 15% of the particles released during CAS are related to crossing the lesion before protection can be initiated (21). In fact, TCD studies performed at the time of carotid stenting procedures have shown high intensity signals (HITS) consistent with embolization during simple manipulation of the guide wire across the lesion (17). In addition, the PAES is separate from the working guide wire and thus allows the operator the advantage of selecting the guide wire appropriate for the specific ICA anatomy encountered.

Flow reversal is unique to the PAES, but arresting flow in the ICA with a distal balloon on a catheter or wire is the most widely studied means of protecting the brain from embolization (22–30). Reflux of particles from the ICA has resulted in paradoxical embolization to the brain or eye via ECA collaterals (31). In contrast to the distal balloon occlusive device, the PAES external balloon prohibits embolization into the ECA, and continuous flow reversal provides constant clearing of the ICA debris. The latter is an important distinction because immediately closing the PBRS and/or deflating the proximal guide catheter balloon can resolve intolerance to ICA flow reversal or arrest. Because the ICA is constantly being cleared, one does not have to complete the additional step of particle removal prior to deflating the balloon and restoring antegrade flow. Even patients with contralateral carotid artery occlusion or an incomplete circle of Willis could potentially undergo carotid stenting with flow reversal using intermittent cerebral protection or by using the PAES to facilitate placement of a distal filter (called "seat belt and airbag protection") (32).

The PAES can be easily distinguished from distal filter protection devices by its ability to collect all particles. The size of particles that can be flushed through the distal arteriolar system in the brain appear to be less than 15 microns based on early studies evaluating cerebral blood flow (33). These animal studies were performed by injecting particles that were labeled with gamma omitting isotopes into the left atrium. It was shown that only 2% of microspheres with a 15-micron cross section diameter injected in the brain shunted to the venous blood; thus, 98% were trapped in the arteriolar system. Therefore, it must be assumed that most particles larger than 15 microns will occlude arterioles in the brain. The average filter pore size is 100 microns, and the consequence of this "controlled embolization," or release of microemboli directly into the ipsilateral hemisphere, has not been clearly defined. Interestingly, Coggia et al. (33), using a coulter technique to evaluate microemboli (less than 100 microns) in an *ex vivo* model, demonstrated that 40,000 microemboli were generated just with guide wire passage, and thousands of microemboli were released during the procedure. Analysis of debris retrieved during CAS with the distal occlusion system (GuardWire, PercuSurge, Medtronic, Inc., Minneapolis, MN) supported the observations of Coggia et al. with particles ranging from 3.6 to 5,262 microns and by number, not volume, 50% were less than 60 microns (22,26). The consequence of releasing a high burden of microemboli simultaneously to the brain is unclear. We have learned from the coronary bypass experience that the effect of microemboli cannot be assessed based on the National Institutes of Health (NIH) coma scale because these patients may have subtle changes in neurocognitive function rather than gross motor and sensory findings. In fact, autopsy studies of the brain in patients with neurocognitive dysfunction after cardiopulmonary bypass revealed that the predominant particle size responsible for occult cerebral injury was in the range of 10 to 70 microns (38). Similarly, patients undergoing CEA who have more than 10 particulate emboli on TCD may have no evidence of stroke on exam but still have significant deterioration in postoperative cognitive function (36). Diffusion-weighted magnetic resonance imaging (DW-MRI) seems to be a very sensitive way to evaluate patients who are at risk for microemboli or subclinical stroke (40,41). Abnormalities on DW-MRI have been reported in 4.2% of patients after CEA and as many as 22% of patients after CAS without protection (42,43). Recent studies have shown abnormalities on DW-MRI after filter-protected carotid stenting, amplifying concerns about silent cerebral injury from microemboli (44).

In summary, the PAES provides several theoretical advantages over current existing Anti-Embolization devices. It allows the operator to initiate cerebral protection prior to interaction with the lesion and also prevents microembolization. There is no panacea in medicine, and this device does have the disadvantage of requiring a 10 French arterial sheath and venous access. However, this may be the only device that will allow true clinical equipoise to surgical results.

REFERENCES

1. Roubin GS, New G, Iyer SS, et al. Immediate and late clinical outcomes of carotid artery stenting in patients with symptomatic and asymptomatic carotid artery stenosis: a 5-year prospective analysis. *Circulation* 2001;103:532–537.
2. Kao HL, Lin LY, Lu CJ, et al. Long-term results of elective stenting for severe carotid artery stenosis in Taiwan. *Cardiology* 2002;97:89–93.
3. Silver MJ, Yadav JS, Wholey M. Intermediate outcome after carotid stenting: what should we expect? *Sem Vasc Surg* 2000;13:130–138.
4. Wholey MH, Wholey M, Bergeron P, et al. Current global status of carotid artery stent placement. *Catheter Cardiovasc Diagn* 1998;44:1–6.
5. Naylor AR, Bolia A, Abbott RJ, et al. Randomized study of carotid angioplasty and stenting versus carotid endarterectomy: a stopped trial. *J Vasc Surg* 1998;28:326–334.
6. Leisch F, Kerschner K, Hofman R, et al. [Carotid stenting: acute results and complications.] *Z Kardiol* 1999;88:661–668.
7. Bettman MA, Katzen BT, Whisnant J, et al. Carotid stenting and angioplasty: a statement for healthcare professionals from the Councils on Cardiovascular Radiology, Stroke, Cardio-Thoracic and Vascular Surgery, Epidemiology and Prevention, and Clinical Cardiology, American Heart Association. *Stroke* 1998;29:336–348.
8. Moore WS, Barnett HJM, Beebe HG, et al. Guidelines for carotid endarterectomy. A multidisciplinary consensus statement from the Ad Hoc Committee, American Heart Association. *Stroke* 1995;26: 188–201.
9. Parodi JC, Bates MC. How to recover emboli and other particles from the middle cerebral artery: will this be valuable in carotid stenting and carotid endarterectomy? *Endovascular Multimedia Magazine* 2001 5:167–174.
10. Tan W, Bates MC, Wholey M. Cerebral protection systems for distal emboli during carotid artery interventions. *J Intervent Cardiol* 2001;14:1–9.
11. Ouriel K, Greenberg RK, Sarac TP. Hemodynamic conditions at the carotid bifurcation during protective common carotid occlusion. *J Vasc Surg* 2001;34:577–580.
12. Kachel R. Results of balloon angioplasty in the carotid arteries. *J Endovasc Surg* 1996;3:22–50.
13. Ohki T, Parodi J, Veith FJ, et al. Efficacy of a proximal occlusion catheter with reversal of flow in the prevention of embolic events during carotid artery stenting: an experimental analysis. *J Vasc Surg* 2001;33:504–509.
14. Davies RP, Blumberg P, Kew J. Parodi anti-emboli brain protection system—effects on the carotid arteries and brain in a swine model. Presented at: Global Endovascular Therapeutics (GET) Conference; 2001.
15. Hagen PT, Scholz DG, Edwards WD. Incidence and size of patent foramen ovale during the first decades of life: an autopsy study of 965 normal hearts. *Mayo Clin. Proc* 1984;59:17–20.
16. Gains PA. Techniques of carotid stenting. In: *Vascular and endovascular surgical techniques*, 4th ed. Greenhalgh RM, ed. London: W.B. Saunders, 2001:49–52.
17. Orlandi G, Fanucchi S, Fioretti C, et al. Characteristics of cerebral microembolism during carotid stenting and angioplasty alone. *Arch Neurol* 2001;58:1410–1413.
18. Parodi JC, Schonolz C, Ferreira M, et al. Parodi Antiembolism System in carotid stenting: the first

100 patients. Presented at Society of Cardiovascular Interventional Radiology 27th Annual Scientific Meeting; April 8, 2002; Baltimore, Maryland.

19. Adami A, Scuro A, Spinamano L, et al. Use of the Parodi Anti-Embolism System in carotid stenting: Italian trial results. *J Endovasc Ther* 2002;9:147–154.

20. Sievert H, Rabe K, Pfeil W, et al. Carotid angioplasty: initial experience with the flow reversal technique for prevention of embolic complications during carotid angioplasty. Presented at Society of Cardiovascular Interventional Radiology 27th Annual Scientific Meeting; April 8, 2002; Baltimore, Maryland.

21. Ohki T, Roubin GS, Veith FJ, et al. Efficacy of a filter in the prevention of embolic events during carotid angioplasty and stenting: an ex vitro study. *J Vasc Surg* 1999;30:1034–1044.

22. Henry M, Henry I, Klonaris C, et al. Benefits of cerebral protection during carotid stenting with the PercuSurge GuardWire system: midterm results. *J Endovasc Ther* 2002;9:1–13.

23. Henry M, Amor M, Henry I, et al. Carotid stenting with cerebral protection: first clinical experience using the PercuSurge GuardWire system. *J Endovasc Surg* 1999;6:321–331.

24. Roubin GS, Mehran R, Iyer SS, et al. Carotid stent-supported angioplasty with distal neuro-protections using the GuardWire: initial results from the carotid angioplasty free of emboli (CAFE-USA) trial. *Circulation* 2000(Suppl);102:II–475.

25. Zanella FE, Berkefeld J. Carotid stenting with embolism prevention *Z Kardiol* 2000;89(Suppl 8): 47–52.

26. Whitlow PL, Lylyk P, Londero H, et al. Carotid artery stenting protected with an emboli containment system. *Stroke* 2002;33:1308–1314.

27. Grego F, Frigatti P, Amista P, et al. Prospective comparative study of two cerebral protection devices in carotid angioplasty and stenting. *J Cardiovasc Surg (Torino)* 2002;43:391–397.

28. Al-Mubarak N, Roubin GS, Vitek JJ, et al. Effect of the distal-balloon protection system on microembolization during carotid stenting. *Circulation* 2001;104:1999–2002.

29. Theron JG, Payelle GG, Coskun O, et al. Carotid artery stenosis: treatment with protected balloon angioplasty and stent placement. *Radiology* 1996;201:627–636.

30. Terada T, Yokote H, Nakamura Y, et al. Newly developed blocking balloon catheter for PTA of internal carotid artery. *No Shinkei Geka* 1993;21:891–895.

31. Al-Mubarak N, Vitek JJ, Iyer S, et al. Embolization via collateral circulation during carotid stenting with the distal balloon protection system. *J Endovasc Ther* 2001;8:354–357.

32. Parodi JC, Schonholz C, Ferreira LM, et al. "Seat belt and air bag" technique for cerebral protection during carotid stenting. *J Endovasc Ther* 2002;9:20–24.

33. Coggia M, Goeau-Brissonniere O, Duval JL, et al. Embolic risk of the different stages of carotid bifurcation balloon angioplasty: an experimental study. *J Vasc Surg* 2000;31:550–557.

34. Wityk RJ, Goldsborough MA, Hillis A, et al. Diffusion- and perfusion-weighted brain magnetic resonance imaging in patients with neurologic complications after cardiac surgery. *Arch Neurol* 2001; 58:549–550.

35. Brown WR, Moody DM, Challa VR, et al. Histologic studies of brain microemboli in humans and dogs after cardiopulmonary bypass. *Echocardiography* 1996;13:559–566.

36. Brown WR, Moody DM, Mills SA, et al. Surrogate tissues for detecting brain microemboli after cardiopulmonary bypass. *Perfusion* 1994;9:389–392.

37. Stump DA, Kon NA, Rogers AT. Emboli and neuropsychological outcome following cardiopulmonary bypass. *Echocardiography* 1996;13:555–558.

38. Moody DM, Brown WR, Challa VR, et al. Brain microemboli associated with cardiopulmonary bypass: a histologic and magnetic resonance imaging study. *Ann Thorac Surg* 1995;59:1304–1307.

39. Gaunt ME, Martin PJ, Smith JL, et al. Clinical relevance of intraoperative embolization detected by transcranial Doppler ultrasonography during carotid endarterectomy: a prospective study of 100 patients. *Br J Surg* 1994;81:1435–1439.

40. Sakai H, Sakai N, Higashi T, et al. Embolic complications associated with neurovascular intervention: prospective evaluation by use of diffusion-weighted MR imaging. *No Shinkei Geka* 2002;30:43–49.

41. Lovblad KO, Pluschke W, Remonda L, et al. Diffusion-weighted MRI for monitoring neurovascular interventions. *Neuroradiology* 2000;42:134–138.

42. Barth A, Remonda L, Lovblad KO, et al. Silent cerebral ischemia detected by diffusion-weighted MRI after carotid endarterectomy. *Stroke* 2000;31:1824–1828.

43. Jaeger HJ, Mathias KD, Drescher R, et al. Diffusion-weighted MR imaging after angioplasty or angioplasty plus stenting of arteries supplying the brain. *AJNR Am J Neuroradiol* 2001;22:1251–1259.

44. Jaeger H, Mathias K, Drescher R, et al. Clinical results of cerebral protection with a filter device during stent implantation of the carotid artery. *Cardiovasc Intervent Radiol* 2001;24:249–256.

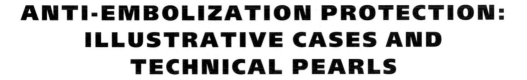

ANTI-EMBOLIZATION PROTECTION: ILLUSTRATIVE CASES AND TECHNICAL PEARLS

FRANCESCO LIISTRO
ANTONIO COLOMBO

The major limitation of the endovascular treatment for obstructive carotid artery disease is the potential risk for distal embolization of plaque fragments or thrombotic materials during the procedure (1–3). These embolic particles may be released during all stages of the procedure including: guiding catheter placement, guide wire manipulation across the stenosis, balloon placement across and lesion dilatation, stent delivery and deployment, and postdilatation (1,2). Embolic neurological events after the stenting procedure is completed are relatively rare. Transcranial Doppler monitoring and diffusion-weighted magnetic resonance imaging performed during carotid artery stenting (CAS) showed that many emboli are asymptomatic (1,4–8). This fact might be partially explained by the presence of adequate collateral flow supplying very small ischemic regions or the lack of appropriate neurological evaluation. Therefore, the clinical significance of the number of embolic particles released during CAS is not completely elucidated, although there is some evidence that patients with a large number of particles generated by the intervention would have higher risk for procedural stroke than patients in whom fewer particles are produced (9–11).

The recent introduction of filter Anti-Embolization devices into the CAS procedure with the objective of minimizing distal embolization and related clinical events has enhanced the safety of the procedure and expanded its indications (12–14). Carotid stent implantation with an Anti-Embolization device aims at the treatment of the obstructive carotid artery lesion by: (a) the achievement of a widely patent carotid artery, (b) containment and exclusion of the plaque segment (stent barrier) preventing its complications (thrombosis, ulceration), and (c) avoiding distal embolization during the procedure.

A variety of filter-based systems that are designed to capture embolic debris released during CAS have recently been introduced. In contrast to the balloon-based Anti-Embolization systems, filters can prevent embolic events without interrupting blood flow distally. This feature is very important when treating patients with occlusion in the circle of Willis and "watershed areas" of the brain extremely sensible to transient ischemia (approximately 5% to 10% of patients undergoing CAS). Another important advantage of filters is the feasibility of angiography during the procedure, hence the possibility of proper verification of the stent position prior to its final deployment. The disadvantages of the filter Anti-Embolization protection are: (a) small particles can still pass through the pores, (b) the fact that the filter may not be completely apposed to the vessel wall, (c) a relatively large crossing profile, resulting in difficulties in crossing tight or tortuous lesions, and (d) the potential risk of spasm and dissection in the distal internal carotid artery (ICA) (15).

TABLE 18-1. FEATURES OF DIFFERENT PROTECTION DEVICES

Device	Pore Size (μm)	Crossing Profile (inches)	Capture Sheath Profile (inches)	Diameters Available (mm)
AngioGuard XP	100	0.042–0.052	0.066	4–8
MedNova III	120	0.048	0.096	4–6
MedNova IV	120	0.037	0.084	3–7
BSc FilterWire	110	0.049	0.049	One size fits 3.5–5.5
Medtronic AVE	100	0.039	0.039	3.5–5.5
Guidant AccuNet	115	0.045–0.048	0.071	4.5–7.5
Microvena TRAP	200	0.037	0.066–0.078	2.5–7.5
Spider ev3	80	0.038	0.054–0.063	3–7
PercuSurge	NA	0.028–0.036	0.042–0.070	3–6

NA, not applicable.

All filter Anti-Embolization systems consist of three basic components: (a) guide wire with a filter at its distal end or a guide wire independent from the filter, (b) delivery catheter (always incorporated with the filter but not necessarily with the guide wire), and (c) retrieval catheter.

The following steps are common to almost all systems. After shaping the tip of the guide wire, the delivery catheter is introduced and gently advanced across the stenosis so that the filter can be deployed at least 2 cm distal to the target lesion. The filter is then deployed by withdrawal of the delivery catheter, and its position is verified by a contrast injection. The same guide wire is then used for the advancement of balloon catheters and stents to the target lesion. There are new, more trackable generation filters, which have a guide wire that moves independently from the filter. Using these filter systems, the guide wire is first advanced through the lesion, followed by the advancement of the filter delivery catheter over this guide wire. Following treatment, the retrieval catheter is advanced towards the filter until the distal end of the catheter completely envelops the filter. Thereafter, the retrieval catheter with its contents is completely withdrawn. The ideal filter Anti-Emboliza-tion device should have the following features: (a) easy positioning of the guide wire, which has to provide consistent support for stent placement, (b) low profile and high flexibility of the system to facilitate the successful passage and application in the severely tortuous carotid arteries, and (c) efficacy in capturing fragments without inducing obstruction of the blood flow.

In this chapter, we present some clinical cases of CAS with various filter Anti-Emboliza-tion systems and discuss the indications, choice, and success of these devices. These examples are selected from our combined experience (Table 18-1) in Columbus Hospital and San Raffaele Hospital since the beginning of carotid stenting (1998) until September 2002.

FILTER PLACEMENT IN TORTUOUS INTERNAL CAROTID ARTERIES WITH SEVERE ANGULATIONS

Case 1

Bilateral carotid angiography was performed in a 68-year-old woman with hypertension and hypercholesterolemia who had suffered a transient ischemic attack (TIA) 3 months earlier with subsequent carotid duplex ultrasound evaluation revealing a high-grade stenosis of the left internal carotid artery (LICA). Selective left carotid angiography (Fig. 18-1A) showed a severe lesion in the proximal segment of the internal carotid artery (ICA). Distal to the stenosis, the vessel was severely tortuous and had a double curve. Following the guiding sheath placement within the common carotid artery (CCA), the AngioGuard filter system (Cordis, Warren, NJ) was selected as the Anti-Embolization device to complete the CAS procedure. This system consists of a filter, a deployment sheath, a capture sheath, one torque device, and one peel-away introducer. The filter is fixed on a 0.014-inch guide wire and is designed as a basket made of polyurethane (with the pore size of 100 μm) and eight nitinol struts (four of them have radiopaque markers). The length of the filter with open basket varies from 8.9 mm to 14.2 mm according to the filter diameters (4.0 to 8.0 mm, with 1 mm increases). The crossing profile ranges from 3.2F (for 4-mm-diameter filter) to 3.9F (for 8-mm-diameter filter). For this specific vessel, we choose a 6.0-mm-diameter filter device. The capture sheath has a crossing profile of 5.1F. The tip of the pod is very flexible in order to facilitate the passage through the implanted stent at the target lesion.

Despite the easy passage through the stenosis, the device could not be advanced beyond the first curve (Fig. 18-1B) of the ICA owing to severe tortuosities and inability to negotiate the second curve located beyond the stenosis. The first maneuver to enhance the system pushability during advancement through these tortuous arterial segments was to ensure adequate guiding sheath backup support. To achieve this goal, the guiding sheath was advanced and positioned at the bifurcation of the carotid artery. It is important to note that sheath advancement should always be performed with the dilator or a diagnostic catheter inserted within, as the sharp sheath tip may traumatize and dissect the CCA (Fig. 18-2). Despite the extra support provided by the distal guiding sheath position, a second attempt to further advance the filter system was unsuccessful. Subsequent control angiography revealed an occlusive flow-limiting vascular dissection at the point where the filter was stuck (Fig. 18-1C). The patient became symptomatic and developed impairment in contralateral motor function. The situation turned into an emergency, and the filter was immediately replaced by a soft 0.014-inch coronary guide wire. An attempt to advance an Easy Wallstent at the point of the occlusive dissection was unsuccessful, and it was implanted in the proximal

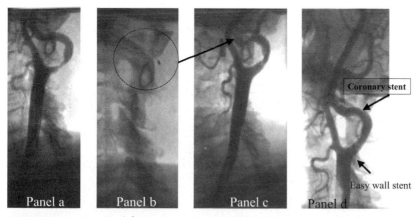

FIGURE 18-1. Selective left carotid angiography (**A**) showing a severe lesion in the proximal segment of the internal carotid artery (ICA). Distal to the stenosis, the vessel appeared severely tortuous with a double curve. The filter could not be advanced beyond the first curve (**B**). Control angiography was performed, and an occlusive vessel dissection appeared at the point where the filter was stuck (**C**). After stent implantation, the angiographic result was good (**D**).

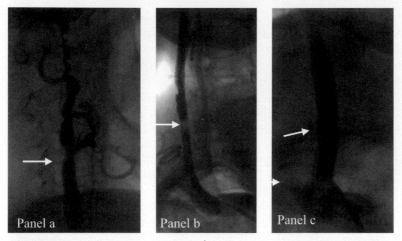

FIGURE 18-2. Stenosis at the right carotid artery bifurcation (**A**). The advancement of the sheath without the dilator or a catheter acting as a protecting system for the sharp tip led to extensive occlusive dissection of the common carotid artery (**B**). Implantation of a long, self-expanding stent was necessary to treat this problem (**C**).

segment of the vessel to cover the original stenotic lesion (Carotid Wallstent was not available at that time). The distal dissection was then successfully sealed by a 5-mm coronary stent (Ultra stent, Guidant Co., Temecula, CA). The angiographic results were good (Fig. 18-1D), and the neurological deficit completely resolved within few minutes.

In retrospect, the best way to handle this problem was to prevent its occurrence. Instead of forcing the filter through the tortuosity, the most rational and safe approach is to exchange this filter device to another more trackable system. The case in Figure 18-3 illustrates an

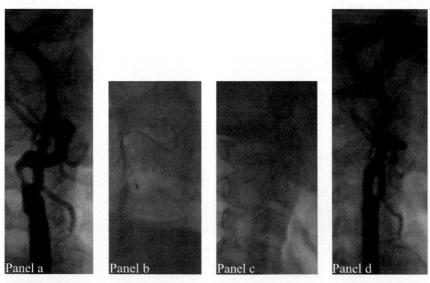

FIGURE 18-3. Stenosis at the proximal segment of the right internal carotid artery, which appears tortuous (**A**). The AngioGuard filter, which could not be negotiated distally to the double curve (**B**). Successful passage of the MedNova EmboShield through the lesion (**C**) and optimal angiographic result after stent implantation (**D**).

AngioGuard filter device that could not be negotiated through a double curve (Fig. 18-3A, 18-3B). In this case, the operator decided to change the filter device to a new filter system in which the bare guide wire is first advanced independently (EmboShield, MedNova Ltd., Abbot Vascular Devices, Galway, Ireland). The initial introduction of the guide wire straightened the vascular double curve and facilitated the subsequent advancement of the stiffer component of the filter system (Fig. 18-3C, 18-3D).

An intermediate solution, particularly for the operator who does not have an alternative system available, is not willing to lose the distal position that is partially achieved with the first filter device, or has economic limitations, is to advance a second coronary wire (buddy wire) parallel to the filter to first straighten the curve and then reattempt the filter advancement.

Case 2

A 74-year-old man underwent bilateral carotid angiography after he was found to have high-grade bilateral ICA stenoses during carotid duplex ultrasound evaluation. The patient's medical history included diabetes, hypertension, hypercholesterolemia, and coronary artery disease with prior coronary artery bypass surgery. He had never experienced any neurological symptoms in the past. The angiography revealed severe stenosis at the ostial right ICA (RICA). The vessel appeared tortuous with a double curve in the proximal midsegment (Fig. 18-4A). A guiding sheath was positioned within the distal ICA, and a 0.014-inch coronary guide wire (BMW, Guidant Co., Temecula, CA) was used to cross the lesion and positioned distal in the vessel. This was then exchanged with a TRAP filter (Fig. 18-4B; *circled*). The TRAP system (Microvena Inc., White Bear Lake, MN) consists of a delivery and capture catheter and a filter. The 0.014-inch filter wire has a nitinol basket at its tip. The delivery catheter (3.5F) is delivered over an ordinary 0.014-inch guide wire. Thereafter,

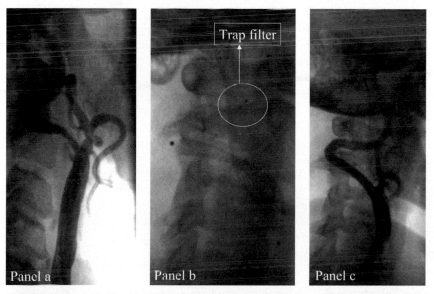

FIGURE 18-4. Carotid angiography showed a significant stenosis at the ostium of the right internal carotid artery. The vessel appeared tortuous with a double curve in the proximal midsegment (**A**). Successful delivery of the TRAP system and implantation of an Easy Wallstent (**B**). Final angiographic result (**C**).

the guide wire is exchanged to the filter wire. This device has a low crossing profile (3.5F) and is designed as a nitinol wire-woven basket on a 0.014-inch extra-support guide wire with a polyurethane filter that allows normal blood flow to the distal vessel. The basket diameter varies between 2.5 and 7 mm. In this case, we used a 6-mm-diameter device. Thereafter, an Easy Wallstent (9 mm × 40 mm) was delivered between the RCCA and the proximal segment of the RICA successfully (Fig. 18-4B). The angiographic result was good, and the TRAP filter was retrieved (Fig. 18-4C).

Vascular tortuosities are one of the major anatomical obstacles that are responsible for delivery failure of various interventional devices in the settings of percutaneous revascularization of the coronary arteries as well as in carotid arteries. In the previous two cases, the presence of severe tortuosity was a challenge for the use of the filter device. To overcome these obstacles, the ideal filter device should have a low crossing profile and enhanced flexibility and pushability in order to facilitate its smooth and safe passage through these tortuous vessels. The AngioGuard filter has the advantage of a good visibility and ease of use. However, the short segment of the floppy wire distal to the mounted filter may not provide enough support to deliver the filter across tortuous vessels. The alternative choice in these settings is a filter device that is delivered over a guiding wire after this is positioned within the distal vessel (TRAP, EmboShield), or a different type of device such as the occlusive balloon systems (PercuSurge GuardWire or Parodi system). Nevertheless, no comparative studies have been performed between these different types of devices, and the choice depends on operator personal experience.

DIFFICULT FILTER RETRIEVAL

Case 3

Carotid angiography was performed on a 56-year-old man with diabetes mellitus and hypercholesterolemia who suffered a TIA 2 months earlier. This revealed a 60% diameter stenosis in the left carotid artery bifurcation involving more the external carotid artery (ECA) than the ICA (Fig. 18-5A). For his symptomatic stenosis, he underwent CAS. Following placement of an 8F guiding sheath, a 7-mm AngioGuard filter was advanced through the lesion without technical difficulties (Fig. 18-5B, *arrow*). Direct stent implantation was successfully performed using an 8-mm × 40-mm Wallstent without complications. During postdilatation of the stent using a 5.5-mm × 20-mm balloon, severe spasm that was resistant to intraarterial nitroglycerin occurred at the filter site (Fig. 18-5B, 18-5C). A vascular dissection was excluded angiographically and filter retrieval was considered. However, the filter retrieval catheter could not be advanced through the stent despite a deep cannulation of the guiding sheath into the ICA (Fig. 18-5D). The crossing profile of the retrieval catheter of the AngioGuard filter is 5.1F, but the flexibility of the device is not optimal. Additionally, this retrieval catheter has a sharp tip that occasionally faces obstacles from the stent struts. To overcome the problem in the filter retrieval, we replaced the filter retrieval catheter with a 6F multipurpose coronary guiding catheter. This catheter was easily advanced through the stent, and the filter was pulled into the guide catheter and was successfully retrieved (Fig. 18-5E, 18-5F). After the filter removal, the spasm resolved completely (Fig. 18-5G). The patient remained asymptomatic during the entire procedure.

Vessel angulation is one of the most challenging anatomical features during the filter application. In some situations, the delivery of the system does not provide particular difficulties, but the filter retrieval can be problematic. In the present case, although we had an optimal backup support from the advanced position of the guiding catheter, the retrieval

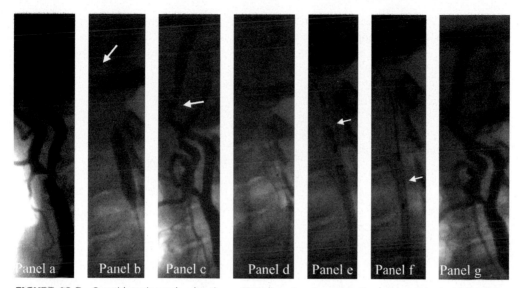

FIGURE 18-5. Carotid angiography showing a 60% diameter stenosis in the left carotid artery bifurcation (**A**). Positioning of a 7-mm AngioGuard filter distal to the lesion and stent implantation (**B**, *arrow*). Optimal angiographic results of the stented segment, whereas a severe spasm that was resistant to intraarterial nitroglycerin is visible at the site of the filter (**C** and **D**). The filter retrieval catheter could not be advanced through the stent despite a deep cannulation of the guiding sheath (**E**). A 6F multipurpose coronary guiding catheter was easily advanced through the stent, and the filter was successfully retrieved (**F** and **G**).

catheter could not be properly advanced through the stent owing to the friction with the stent struts that was exacerbated by the vessel angulation. The multipurpose catheter was successful in retrieving the filter despite being 1F larger.

STRING SIGN

Case 4

The case that follows highlights the risk in performing a percutaneous carotid intervention in the presence of a subtotal occlusion of the ICA (string sign). Figure 18-6 illustrates the baseline angiogram of a 75-year-old man who had suffered recurrent minor strokes. The baseline angiogram showed a subtotal occlusion of the carotid artery (Fig. 18-6A). An EmboShield protection device (Fig. 18-6B, *circled*) was easily advanced into the ICA, and, following predilatation, the lesion was successfully stented (Fig. 18-6B). Angiography at the end of the procedure revealed absent distal flow in the ICA with a large angiographic filling defect visible distal to the subocclusive stenosis (Fig. 18-6C, *arrows*). A few hours later, the patient experienced a major stroke probably related to the distal migration of the thrombotic material. The risk of thrombus layered distally to a subocclusive stenosis is a serious consideration, which may be regarded as a contraindication to perform carotid stenting in this specific setting. The usage of flow reversion with the Parodi system could theoretically overcome this problem, but the question remains open for how long the flow reversal should be maintained to remove all the thrombotic material, which eventually could migrate distally when forced by a higher forward arterial pressure.

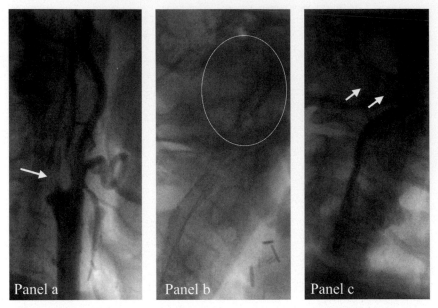

FIGURE 18-6. Baseline angiogram showing a subtotal occlusion string sign of the carotid artery (**A**). The EmboShield protection device was positioned distal to the lesion (**B**, *circled*). Following dilatation and stent placement, the internal carotid artery appeared without any distal flow owing to a large thrombus present distally to the suboclusive stenosis (**C**, *arrows*). A few hours later, the patient suffered a disabling stroke.

ANTI-EMBOLIZATION DEVICES IN THE EMERGENCY SETTING

Case 5

The patient in this case was a 67-year-old man with coronary artery disease and bilateral carotid artery disease who suffered a TIA on the left cerebral hemisphere. The patient underwent left carotid endarterectomy (CEA), which was complicated by the occurrence of an early (1 hour from the end of the surgical procedure) ischemic event contralateral to the treated artery. Emergency carotid angiography revealed angiographic evidence of thrombus at the endarterectomy site involving the bifurcation as well as the ICA and ECA (Fig. 18-7A, *arrows*). As previously reported by our center (16), we decided to perform direct carotid stenting. In order to prevent distal embolization of the large thrombotic materials present at the atherectomy site, we decided to use a filter Anti-Embolization system. An AngioGuard filter 6.0 mm large (Fig. 18-7B, *circled*) was gently advanced through the lesion and the basket opened in the distal segment. Direct stenting was performed with an Easy Wallstent (8.0 × 40 mm) covering the entire atherectomy site. The final angiography showed an optimal result (Fig. 18-7C, *arrow*), and the patient's neurological status completely recovered. The retrieved AngioGuard filter showed one macroscopically visible particle consistent with a thrombus captured in the basket (Fig. 18-7D).

In the settings of emergency stenting for stroke complicating CEA, the main problem concerns the presence of thrombus, which might be caused by rough endarterectomy surface, the use of synthetic patch material, the presence of unremoved plaque parts at the endarterectomy site, or stenosis from the endarterectomy closure (17,18). If the use of Anti-Embolization devices in these settings should be mandatory, the choice of device is controversial. The occlusive devices such as the PercuSurge GuardWire (Medtronic Inc., Santa Rosa, CA)

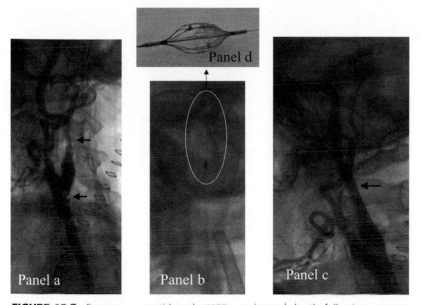

FIGURE 18-7 Emergency carotid angiography, performed shortly following an acute neurological event that complicated carotid endarterectomy, showing the presence of thrombus at the endarterectomy site involving the bifurcation as well as the internal and external carotid arteries (**A**, *arrows*). An AngioGuard filter was positioned distal to the lesion (**B**, *circled*). The final angiography showed an optimal result (**C**, *arrow*). Thrombotic materials visible inside the AngioGuard basket (**D**).

or Parodi (ArteriA, San Francisco, CA) device might be the best choice if well tolerated by the patient. In our experience of 26 cases of emergency carotid stenting for stroke complicating CEA, we used an Anti-Embolization device in 61% of the procedures, and the most frequently used device was the distal occlusion balloon. This device was not tolerated in the majority of the patients, and it had to be deflated several times during the procedure. Bilateral carotid disease, contralateral carotid occlusion, or diffuse intracerebral spasm caused by ongoing ischemia (common in patients experiencing ischemic CEA-related complications) may be responsible for the low tolerance of occlusive balloon devices observed in emergency settings.

REFERENCES

1. Al-Mubarak N, Roubin GS, Vitek JJ, et al. Effect of the distal-balloon protection system on microembolization during carotid stenting. *Circulation* 2001;104:1999–2002.
2. Manninen HI, Rasanen HT, Vanninen RL, et al. Stent placement versus percutaneous transluminal angioplasty of human carotid arteries in cadavers in situ: distal embolization and findings at intravascular US, MR imaging and histopathologic analysis. *Radiology* 1999;212:483–492.
3. Ohki T, Marin ML, Lyon RT, et al. Ex vivo human carotid artery bifurcation stenting: correlation of lesion characteristics with embolic potential. *J Vasc Surg* 1998;27:463–471.
4. Imparato AM, Riles TS, Gorstein F. The carotid bifurcation plaque: pathologic findings associated with cerebral ischemia. *Stroke* 1979;10:238–245.
5. Roubin GS, Yadav S, Iyer SS, et al. Carotid stent-supported angioplasty: a neurovascular intervention to prevent stroke. *Am J Cardiol* 1996;78:8–12.
6. Veith FJ, Amor M, Ohki T, et al. Current status of carotid bifurcation angioplasty and stenting based on a consensus of opinion leaders. *J Vasc Surg* 2001;33:S111–S116.

7. Ohki T, Roubin GS, Veith FJ, et al. Efficacy of a filter device in the prevention of embolic events during carotid angioplasty and stenting: an ex vivo analysis. *J Vasc Surg* 1999;30:1034–1044.

8. Martin JB, Pache JC, Treggiari-Venzi M, et al. Role of the distal balloon protection technique in the prevention of cerebral embolic events during carotid stent placement. *Stroke* 2001;32:479–484.

9. Tubler T, Schluter M, Dirsch O, et al. Balloon-protected carotid artery stenting: relationship of periprocedural neurological complications with the size of particulate debris. *Circulation* 2001;104: 2791–2796.

10. Jaeger HJ, Mathias KD, Hauth E, et al. Cerebral ischemia detected with diffusion-weighted MR imaging after stent implantation in the carotid artery. *AJNR Am J Neuroradiol* 2002;23:200–207.

11. Burdette JH, Ricci PE, Petitti N, et al. Cerebral infarction: time course of signal intensity changes on diffusion-weighted MR images. *AJR Am J Roentgenol* 1998;171:791–795.

12. Reimers B, Corvaja N, Moshiri S, et al. Cerebral protection with filter devices during carotid artery stenting. *Circulation* 2001;104:12–15.

13. Al-Mubarak N, Colombo A, Gaines PA, et al. Multicenter evaluation of carotid artery stenting with a filter protection system. *J Am Coll Cardiol* 2002;39:841–846.

14. Roubin GS, New G, Iyer SS, et al. Immediate and late clinical outcomes of carotid artery stenting in patients with symptomatic and asymptomatic carotid artery stenosis: a 5-year prospective analysis. *Circulation* 2001;103:532–537.

15. Ohki T, Veith FJ. Carotid artery stenting: utility of cerebral protection devices. *J Invasive Cardiol* 2001;13:47–55.

16. Anzuini A, Briguori C, Roubin GS, et al. Emergency stenting to treat neurological complications occurring after carotid endarterectomy. *J Am Coll Cardiol* 2001;37:2074–2079.

17. Riles TS, Imparato AM, Jacobowitz GR, et al. The cause of perioperative stroke after carotid endarterectomy. *J Vasc Surg* 1994;19:206–216.

18. Rockman CB, Jacobowitz GR, Lamparello PJ, et al. Immediate reexploration for the perioperative neurologic event after carotid endarterectomy: is it worthwhile? *J Vasc Surg* 2000;32:1062–1070.

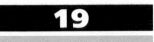

RESTENOSIS FOLLOWING CAROTID ARTERY STENTING

FAYAZ SHAWL

Restenosis is the Achilles heel of percutaneous interventions. Although stenting has dramatically lowered the restenosis rate seen with balloon angioplasty, in-stent restenosis remains an important clinical problem (1–3). The in-stent restenosis rate also varies with the vascular bed stented. Although in-stent restenosis has been reported in 16% to 59% of coronary stents and 13% to 39% of iliac stents, it occurs in only 2% to 5% of carotid stents (4–13). Although this figure is low, the absolute number of restenoses will increase as the number of carotid stent procedures increases. The purpose of this chapter is to discuss the incidence, pathophysiology, diagnosis, and treatment of carotid in-stent restenosis.

INCIDENCE OF IN-STENT RESTENOSIS

In a multicenter study involving 4,757 patients, the incidence of in-stent restenosis 12 months after carotid artery stenting (CAS) was 3.5% (10). Similarly, other studies have reported restenosis rates of 2% to 5% (Table 19-1) (10–16). In the Carotid and Vertebral Artery Transluminal Angioplasty Study (CAVATAS), a randomized trial in which carotid endarterectomy (CEA) and carotid angioplasty treatment for carotid stenosis were compared, restenosis was noted in 18% of patients treated by carotid balloon angioplasty (14). This high rate of restenosis could be due to the fact that only 26% of patients who had carotid angioplasty received a stent.

Although most studies have used more than or equal to 50% diameter obstruction as a definition of restenosis, some have used more severe narrowing (11,13,15,17,18). Certain clinical and angiographic characteristics have been associated with an increased restenosis rate. In peripheral interventions, restenosis is increased in smokers, small diameter vessels, and with the use of multiple stents (9). In the coronary system, the use of multiple stents, diabetes mellitus, and a small final luminal diameter have been strongly associated with increased risk of in-stent stenosis (19). In the carotid circulation, in-stent restenosis appears to be increased in patients with previous CEA (20). In this small study of eight patients, the incidence was noted at 75%, but this has not been seen in a large multicenter trial (20,21).

It is interesting to note that CAS is associated with the lowest rate of restenosis. It is possible that the carotid artery's high flow rate and the low resistance in the cerebral vessels may result in less myointimal hyperplasia than in other vascular beds.

TABLE 19-1. INCIDENCE OF RESTENOSIS AFTER CAROTID STENTING

Author	Year	Patients, n	Method of Follow-up	Restenosis No. (%)
Yadav et al. (11)	1997	107	Angioplasty/duplex	5 (4.9)
Wholey et al. (12)	1998	2048	Angioplasty/duplex	98 (4.8)
Shawl et al. (13)	2000	170	Angioplasty/duplex	3 (1.8)
Wholey et al. (10)	2000	4757	Angioplasty/duplex	165 (3.5)
CAVATAS (14)	2001	173	Angioplasty/duplex	32 (18)[a]
Wilfort-Ehringer et al. (15)	2002	279	Angioplasty/duplex	9 (3.0)
Shawl (16)	2002	299	Angioplasty/duplex	8 (2.7)

[a] Only 26% of patients received stent.
CAVATAS, Carotid and Vertebral Artery Transluminal Angioplasty Study.

PATHOPHYSIOLOGY OF CAROTID IN-STENT RESTENOSIS

The pathophysiology of carotid in-stent restenosis can be inferred from what has been reported about carotid restenosis after CEA as well as lessons learned about coronary and peripheral vascular in-stent restenosis. Restenosis (defined as more than or equal to 50% diameter obstruction) has been documented to occur in 3% to 26% of patients following CEA (Table 19-2) (22–33). In patients with recurrent carotid stenosis following CEA, neurological events have been reported in only 1% to 5% of these patients. After CEA, restenosis that occurs within the first 2 years has been attributed to intimal hyperplasia, and recurrent stenosis that occurs after 2 years is due to atherosclerosis (34). Washburn et al. (35) demonstrated that early restenosis, presumably resulting from myointimal hyperplasia, leads to significantly fewer neurological events than late restenosis resulting from atherosclerosis. Sterpetti et al. (36) also observed different clinical outcomes among patients with recurrent stenosis at different times in the postoperative period. These investigators evaluated ultrasonographic and pathologic data and demonstrated that homogeneous soft plaque, homogeneous hard plaque, and heterogeneous plaque correlate with myointimal hyperplasia, fibrous atherosclerotic plaque, and complex atherosclerotic plaque, respectively. The homogeneous plaque occurred earlier in the postoperative course, whereas symptoms of cerebral

TABLE 19-2. INCIDENCE OF RESTENOSIS AFTER CAROTID ENDARTERECTOMY

Source	Year	Patients, n	Method of Follow-up	Restenosis, (%)
Hansen et al. (22)	1993	232	Dop/Dpx	9.8
Harker et al. (23)	1992	163	Dpx	12.9
Archie (24)	1986	181	OPG/Dop	2.7
Strawn et al. (25)	1990	146	Dpx	6.1
Ten Holter et al. (26)	1990	304	Dpx	13.5
DeGroote et al. (27)	1987	265	OPG/Dop	13.3
Keagy et al. (28)	1985	106	Dop/Dpx	22.1
Kinney et al. (29)	1993	430	Dpx	7.6
Rosenthal et al. (30)	1990	849	Dop	3.4
Healy et al. (31)	1989	301	Dpx	25.9
Zbornikova et al. (32)	1986	143	Dpx	23.9
Salenius et al. (33)	1989	116	Dpx	21.8

Dop, Doppler; Dpx, duplex; OPG, Ocular plethysmography.

ischemia were more common at the later stage with heterogeneous plaque. By analogy, it is presumed that carotid in-stent restenosis that develops within the first year or two is most likely caused by intimal hyperplasia.

Dangas and Fuster (37) described the pathophysiology of coronary in-stent stenosis in three phases: (a) early elastic recoil, first day, (b) formation and organization of mural thrombus, first 2 weeks, and (c) neointimal proliferation, first 3 months. Elastic recoil is believed to be a mechanical phenomenon and is clearly eliminated by stenting. Mural thrombus formation is related to tissue injury. Several studies have associated coronary angioplasty restenosis with neutrophil activation (38–40). Activated neutrophils release a number of inflammatory mediators that can aggravate endothelial damage and therefore stimulate platelet aggregation (41). Organization of mural thrombus involves smooth muscle cell proliferation and extracellular matrix deposition leading to neointimal hyperplasia (37,41,42). The final result is fibrous tissue buildup within the stent. The extent of tissue formed is proportional to the amount of injury.

NATURAL HISTORY

Given the paucity of long-term follow-up data regarding carotid in-stent stenosis, inferences regarding treatment must be made using data about CEA and coronary and peripheral vascular in-stent restenosis for the time being. Critical recurrent stenosis after CEA has been associated with carotid occlusion and stroke (43). Although the natural history of in-stent stenosis in the carotid artery is not well defined, the carotid surgery experience indicates that treatment should be considered for high-grade and symptomatic restenotic lesions. But there is a lack of compelling data to justify operative treatment (31,44). However, O'Donnell et al. (45) observed a 7.5% stroke rate in high-grade recurrent stenosis (more than or equal to 75% diameter obstruction) managed medically, compared with 2.1% in surgically treated patients. This has led to some enthusiasm for treatment of high-grade recurrent stenosis following CEA even if patients are asymptomatic.

Recurrent carotid artery stenosis after CEA, particularly when attributed to myointimal hyperplasia, is optimally treated by CAS (46,47). The rationale for this is two-fold. First, reoperative carotid surgery carries a higher risk of technical complications, including cranial nerve injury and problems with wound healing. Secondly, the smooth nature of the myointimal hyperplasia makes it much less prone to embolic sequelae caused by endoluminal manipulation.

This approach is valid only if it results in fewer clinical events, specifically fewer ipsilateral cerebral ischemic events. Such data regarding CAS are unknown at the present moment. In the absence of such data, studies have, instead, used the available information from coronary and peripheral in-stent restenosis. Symptoms caused by blockages in the peripheral circulation are related to the severity of arterial blockage. Therefore, restenosis results in the return of ischemic symptoms. The same is true for the coronary arteries. Both coronary and peripheral arteries serve primarily muscular distribution, which at times of physiologic stress require greater amounts of arterial flow than the stenotic and collateral arteries can readily provide. However, the internal carotid artery supplies a neural distribution, and the satisfactory nutrition of this neuronal distribution depends on a fairly stable arterial flow requirement, and ischemic symptoms appear to develop more often from embolization than from a lack of flow reserve. This is true about carotid artery disease in general, as the symptoms are mostly due to embolization, whereas symptoms in peripheral and coronary arteries are due to occlusion. It is, therefore, uncertain at this moment that the severity of a restenotic lesion following carotid artery stent implantation will be important. Until more data become available, the current consensus is to treat asymptomatic patients who have more than or equal to 80% in-stent restenosis following CAS and those patients who have symptoms along with more than or equal to 50% in-stent restenosis.

DIAGNOSIS

Because of the limited number of patients and the heterogenity of lesions, diagnostic criteria for quantifying in-stent restenosis are still being developed. Although carotid angiography remains the gold standard for the diagnosis of significant restenosis, it is difficult to justify liberal application of routine carotid angiography, particularly in asymptomatic patients.

The use of duplex ultrasound scans for evaluation of in-stent restenosis following CAS is evolving. Robbin et al. (48) prospectively compared the diagnosis of carotid in-stent restenosis with duplex scanning criteria and carotid angiography. The results were promising; however, in another study, Ringer et al. (49) revealed that a stent, per se, does indeed alter the blood flow velocity. In their study, both standard blood flow velocity criteria and customized criteria led to a high rate of false-positive studies. No patient with Doppler criteria for significant stenosis had greater than 50% in-stent restenosis. Three of the nine patients who underwent follow-up angiography had stenosis of 50% or more. The peak in-stent velocity or internal carotid artery to common carotid artery velocity ratio of each of the three patients with restenosis, but not for the six other patients, had increases of more than 80% since the immediate poststenting Doppler study. A single blood flow velocity criteria of the CAS was less reliable than changes in velocity over time. In a study by the author and colleagues (50), no patient with duplex criteria for significant stent restenosis had significant angiographic restenosis (Figs. 19-1, 19-2), except for those with marked increase in the peak systolic velocity (Fig. 19-3C, 19-3G,

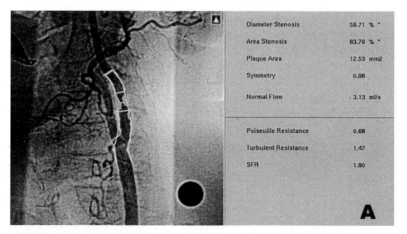

Diameter Stenosis	59.71 % *
Area Stenosis	83.76 % *
Plaque Area	12.53 mm2
Symmetry	0.98
Normal Flow	- 3.13 ml/s
Poiseuille Resistance	0.68
Turbulent Resistance	1.47
SFR	1.90

FIGURE 19-1. 64-year-old female with a history of transient ischemic attacks and right (**A**) internal carotid artery stenosis (59.7%) underwent successful stenting (residual of −15.5%) (**B**). Subsequent follow-up angiogram at 9 months revealed patent right carotid stent [minimal luminal diameter (MLD) = 5.4 mm] with no restenosis (**C**). Carotid angiogram was undertaken because of an abnormal carotid duplex ultrasound that showed peak systolic velocity = 256 cm per second, end diastolic velocity = 72 cm per second, and internal carotid artery (ICA)/common carotid artery (CCA) ratio = 3.2. (*Continues.*)

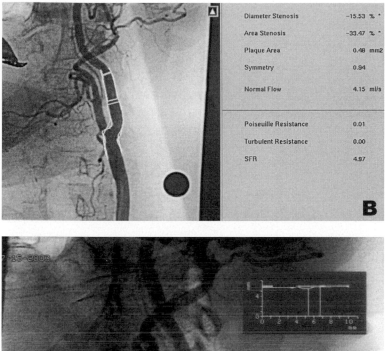

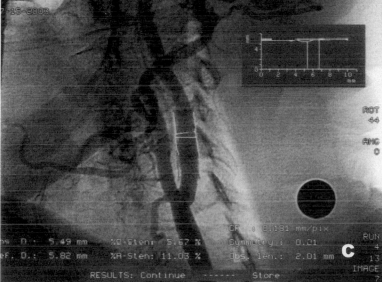

FIGURE 19-1. *(Continued.)*

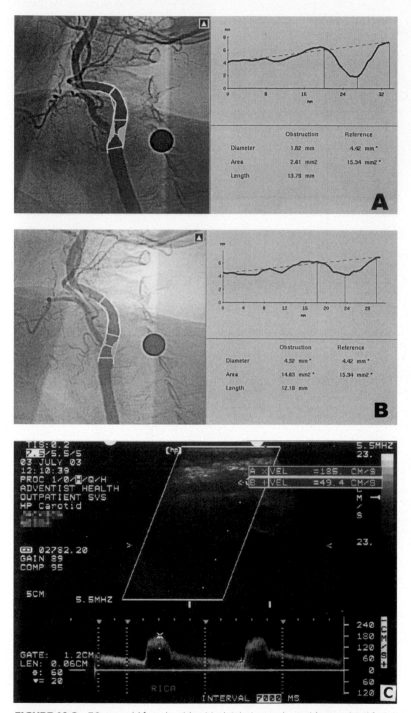

FIGURE 19-2. 76-year-old female with critical right internal carotid artery (ICA) [minimal luminal diameter (MLD) = 1.82 mm] stenosis (**A**) underwent successful (MLD = 4.32 mm) right ICA stenting (**B**). Follow-up carotid duplex ultrasound study at 10 months revealed peak systolic velocity (PSV) = 185 cm per second, end diastolic velocity (EDV) = 92 cm per second, and ICA/common carotid artery (CCA) ratio = 2.0 (**C**) and **D**). Subsequent follow-up carotid angiogram revealed (**E**) no restenosis (MLD = 4.14 mm; late loss = 0.18 mm). (*Continues*)

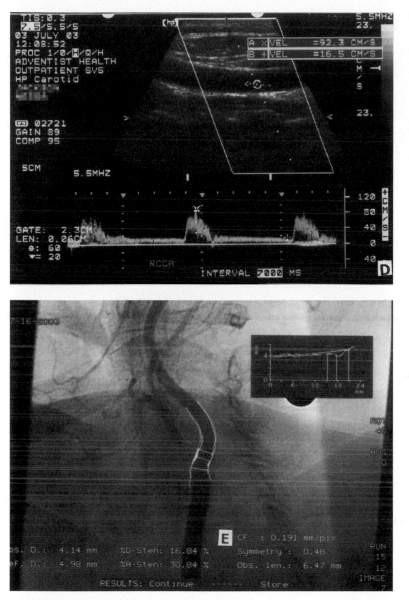

FIGURE 19-2. (Continued)

19-3H) compared to peak systolic velocity obtained within 4 weeks of stenting (Fig. 19-3A, 19-3B). Therefore, an immediate poststenting Doppler study should be obtained to serve as a reference value for future follow-up evaluation.

As a matter of fact, in a recent study by Qureshi et al. (51), the accuracy of carotid Doppler ultrasound in general did not justify its use as the sole basis for selecting appropriate patients for carotid surgery in patients with atherosclerotic carotid disease. Given the relatively low rate of associated morbidity with present-day techniques, confirmatory studies such as angiography should be performed in every patient before a decision regarding intervention is made, even in patients considered for intervention or surgery (51).

Text continues on p. 233

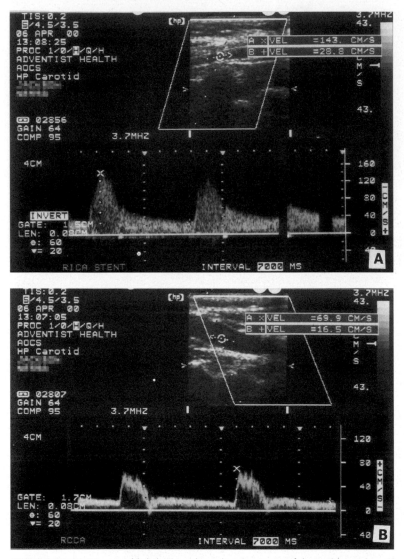

FIGURE 19-3. 68-year-old diabetic male underwent successful carotid stenting. At 4 weeks postprocedure, carotid duplex ultrasound revealed peak systolic velocity (PSV) = 143 cm per second, end diastolic velocity (EDV) = 28 cm per second, and internal carotid artery (ICA)/common carotid artery (CCA) ratio = 2.0 (**A** and **B**). Five months later, the patient had follow-up carotid duplex ultrasound that revealed PSV = 611 cm per second, EDV = 271 cm per second, and ICA/CCA = 10.5 (**C** and **D**). Subsequent angiogram confirmed restenosis (**E**). Successful balloon angioplasty was done using a 4.5-mm x 20-mm symmetry balloon with excellent angiographic results (**F**). Follow-up ultrasound 1 month later revealed no significant change from (**A** and **B**); however, subsequent follow-up ultrasound at 3 months revealed PSV = 367 cm per second, EDV = 88 cm per second, and ICA/CCA = 6.6 (**G** and **H**). Repeat carotid angiogram confirmed critical restenosis (**I**), which was successfully redilated (**J**). Follow-up carotid ultrasound 13 months later revealed patent right carotid stent, PSV = 145 cm per second, EDV = 43 cm per second, and ICA/CCA = 2.6 (**K** and **L**). (*Continues.*)

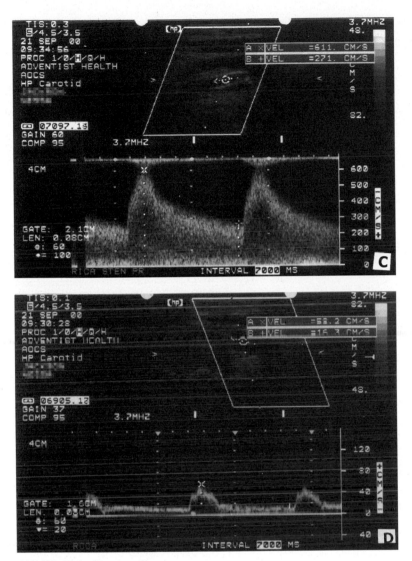

FIGURE 19-3. *(Continued.)*

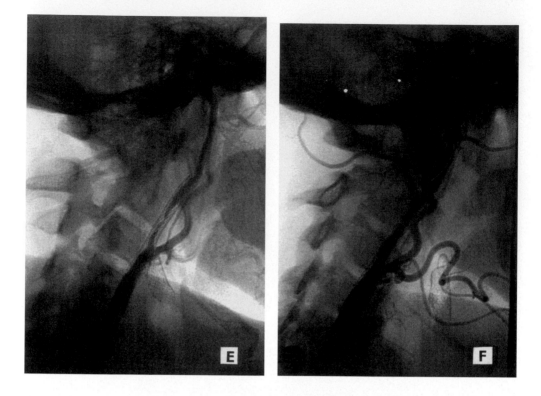

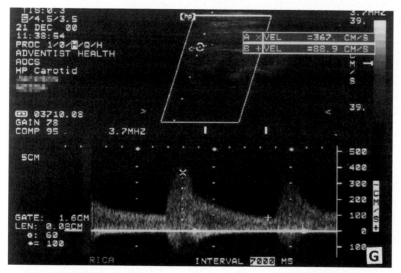

FIGURE 19-3. *(Continued.)*

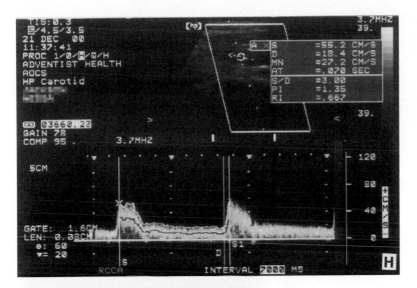

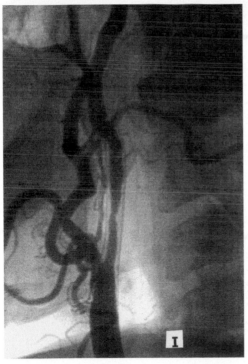

FIGURE 19-3. *(Continued.)*

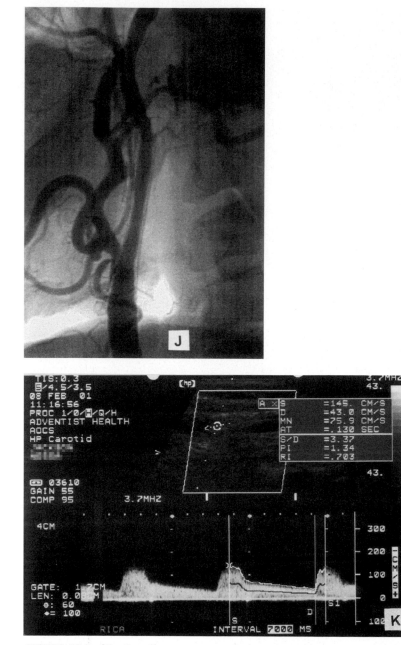

FIGURE 19-3. *(Continued.)*

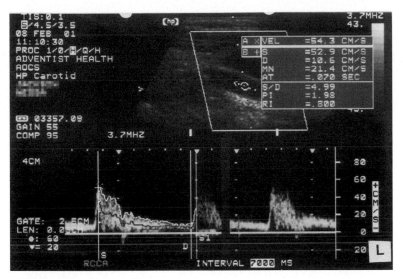

FIGURE 19-3. *(Continued.)*

LONG-TERM ANGIOGRAPHIC FOLLOW-UP

The author and colleagues (13,52) reported the extent of late angiographic lumen loss following CAS. In 130 patients, angiographic follow-up at a mean of 8 ± 3 months was available (Fig. 19-4). The cumulative frequency distribution for minimal luminal diameter revealed a late luminal loss of 0.43 mm (Fig. 19-5). This high rate of angiographic follow-up is partly due to frequent angiographic evaluation in such patients who have high incidence of concomitant coronary and noncoronary obstructive disease. In another study by the author and colleagues (50), serial carotid angiograms were available in 23 patients (Table 19-3). As noted, there was significant improvement in the minimal luminal diameter (late luminal gain) at a mean follow-up of 28 months compared with angiographic follow-up at mean of 7 months (Fig. 19-4E–H). Odashiro et al. (53) reported similar favorable angiographic outcomes. It is of interest to note that late improvement of intimal hyperplasia that occurred after 6 months has also been reported following coronary stenting. These angiographic data indicate that the long-term patency is very favorable following CAS if no restenosis is demonstrated after 9 to 12 months. In another study by the author (16), a restenosis rate of 2.7% was noted at a mean follow-up of 26 ± 13 months among 299 patients who underwent successful CAS. Repeat balloon angioplasty was successful in all of these patients without any complications

TABLE 19-3. SERIAL ANGIOGRAPHIC RESULTS (N = 23)

	Preprocedure	Post procedure	Mean Follow-up 7 MO	Mean Follow-up 28 MO
MLD	1.67 ± 0.5	4.8 ± 0.6	3.5 ± 0.9	3.89 ± 0.8

MLD, minimal luminal diameter.

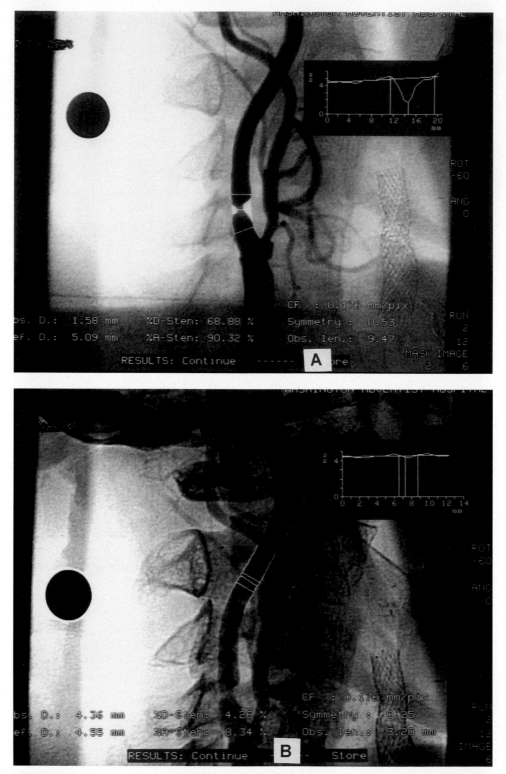

FIGURE 19-4. A: A carotid angiogram in the right internal carotid artery (ICA) shows significant (63.8%) stenosis [minimal luminal diameter (MLD) = 1.58 mm] with (**B**) reference MLD of 4.36 mm prior to stenting. (*Continues.*)

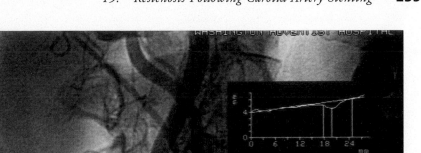

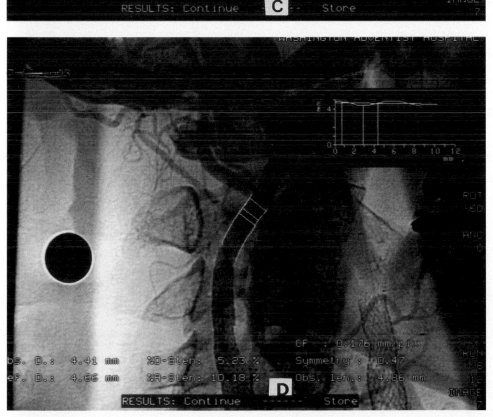

FIGURE 19-4. (*Continued.*) **C:** A carotid angiography after angioplasty and stent placement shows excellent results (residual stenosis of −3%) with marked improvement (MLD = 4.58 mm) and reference MLD of 4.41 mm (**D**).

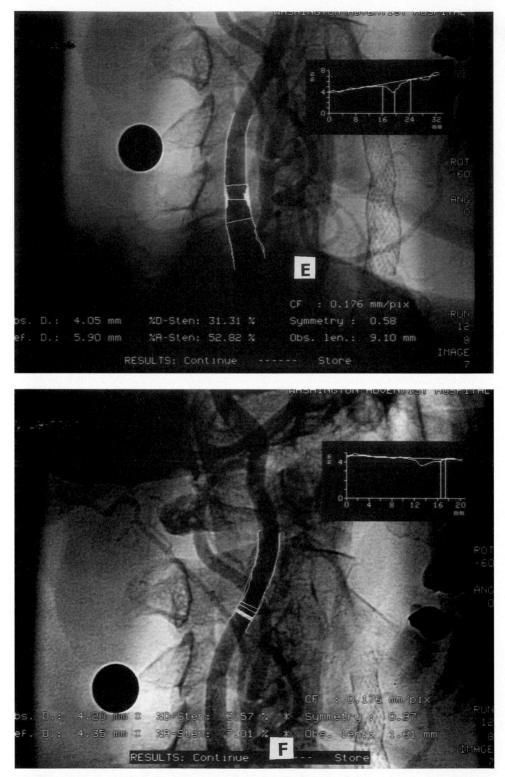

FIGURE 19-4. *(Continued.)* (**E** and **F**) Follow-up carotid angiogram at 6 months reveals residual stenosis (MLD = 4.05 mm) of 4%.

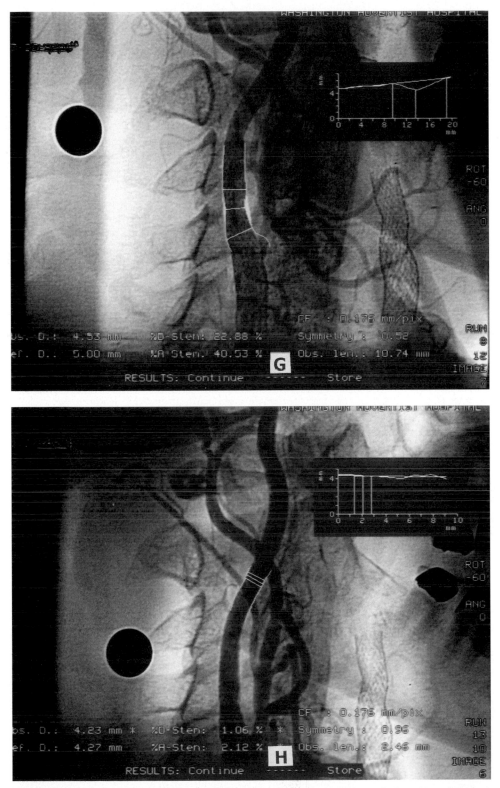

FIGURE 19-4. (*Continued.*) Subsequent follow-up carotid angiograms 18 months later (**G** and **H**) show reduction (0.30 mm) in intimal hyperplasia (MLD = 4.35 mm) with improved residual stenosis of −7%.

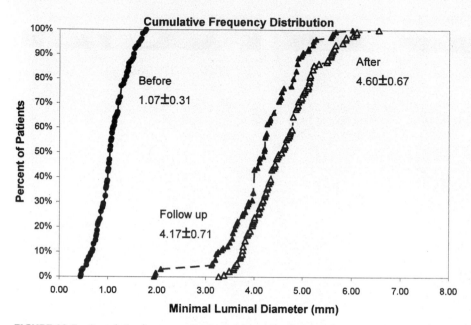

FIGURE 19-5. Cumulative frequency distribution for minimal luminal diameter before, immediately after, and at an average of 8 months postprocedure.

(Fig. 19-6). However, subsequent angioplasty was required for recurrent in-stent stenosis in four patients, all of whom had diffuse in-stent disease at their initial presentation for in-stent restenosis (Fig. 19-3I, 19-3J).

Wilfort-Ehringer et al. (15) reported a restenosis rate of 3% within 12 months after CAS in 279 patients. Two types of restenosis were described. In the more common form (six patients), the stenosis was not only seen at the site of the original stenosis, but was also noted proximal and at the distal end of the stent. All of the six patients were treated with repeat CAS. However, two of these patients had recurrent in-stent restenosis that was treated with repeat intervention. In the remaining three patients of this series, the stenosis was more at the "end of the stent," all at sites of kinks or bending distal to the stent. These three patients were treated with percutaneous transluminal angioplasty (PTA) along with no further restenosis observed at more than 12 months' follow-up.

MANAGEMENT OF IN-STENT RESTENOSIS

The most common treatment is balloon angioplasty. Although the acute results are usually acceptable, certain cases of in-stent restenosis have unfavorable long-term results when treated with balloon angioplasty. In the study presented by Yokoi et al. (54), the recurrence rate in coronary in-stent restenosis for diffuse in-stent restenosis was 85% after balloon angioplasty compared to 12% when the lesion was focal and 19% when the lesion was at the stent border. Similarly, other investigators have found significantly worse clinical outcomes when lesions longer than 20 mm are treated with a repeat intervention using balloon angioplasty or laser atherectomy (55,56). Whether a similar outcome occurs following carotid intervention remains to be seen. There have also been reports of cutting balloon angioplasty as well as reports of brachytherapy for carotid in-stent restenosis (57,58).

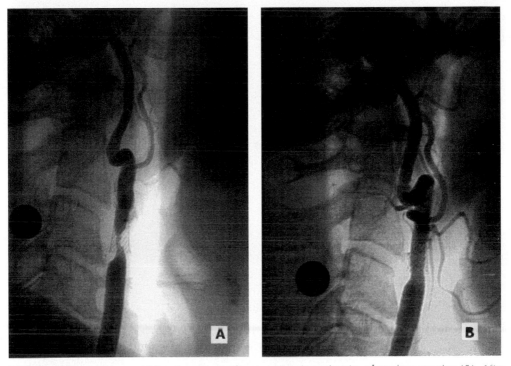

FIGURE 19-6. A 72-year-old female with significant restenosis at the site of previous stenting (**A**). After positioning a 6F multipurpose coronary guide (Cordis) in the mid common carotid artery, over a 0.014-inch coronary guide wire (Supersoft Wisdom, Cordis), a 4-mm x 10-mm cutting balloon was positioned within the stent and inflated gradually to 8 atmospheres (atm) of pressure (inflation time = 120 seconds). The balloon was then positioned over the proximal portion of stenosis and inflated again to 8 atm for 2 minutes. The balloon was then withdrawn and postangioplasty showed excellent immediate result (**B**). This patient continues to show stent patency at 1-year follow-up.

The technique of angioplasty for in-stent restenosis is essentially identical to that used for carotid stenting, except that one can do the entire procedure using a 6F coronary guide (Fig. 19-6). Other options besides catheter-based interventions include standard endarterectomy, bypass with prosthetic or vein conduit, and reversed saphenous common carotid to internal carotid bypass (59–62).

In our experience, the restenosis is very high following balloon angioplasty as well as following cutting balloon for diffuse in-stent restenosis (16). The role of brachytherapy, particularly beta radiation in such cases, may have to be evaluated because of its short dwelling times. Brachytherapy may also be useful in patients with small diameter carotid vessels and for patients with restenosis following CEA, where restenosis appears high. Although the use of drug-coated stents in the coronary circulation has been very successful in preventing neointimal proliferation, the use of drug-coated stents in the carotid system remains to be determined (63).

SUMMARY AND CONCLUSIONS

In conclusion, restenosis following carotid stenting is uncommon and can be treated easily with balloon angioplasty. The symptomatic presentation is rare. However, once restenosis occurs, particularly in small diameter internal carotid vessels and those with diffuse in-stent restenosis, the likelihood of recurrent restenosis is high. Duplex ultrasound with standard criteria can lead to a high incidence of false positives. Duplex ultrasound performed within 4 weeks of stenting should be done routinely and will act as a baseline for subsequent follow-up.

Because some cases of in-stent restenosis are refractory to effective long-term management with balloon angioplasty, increased attention has recently been directed to strategies for treating in-stent restenosis. These strategies have focused on cutting balloons, the placement of additional stents, or inhibiting further intimal proliferation with radiation or drug-coated stents, as well as a combination of techniques.

ACKNOWLEDGMENT

I am deeply grateful to my friend and colleague Dr. Michael J. Domanski for his critical review and invaluable suggestions for this chapter. The excellent contribution of my interventional fellow team, particularly Dr. Tarek Abou-Ghazala, with preparation of angiographic figures is greatly recognized. The contributions of Cathy Garey, Research Coordinator, in the preparation of this manuscript and illustrations by David Shawl are also very much appreciated.

REFERENCES

1. Serruys PW, de Jaegere P, Kiemeneij F, et al. A comparison of balloon-expandable-stent implantation with balloon angioplasty in patients with coronary artery disease. Benestent Study Group. *N Engl J Med* 1994;331:489–495.
2. Fischman DL, Leon MB, Baim DS, et al. Continued benefit of coronary stenting versus balloon angioplasty in the treatment of coronary artery disease. Stent Restenosis Study Investigators. *N Engl J Med* 1994;331:496–501.
3. Kimura T, Nosaka H, Yokoi H, et al. Serial angiographic follow-up after Palmaz-Schatz stent implantation: comparison with conventional balloon angioplasty. *J Am Coll Cardiol* 1993;21:1557–1563.
4. Laham RJ, Carrozza JP, Berger C, et al. Long-term (4- to 6-year) outcome of Palmaz-Schatz stenting: paucity of late clinical stent-related problems. *J Am Coll Cardiol* 1996;28:820–826.
5. Edelman ER, Rogers C. Hoop dreams: stent without restenosis. *Circulation* 1996; 94:1199–1202.
6. Kastrati A, Schomig A, Elezi S, et al. Predictive factors of restenosis after coronary stent placement. *J Am Coll Cardiol* 1997;30:1428–1436.
7. Cikrit DF, Gustafson PA, Dalsing MC, et al. Long-term follow-up of the Palmaz stent for iliac occlusive disease. *J Vasc Surg* 1995;118:608–613.
8. Becquemin JP, Allaire E, Qvarfordt P, et al. Surgical transluminal iliac angioplasty with selective stenting: long-term results assessed by means of duplex scanning. *J Vasc Surg* 1999;23:422–429.
9. Sapoval MR, Chatellier G, Long AL, et al. Self-expandable stents for the treatment of iliac artery obstructive lesions: long-term success and prognostic factors. *AJR Am J Roentgenol* 1996;165:1173–1779.
10. Wholey MH, Wholey M, Mathias K, et al. Global experience in cervical carotid artery stent placement. *Catheter Cardiovasc Interv* 2000;50:160–167.
11. Yadav JS, Roubin GS, Iyer S, et al. Elective stenting of the extracranial carotid arteries. *Circulation* 1997;95:376–381.
12. Wholey MH, Wholey M, Bergeron P, et al. Current global status of carotid artery stent placement. *Cathet Cardiovasc Diag* 1998;44:1–6.
13. Shawl F, Kadro W, Domanski MJ, et al. Safety and efficacy of elective carotid artery stenting in high-risk patients. *J Am Coll Cardiol* 2000;35:1721–1728.
14. Endovascular versus surgical treatment in patients with carotid stenosis in the Carotid and Vertebral Artery Transluminal Angioplasty Study (CAVATAS): a randomised trial. *Lancet* 2001:357:1729–1737.

15. Wilfort-Ehringer A, Ramazanali A, Gschwandter ME, et al. Single-center experience with carotid stent restenosis. *J Endovasc Ther* 2002;9:299–307.
16. Shawl FA. Carotid artery stenting: acute and long-term results. *Curr Opin Cardiol* 2002;17:671–676.
17. Roubin GS, New G, Iyer SS, et al. Immediate and late clinical outcomes of carotid artery stenting in patients with symptomatic and asymptomatic carotid artery stenosis. *Circulation* 2001;103:532–537.
18. Chakhtoura EY, Hobson RW II, Goldstein J, et al. In-stent restenosis after carotid angioplasty stenting: incidence and management. *J Vasc Surg* 2001;33:220–226.
19. Kastrati A, Schomig A, Elezi S, et al. Predictive factors of restenosis after coronary stent placement. *J Am Coll Cardiol* 1997;30:1428–1436.
20. Leger AR, Neale M, Harris JP. Poor durability of carotid angioplasty and stenting for treatment of recurrent artery stenosis after carotid endarterectomy: an institutional experience. *J Vasc Surg* 2001; 33:1008–1014.
21. New G, Roubin GS, Iyer SS, et al. Safety, efficacy, and durability of carotid artery stenting for restenosis following carotid endarterectomy: a multi-center study. *J Endovasc Ther* 2000; 7:345–352.
22. Hansen F, Lindblad B, Persson NH, et al. Can recurrent stenosis after carotid endarterectomy be prevented by low-dose acetylsalicylic acid? A double-blind, randomized and placebo-controlled study. *Eur J Vasc Surg* 1993;7:380–385.
23. Harker LA, Bernstein EF, Dilley RB, et al. Failure of aspirin plus dipyridamole to prevent restenosis after carotid endarterectomy. *Ann Intern Med* 1992;116:731–736.
24. Archie JP Jr. Prevention of early restenosis and thrombosis-occlusion after carotid endarterectomy by saphenous vein patch angioplasty. *Stroke* 1986;17:901–905.
25. Strawn DJ, Hunter GC, Guernsey JM, et al. The relationship of intraluminal shunting to technical results after carotid endarterectomy. *J Cardiovasc Surg (Torino)* 1990;31:424–429.
26. Ten Holter JB, Ackerstaff RG, Thoe Schwartzenberg GW, et al. The impact of vein patch angioplasty on long-term surgical outcome after carotid endarterectomy; a prospective follow-up study with serial duplex scanning. *J Cardiovasc Surg (Torino)* 1990;31:58–65.
27. DeGroote RD, Lynch TG, Jamil Z, et al. Carotid restenosis: long-term noninvasive follow-up after carotid endarterectomy. *Stroke* 1987;18:1031–1036.
28. Keagy BA, Edrington RD, Poole MA, et al. Incidence of recurrent or residual stenosis after carotid endarterectomy. *Am J Surg* 1985;149:722–725.
29. Kinney EV, Seabrook GR, Kinney LY, et al. The importance of intraoperative detection of residual flow abnormalities after carotid artery endarterectomy. *J Vasc Surg* 1993;17:912–922.
30. Rosenthal D, Archie JP Jr, Garcia-Rinaldi R, et al. Carotid patch angioplasty: immediate and long-term results. *J Vasc Surg* 1990;12:326–333.
31. Healy DA, Zierler RE, Nicholls SC, et al. Long-term follow up and clinical outcome of carotid restenosis. *J Vasc Surg* 1989;10:662–668.
32. Zbornikova V, Elfstrom J, Lassvik C, et al. Restenosis and occlusion after carotid surgery assessed by duplex scanning and digital subtraction angiography. *Stroke* 1986;17:1137–1142.
33. Salenius JP, Haapanen A, Harju E, et al. Late carotid restenosis: etiologic factors for recurrent carotid artery stenosis during long-term follow-up. *Eur J Vasc Surg* 1989;168:217–223.
34. Frericks H, Kievit J, van Baalen JM, et al. Carotid recurrent stenosis and risk of ipsilateral stroke: a systematic review of the literature. *Stroke* 1998;29:244–250.
35. Washburn WK, Mackey WC, Belkin M, et al. Late stroke after carotid endarterectomy: the role of recurrent stenosis. *J Vasc Surg* 1992;15:1032–1037.
36. Sterpetti AV, Schultz RD, Feldhaus RJ, et al. Natural history of recurrent carotid artery disease. *Surg Gynecol Obstet* 1989;168:217–223.
37. Dangas G, Fuster V. Management of restenosis after coronary intervention. *Am Heart J* 1996;132: 428–436.
38. De Servi S, Mazzone A, Ricevuti G, et al. Granulocyte activation after coronary angioplasty in humans. *Circulation* 1990;82:140–146.
39. Ikeda H, Nakayama H, Oda T, et al. Neutrophil activation after percutaneous transluminal coronary angioplasty. *Am Heart J* 1994;128:1091–1098.
40. Ricevuti G, Mazzone A, Pasotti D, et al. Role of granulocytes in endothelial injury in coronary heart disease in humans. *Atherosclerosis* 1991;91:1–14.
41. Inoue T, Sakai Y, Hoshi K, et al. Lower expression of neutrophil adhesion molecule indicates less vessel wall injury and might explain lower restenosis rate after cutting balloon angioplasty. *Circulation* 1998;97:2511–2518.
42. Kearney M, Pieczek A, Haley L, et al. Histopathology of in-stent restenosis in patients with peripheral artery disease. *Circulation* 1997;95:1998–2002.

43. Carballo RE, Towne JB, Seabrook GR, et al. An outcome analysis of carotid endarterectomy: the incidence and natural history of recurrent stenosis. *J Vasc Surg* 1996;23:749–754.
44. Lattimer C, Burnand KG. Recurrent carotid stenosis after carotid endarterectomy. *Br J Surg* 1997;84: 1206–1219.
45. O'Donnell T, Rodriquez A, Fortunato J, et al. Management of recurrent carotid stenosis: should asymptomatic lesions be treated surgically? *J Vasc Surg* 1996;24:207–212.
46. Lanzino G, Mericle RA, Lopes DK, et al. Percutaneous transluminal angioplasty and stent placement for recurrent carotid stenosis. *J Neurosurg* 1999;90:688–694.
47. Bergeron P, Chambran P, Benichou H, et al. Recurrent carotid disease: will stents be an alternative to surgery? *J Endovasc Surg* 1996;3:76–79.
48. Robbin RL, Lockhart ME, Weber TM, et al. Carotid artery stents: early and intermediate follow-up with Doppler US. *Radiology* 1997;205:749–756.
49. Ringer AJ, German JW, Guterman LR, et al. Follow-up of stented carotid arteries by Doppler ultrasound. *Neurosurgery* 2002;51:639–643.
50. Shawl FA, Lapetina F, Kadro WY, et al. Long-term outcome following carotid artery stenting. *J Am Coll Cardiol* 2000;35:69A.
51. Qureshi AI, Suri FK, Ali Z, et al. Role of conventional angiography in evaluation of patients with carotid artery stenosis demonstrated by Doppler ultrasound in general practice. *Stroke* 2001;32:2287–2291.
52. Shawl FA, Lapetina F, Kadro WY, et al. Extent of late luminal angiographic loss following carotid artery stenting. *J Am Coll Cardiol* 2000;35:15A.
53. Odashiro K, Yokoi H, Kimura T, et al. Serial changes of intimal hyperplasia of carotid artery after carotid stenting. *J Am Coll Cardiol* 2001;37:50A.
54. Yokoi H, Kimura T, Nakagawa Y, et al. Long-term clinical and quantitative angiographic follow-up after the Palmaz-Schatz stent restenosis. *J Am Coll Cardiol* 1996;27:224A (abst).
55. Mehran R, Ito S, Abizaid A, et al. Does lesion length affect late outcome of patients with in-stent restenosis? Results of the multicenter Laser Angioplasty for Stent Restenosis (LARS) registry. *J Am Coll Cardiol* 1998;31(Suppl):142A.
56. Sharma SK, Rjawat Y, Kakarala V, et al. Angiographic pattern of in-stent restenosis after Palmaz-Schatz stent implantation. *J Am Coll Cardiol* 1997;29(Suppl):313A.
57. Bendok BR, Roubin GS, Katzen BT, et al. Cutting balloon to treat carotid in-stent stenosis: technical note. *J Invas Cardiol* 2003;15:227–232.
58. Chan AW, Roffi M, Mukherjee D, et al. Carotid brachytherapy for in-stent restenosis. *Cathet Cardiovasc Interv* 2003;58:86–92.
59. Yale FL, Fisher WS 3rd, Jordan WD Jr, et al. Carotid endarterectomy performed after progressive carotid stenosis following angioplasty and stent placement: case report. *J Neurosurg* 1997;87:940–943.
60. Coumans JV, Warson VF, Picken CA, et al. Saphenous vein interposition graft for recurrent carotid stenosis after prior endarterectomy and stent placement: case report. *J Neurosurg* 1999;90:567–570.
61. Johnson SP, Fujltanl RM, Leyendecker JR, et al. Stent deformation and intimal hyperplasia complicating treatment of a post-carotid endarterectomy intimal flap with a Palmaz stent. *J Vasc Surg* 1997;25: 764–768.
62. Owens EL, Kumins N II, Bergan JJ, et al. Surgical management of acute complications and critical restenosis following carotid artery stenting. *Ann Vasc Surg* 2002;16:168–175.
63. Regar E, Serruys PW, Bode C, et al. Angiographic findings of the multicenter randomized study with the sirolimus-eluting Bx Velocity balloon-expandable stent (RAVEL): sirolimus-eluting stents inhibit restenosis irrespective of the vessel size. *Circulation* 2002;106:1949–1956.

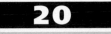

LIMITATIONS OF CURRENT EQUIPMENT AND THE FUTURE CAROTID ARTERY STENTING DEVICE

HORST SIEVERT
KASJA RABE

The editors asked us to focus on the limitations of the currently available equipment including carotid access, balloons, stents, and embolic protection devices and to address our view of the ideal future device. In doing so, we will try to avoid discussing advantages and drawbacks of the particular devices from individual companies. Instead, because all kinds of problems and limitations may occur or be present with all devices from all companies, we will give a general overview about the limitations of the currently available devices. We also will try to give an idea about what we think will be the future of the technical equipment.

In preparing the manuscript, we realized that it is not an easy task to write about problems of carotid artery stenting (CAS). That is because today we already have excellent results not only acutely but also regarding long-term follow-up (1). Carotid angioplasty is not a new procedure. The first balloon angioplasty of a carotid stenosis was already performed over two decades ago (in 1979) (2). However, only within the last 5 to 10 years has it become a procedure that is performed routinely in many centers worldwide. Fifteen years ago, coronary angioplasty was performed as routinely as CAS today. The results of coronary angioplasty were rather poor at that time. We had a technical failure rate of more than 30%; emergency surgery, myocardial infarction or death in 5% to 10%; and a high restenosis rate (3,4). It was easy to talk about limitations of coronary angioplasty equipment at that time. In contrast, the results of CAS today are already excellent. In our own experience, the technical failure rate has been only 0.6%. This is consistent with the experience in other centers and the world registry of CAS, where the technical success rate was 98.4% (5). Emergency surgery almost never becomes necessary. Cerebral infarction occurs in less than 3% in most experienced centers, mortality rates are below 1%, and re-stenosis rates are far below 10% (6–12).

So what are the remaining problems? In discussing this, we should concentrate not only on problems that may lead to a failure or a complication, but also on those minor problems that can usually be solved and may cause complications if the number of procedures increases further.

VASCULAR ACCESS AND ACCESS TO THE CAROTID ARTERIES

All problems associated with vascular access, such as hematoma, bleeding, local thrombosis, pseudoaneurysm, etc., are obviously not specific for CAS. They also occur in coronary and peripheral interventions. However, we have to keep in mind that the patients referred for CAS are on average 10 years older than those referred for coronary procedures; in our practice, 70 years versus 62 years. Elderly patients do not tolerate all kinds of local vascular complications as well as the younger ones. Therefore, decreasing the French size of sheaths and catheters will play an important role in the future. This may also allow the use of brachial or radial access more frequently (13). The use of closure devices may be an alternative. With most of these devices, increased patient comfort and earlier ambulation could be demonstrated (14–18). Unfortunately, this did not lead to a decrease of complication rates (19,20). However, new device generations may lead to better results.

Access to the carotid artery is rarely a cause of procedural failure. However, access difficulties may unnecessarily prolong the procedure and increase the amount of contrast medium that, in turn, may result in further problems and complications, especially in cerebral procedures. Furthermore, the risk of scraping the vessels of the aortic arch leading to embolism increases with multiple catheter exchanges.

Today, access to the carotid arteries is obtained usually with a diagnostic 5F catheter. This is then exchanged over a stiff wire to a long sheath or a guiding catheter. Although this works well in the majority of the cases, a single-step procedure would be preferable. Some investigators prefer to advance a 6F or 7F sheath together with a 5F catheter to the aortic arch, to cannulate the external carotid artery with the 5F catheter, and thereafter to advance the sheath over this diagnostic catheter. The sheath of the future will probably have a dilator that is shaped and steerable like a diagnostic catheter. The tip will probably be

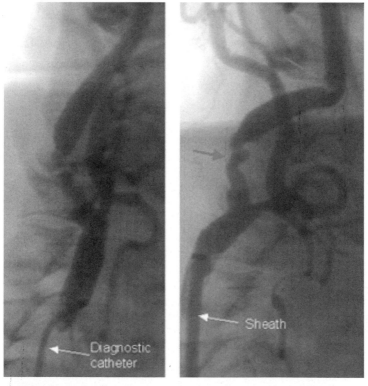

FIGURE 20-1. A stiff sheath may lead to straightening of the common carotid artery and consecutive kinking of the internal artery even before crossing the lesion.

softer than the tip of the currently available guiding catheters, and it will have a smooth transition to the rest of the shaft. This will make cannulation of the external carotid artery unnecessary, which today is often required to achieve a stable position of the exchange wire. A softer tip of the sheath or guiding catheter also avoids straightening of the common carotid artery, which may lead to kinking of the internal carotid artery (Fig. 20-1).

CROSSING OF THE LESION

Procedural failure due to the inability to cross the lesion is also extremely rare. Figure 20-2 gives the only example of a lesion with bizarre intraluminal calcifications that we could not cross. With all the wires that have been developed for coronary interventions, it is very unlikely that we will see much improvement in the near future. This may be different for intracranial angioplasty, where the tip of the guiding catheter may be several vessel curves and bends away from the lesion. Currently, a new technology—stereotaxis—is being developed, which allows navigation of a guide wire and a catheter with the help of a magnetic field (21). This seems to be a promising tool for all kinds of intracranial procedures.

STENT DELIVERY DEVICES AND STENTS

Balloon expandable stents have a risk of fracture or compression whenever they are implanted in vessels that may bend or be compressed by external forces. This may cause a disaster in

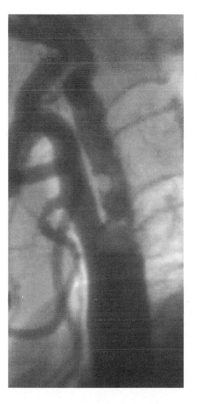

FIGURE 20-2. Bizarre lesion with intraluminal calcifications: Crossing was not possible.

the cerebral circulation. Therefore, in almost all centers, only self-expandable stents are used for carotid angioplasty. However, with self-expanding stents, we are facing a number of new problems, mainly regarding the implantation technique. A major disadvantage of self-expanding stents is the delivery system, which has a larger profile than a balloon. It is stiffer than a balloon, it may be difficult to retrieve, and compared with the balloon-expandable stents, it requires an additional step, i.e., insertion and inflation of a balloon catheter. Initially, all the self-expanding stents were mounted on over-the-wire devices. It is needless to mention that rapid exchange (monorail) devices are superior, and therefore, new stent generations will have this design.

Currently, most of the carotid stents are mounted on a 6F delivery catheter, but there are already 5F devices on the market. Technically, 4F delivery devices are possible and currently being developed. As discussed earlier, a reduction in French size is always an advantage.

Hopefully, a reduction in diameter will also increase flexibility of the delivery catheters. Today, elongated vessels are straightened during stent implantation owing to the stiffness of the stent and delivery catheter (Fig. 20-3). It not only makes exact placement of the stent more difficult, but it also leads to enfolding of the intima proximal and/or distal to the stenosis, which is certainly undesirable.

Sometimes it is difficult to retrieve the delivery catheter, especially if no predilatation has been performed. Usually this problem is caused by the distal tip of the delivery catheter, which may be caught within the stent. Some new generation devices are designed without

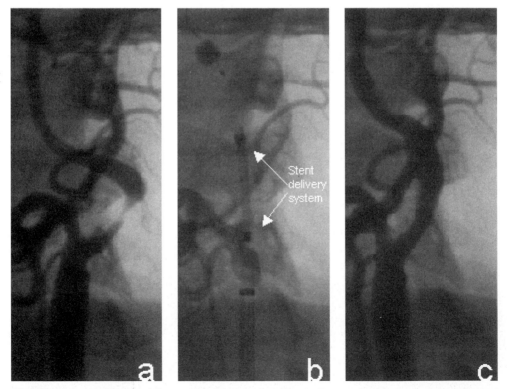

FIGURE 20-3. A stiff stent delivery system does not conform to the vessel anatomy. **A**: Before, **B**: stent delivery system introduced, and **C**: after stent implantation and balloon angioplasty.

distal tip, i.e., the distal tip is formed by the sheath that covers the stent, and this certainly will be the future.

All self-expanding nitinol stents can be compressed only a certain extent. This automatically leaves some space for the shaft of the delivery catheter. Keeping in mind that the profile of the balloons becomes smaller and smaller, it may become possible in the future to implement a balloon inside the stent delivery catheter. This would eliminate the additional step required with self-expanding stents, i.e., exchange for a balloon angioplasty catheter.

As with the delivery catheters, stiffness is a problem of many stents currently available. This leads to a straightening of the vessel, which may result in distal kinking with an immediate stenosis and/or late restenosis at the distal end of the stent (Figs. 20-4–20-6). The ideal stent of the future will completely follow all curves of the vessels. This will be a challenge for the engineers because at the same time they will have to increase the radial strength of the stent to avoid recoil. This problem occurs especially in calcified lesions (Fig. 20-7). To make it even more complex for the engineers, we would like to have stents with a very fine mesh, which means smaller gaps between the stent struts. Large gaps between the stent struts usually do not cause obvious clinical problems, but it may happen that debris protruding through the stent struts into the lumen (Fig. 20-8) may embolize or trigger thrombus formation. In the early days of CAS, complications occurring hours or even days after the procedure were almost unknown because of the small numbers of procedures and because we were busy with those complications occurring during the procedure. These days, the late complications are increasingly getting more attention.

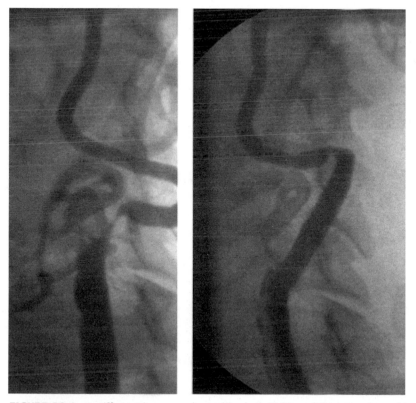

FIGURE 20-4. A stiff stent in a curved vessel leads to kinking of the internal carotid artery distal to the stent.

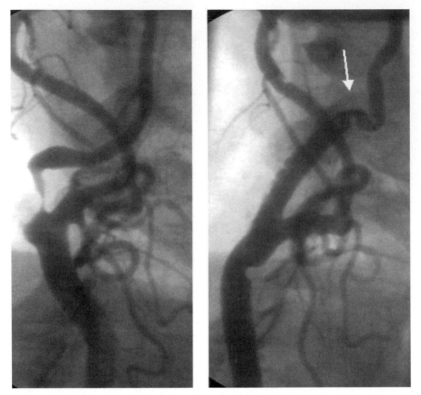

FIGURE 20-5. A stiff stent in a curved vessel leads to kinking of the internal carotid artery distal to the stent.

Late restenosis is also a problem, which is not on the priority list today because it is so rare—less than 5% in our experience. However, in the future, we (and the patients) hope to avoid this completely. Currently, drug-eluting stents most likely will be the winner, but radiation may also have its place. In the carotid arteries, radiation could be performed percutaneously within some hours after procedure, thereby eliminating all the logistical problems this treatment has in the coronaries.

EMBOLI PROTECTION DEVICES

Distal Embolic Protection

This can be performed with occlusion balloons and with filters that are described in detail elsewhere. The distal occlusion balloons have some disadvantages, mainly intolerance in some patients and inability to perform angiography during the procedure (22–25). Therefore, filters are becoming more and more popular (26–28).

What are the problems with the currently available filters? As with all devices in interventional procedures, profile and flexibility is always an issue. Today, the third-generation and fourth-generation devices are available, and they have improved tremendously compared to the first generation. However, it still happens that the lesion and/or tortuous vessels can only be crossed with the help of a "buddy-wire" or not at all.

Another issue is malapposition to the vessel wall. In filter devices with an eccentric

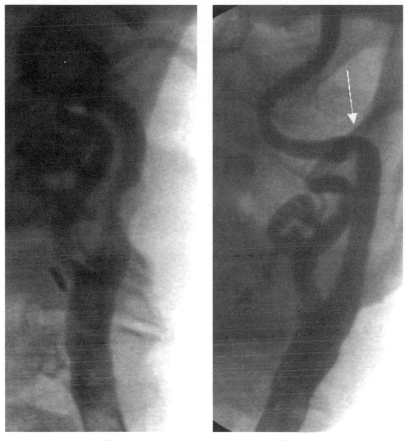

FIGURE 20-6. A stiff stent in a curved vessel leads to kinking of the internal carotid artery distal to the stent.

opening, like the Boston Scientific Filterwire (formerly EPI Filter, Boston Scientific, Natick, MA) or the Spider-Filter, this phenomenon can sometimes be observed during the procedure (Figs. 20-9, 20-10). Malapposition may also occur when using filters with a rounded concentric design (Fig. 20-11). In these cases, malapposition cannot be detected during the procedure.

We all do believe that particles smaller than 100 microns do not harm. Why do we believe this? Maybe because the pore size of the currently available filters is between 80 and 100 microns! The majority of particles are smaller than 100 microns (29–31). It has been shown in animal experiments that they may cause damage to the brain (32). The same has already been demonstrated in humans after cardiopulmonary bypass (33,34), and it is probably also true for carotid angioplasty (35–37).

So why not make the pores smaller? Currently, this may result in filter occlusion due to fibrin or thrombocytes. But this problem may be solved in the future by other filter material or drug coating of the filter.

The primary function of embolic protection devices is to add safety. However, if this is achieved, ease of use also becomes important. Having this in mind, rapid exchange devices will be advantageous. Filters that adapt to different vessel sizes are easier to use than filters that have to match exactly the vessel diameter. They also add some safety because exact

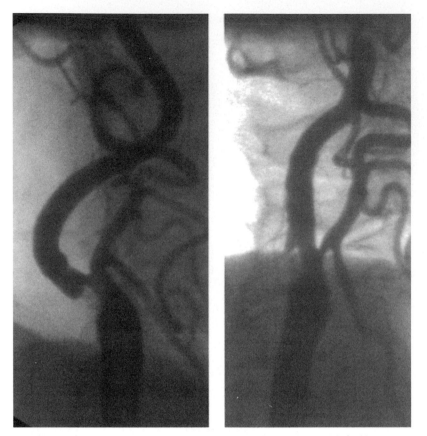

FIGURE 20-7. Residual stenosis due to stent recoil in an eccentric calcified lesion.

measurements of the vessel diameter may be difficult, and the vessel diameter may also change during the procedure. Also, some of the currently available filters require a certain distance between the distal stent end and the filter, which may make placement more difficult.

New devices that do not need a delivery catheter are currently being developed, thereby avoiding one step of the procedure. The next step will be a filter that does not require a retrieval catheter to be removed. It should be possible to design a filter that can be collapsed either remotely or with the help of a balloon catheter. This would eliminate another step of the procedure.

Proximal Protection Devices

Currently, there are only two devices for proximal occlusion available: the ArteriA device (San Francisco, CA) and the MO.MA device (Invatec Srl, Rocadelle, Italy). The major advantage compared with the filter devices is that the protection starts already before crossing the lesion, and even the very small particles are contained (38,39). The operator may use the wire of his choice, and there are no problems related to the device retrieval. The major drawback, however, is the large French size of 10F to 11F, which is necessary to introduce the device. We may expect some improvement in the future, but this will be limited because

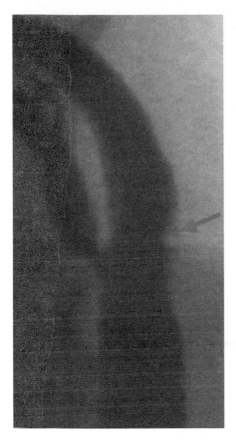

FIGURE 20-8. Arteriosclerotic debris, protruding through the stent struts.

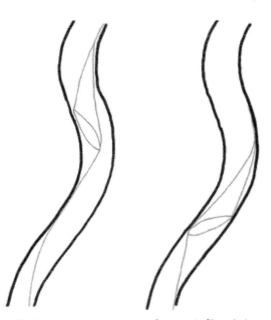

FIGURE 20-9. Malapposition of eccentric filter design.

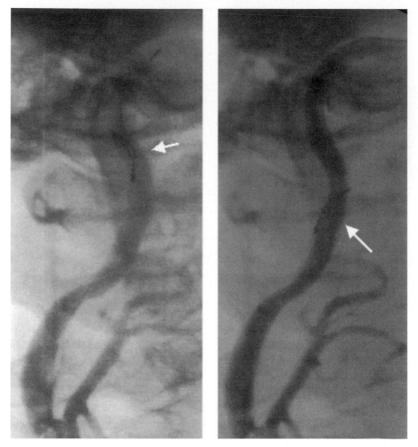

FIGURE 20-10. Malapposition of eccentric filter design.

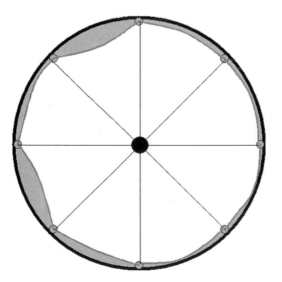

FIGURE 20-11. Malapposition may also occur
with a round filter design.

there has to be some residual space in the guiding catheter to allow blood flow reversal (ArteriA) or blood aspiration (MO.MA).

ANGIOPLASTY BALLOONS

In the early days of CAS, balloon rupture was not uncommon. This, however, was mainly a problem of the stents and not of the balloons. The new generation stents do not have sharp wire ends pointing towards the vessel lumen that would lead to balloon rupture.

There is no question that the profile of the balloon will decrease and the flexibility will increase. Up to a balloon size of 5 mm, we can use coronary angioplasty balloons, which are already very good. The larger balloons (6 to 8 mm) still need some improvement.

Besides all these procedural issues, we are waiting for achievements regarding preprocedural and postprocedural care. Some of these improvements will be related to medical treatment, which may reduce the risk of emboli as well as intracranial hemorrhage. Other improvements and achievements will be related to imaging. We still face the problem of magnetic resonance imaging (MRI)/angiography and duplex overestimating the severity of the lesion. Of course, it may also be that angiography underestimates the severity. The same holds true for stent follow-up investigations, where duplex ultrasound is often unreliable, and the MRI cannot be used at all because the currently available stents are not compatible with MRI. Finally, and probably most important, we need imaging techniques that allow us to differentiate those lesions that need to be treated from those that do not require treatment.

REFERENCES

1. Roubin GS, New G, Iyer SS, et al. Immediate and late clinical outcomes of carotid artery stenting in patients with symptomatic and asymptomatic carotid artery stenosis. A 5-year prospective analysis. *Circulation* 2001;103:532–537.
2. Mathias K, Steiger J, Thron A, et al. Perkutane Katheterangioplastik supraaortaler Arterienobstruktionen. *Angio* 1981;3:47.
3. Dorros G, Cowley MJ, Simpson J, et al. Percutaneous transluminal coronary angioplasty: report of complications from the National Heart, Lung, and Blood Institute PTCA Registry. *Circulation* 1983; 67:723–730.
4. Detre KM, Holmes DR Jr, Holubkov R, et al. Incidence and consequences of periprocedural occlusion. The 1985-1986 National Heart, Lung, and Blood Institute Percutaneous Transluminal Coronary Angioplasty Registry. *Circulation* 1990;82:739–750.
5. Wholey MH, Wholey M, Mathias K, et al. Global experience in cervical carotid artery stent placement. *Catheter Cardiovasc Interv* 2000;50:160–167.
6. Al Mubarak N, Roubin GS, Vitek JJ, et al. Carotid artery stenting: current status and future prospects. *Indian Heart J* 2001;53:445–450.
7. Reimers B, Corvaja N, Moshiri S, et al. Cerebral protection with filter devices during carotid artery stenting. *Circulation* 2001;104:12–15.
8. Shawl FA. Carotid artery stenting: acute and long-term results. *Curr Opin Cardiol* 2002;17:671–676.
9. Wholey MH, Wholey M, Bergeron P, et al. Current global status of carotid artery stent placement. *Catheter Cardiovasc Interv* 1998;44:1–6.
10. Mathias KD, Jaeger MJ, Sahl H. Internal carotid stents—PTA: 7 year experience. *Cardiovasc Interv Radiol* 1997;20(Suppl I):46.
11. Mathias KD. Angioplasty and stenting for carotid lesions: an argument for. In: *Advances in surgery*. Mosby Inc, 1999:225–248.
12. Parodi JC, La Mura R, Ferreira LM, et al. Initial evaluation of carotid angioplasty and stenting with three different cerebral protection devices. *J Vasc Surg* 2000;32:1127–1136.

13. Sievert H, Ensslen R, Fach A, et al. Brachial artery approach for transluminal angioplasty of the internal carotid artery. *Cathet Cardiovasc Diagn* 1996;39:421–423.
14. Slaughter PM, Chetty R, Flintoft VF. A single center randomized trial assessing use of a vascular hemostasis device vs. conventional manual compression following PTCA: what are the potential resource savings? *Cathet Cardiovasc Diagn* 1995;34:210–214.
15. Silber S. [10 years of arterial closure devices: a critical analysis of their use after PTCA]. *Cathet Cardiovasc Diagn* 2000;89:383–389.
16. Rickli H, Unterweger M, Sutsch G, et al. Comparison of costs and safety of a suture-mediated closure device with conventional manual compression after coronary artery interventions. *Cathet Cardiovasc Interv* 2002;57:297–302.
17. Kahn ZM, Kumar M, Hollander G, et al. Safety and efficacy of the Perclose suture-mediated closure device after diagnostic and interventional catheterizations in a large consecutive population. *Cathet Cardiovasc Interv* 2002;55:8–13.
18. Di Mario C. Closure devices: case closed? *Cathet Cardiovasc Interv* 2002;55:14–15.
19. Gonze MD, Sternbergh WC, Salartash K, et al. Complications associated with percutaneous closure devices. *Am J Surg* 1999;178:209–211.
20. Carey D, Martin JR, Moore CA, et al. Complications of femoral artery closure devices. *Cathet Cardiovasc Interv* 2001;52:3–7.
21. Grady MS, Howard MA 3rd, Dacey RG Jr, et al. Experimental study of the magnetic stereotaxis system for catheter manipulation within the brain. *J Neurosurg* 2000;93:282–288.
22. Al-Mubarak N, Roubin GS, Vitek JJ, et al. The effect of the distal-balloon protection system on microembolization during carotid stenting. *Circulation* 2001;104:1999–2002.
23. Al-Mubarak N, Colombo A, Gaines P, et al. Multicenter evaluation of carotid artery stenting with filter protection system. *J Am Coll Cardiol* 2002;39:841–846.
24. Théron J, Courtheoux P, Alachkar F, et al. New triple coaxial catheter system for carotid angioplasty with cerebral protection. *Am J Neuroradiol* 1990;11:869–874.
25. Théron J, Payelle G, Coskun O, et al. Carotid artery stenosis: treatment with protected balloon angioplasty and stent placement. *Radiology* 1996;201:627–636.
26. Ohki T, Roubin GS, Veith FJ et al. Efficacy of a filter device in the prevention of embolic events during carotid angioplasty and stenting: an ex vivo analysis. *J Vasc Surg* 1999;30:1034–1044.
27. Ohki T, Veith FJ. Carotid artery stenting: utility of cerebral protection devices. *J Invasive Cardiol* 2001;13:47–55.
28. Henry M, Amor M, Klonaris C, et al. Endovascular management of carotid artery stenosis. The impact of cerebral protection. In: Veith FH, Amor M, eds. *Endovascular therapies: current status of carotid bifurcation angioplasty and stenting*. New York: Marcel Dekker, 2001:95–117.
29. Ohki T, Marin ML, Lyon RT, et al. Ex vivo human carotid artery bifurcation stenting: correlation of lesion characteristics with embolic potential. *J Vasc Surg* 1998;27:463–471.
30. Coggia M, Goeau-Brissonniere O, Duval JL, et al. Embolic risk of the different stages of carotid bifurcation balloon angioplasty: an experimental study. *J Vasc Surg* 2000;31:550–557.
31. Rapp JH, Pan XM, Sharp FR, et al. Atheroemboli to the brain: size threshold for causing acute neuronal cell death. *J Vasc Surg* 2000;32:68–76.
32. Heistad DD, Marcus ML, Busija DW. Measurement of cerebral blood flow in experimental animals with microspheres: applications of the method. In: *Cerebral metabolism and neural function*. Baltimore: Williams and Wilkins, 1980:202–211.
33. Moody DM, Brown WR, Challa VR, et al. Brain microemboli associated with cardiopulmonary bypass: a histologic and magnetic resonance imaging study. *Ann Thorac Surg* 1995;59:1304–1307.
34. Pugsley W, Klinger L, Paschalis C, et al. The impact of microemboli during cardiopulmonary bypass on neuropsychological functioning. *Stroke* 1994;25:1393–1399.
35. Jordan WD, Voellinger DC, Doblar DD, et al. Microemboli detected by transcranial Doppler monitoring in patients during carotid angioplasty versus carotid endarterectomy. *Cardiovasc Surg* 1999;7:33–38.
36. Ringelstein B, Droste D, Babikian V, et al. Consensus on microembolus detection by TCD. *Stroke* 1998;29:725–729.
37. Tübler T, Schlüter M, Dirsch O, et al. Balloon-protected carotid artery stenting: relationship of periprocedural neurological complications with the size of particulate debris. *Circulation* 2001;104:2791–2796.
38. Parodi JC, Bates MC, Schonholz C, et al. International multi-center Parodi Anti-Embolic System study: preliminary results. *Am J Cardiol* 2000;86(Suppl 1 8A):33i.
39. Adami CA, Scuro A, Spinamano L, et al. Use of the Parodi Anti-Embolism system in carotid stenting: Italian trial results. *J Endovasc Ther* 2002;9:147–154.

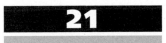

ELECTIVE ANGIOPLASTY AND STENTING FOR INTRACRANIAL ATHEROSCLEROTIC STENOSES

H. CHRISTIAN SCHUMACHER
PHILIP M. MEYERS
J. P. MOHR
RANDALL T. HIGASHIDA

Stroke is the most common life-threatening neurological disease and the third leading cause of death in the United States (1). Approximately 750,000 people suffer a stroke annually, costing an estimated $45 billion in treatment and lost productivity. Intracranial atherosclerosis accounts for about 8% to 9% of all ischemic strokes in population-based (2) or hospital-based studies (3,4). It is estimated that approximately 40,000 strokes annually are due to intracranial atherosclerosis in the United States. In general, intracranial atherosclerosis occurs in the setting of widespread atherosclerosis (5,6). Asians (Japanese, Chinese, Korean) (7–9), African-Americans (4), and Hispanics (2) appear more likely to have intracranial atherosclerosis compared to Caucasians. Besides race and ethnicity, risk factors associated with intracranial atherosclerosis include insulin-dependent diabetes mellitus, hypercholesterolemia, cigarette smoking, and hypertension (2,10,11).

DYNAMICS OF INTRACRANIAL ARTERIAL STENOSES

Intracranial stenoses are usually detected in patients presenting with acute ischemic events, that is, stroke or transient ischemic attacks (TIA). Most published data on the natural history of intracranial atherosclerosis are from patients examined either by conventional angiography or transcranial Doppler sonography (TCD). Intracranial stenoses may undergo progression, regression, or remain stable during the follow-up period. Initial evidence for the dynamic nature of intracranial stenoses comes from case reports and has been confirmed later by larger case series.

In a small series published by Allcock (12), two out of four patients showed changes after the initial angiography: A follow-up angiogram 10 days after an initial study demonstrated complete regression of the middle cerebral artery (MCA) stenosis, and in another patient, a repeat study on the same day revealed some improvement at the site of stenosis with some narrowing in the arterial segments next to it. Hinton et al. (13) examined two patients with MCA stenosis by angiography and demonstrated disease progression in one artery and improvement in the second. No change was observed in another case published by Lascelles and Burrows (14). In a series of 21 patients with a total of 45 intracranial stenoses examined by serial angiography over an average follow-up period of 26.7 months, 40% of the stenoses were stable, 40% progressed, and 20% regressed (15). In this study, carotid siphon stenosis was the most frequent site of intracranial stenosis, accounting for 49% of all stenoses. However, mean stenosis grade remained stable over time. On the other hand, mean stenosis for lesions of the MCA, anterior cerebral artery (ACA), or posterior cerebral artery (PCA), accounting for 40% of all lesions detected, tended to progress. Data for vertebrobasilar stenoses were inconclusive owing to the low number detected in this study.

The dynamic nature of intracranial stenoses has been confirmed by TCD. Schwarze et al. (16) conducted a retrospective study of TCDs in 22 patients with a total of 29 stenoses diagnosed by angiography. At follow-up, a total of ten lesions (35%) were considered to have progressed, whereas two lesions (7%) demonstrated significant decrease in flow velocity, suggesting regression of stenosis. In a prospective series of 100 consecutive acute Chinese stroke patients, Wong et al. (9) examined by TCD 17 patients with intracranial stenosis within 48 hours after stroke onset (14 with MCA stenosis and three with intracranial ICA stenosis), and three of these had tandem stenosis. These 17 cases represented 26% of all examined ischemic stroke patients. In repeat examinations within 3 months poststroke, either by magnetic resonance angiography (MRA) or TCD, three (18%) of 17 stenoses had resolved. In a subsequent paper, Wong et al. (17) examined a total of 143 patients from a prospective cohort of 345 patients with acute ischemic stroke. MCA stenosis was found in 107 (75%) cases. TCD follow-up at 6 months demonstrated complete resolution of the MCA stenosis in 27 (25%), whereas MCA stenosis was still present in 77 (70%) or had progressed to occlusion in five (5%) patients. Segura et al. (3) examined 24 patients with a total of 28 MCA stenoses diagnosed by TCD in the setting of an acute ischemic stroke. At 6 months after the initial evaluation, 25% of the MCA stenoses had completely disappeared on the follow-up TCD examination. Similar TCD studies for the vertebrobasilar artery and PCA have not been published thus far.

In summary, intracranial stenoses are dynamic lesions, and a significant portion of intracranial stenoses diagnosed in the setting of acute ischemic events will regress with medical treatment only. However, current imaging does not establish the future course of a given lesion, and the precise nature of the underlying lesion, that is, local thrombosis or stenotic atherosclerosis, is difficult to distinguish with current imaging techniques. Available evidence suggests that progression of intracranial stenoses might be dependent on the lesion site, with internal carotid artery (ICA) stenoses less likely to progress compared to other intracranial sites, but overall the factors associated with progression, stabilization, or regression remain to be established.

PATHOLOGY AND CHARACTERISTICS OF ATHEROSCLEROTIC PLAQUES

Most of our knowledge about the pathology of intracranial atherosclerosis and associated stenoses is based on autopsy studies (6,18–26). Currently, the *in vivo* disease process of intracranial luminal narrowing of intracranial arteries can be inferred only from *in vivo* observations of atherosclerotic lesions in coronary and extracranial carotid arteries. In most cases, the narrowing is due to atherosclerotic plaque, and pathologic evidence exists that plaque morphology in intracranial vessels resembles those of other vascular territories.

Plaque morphology seems to be important in the setting of acute coronary syndromes, and, by extension, this might apply also to acute cerebrovascular syndromes. Angioscopy of coronary and carotid arteries reveals two types of plaques, white and yellow plaques. White plaques are also named stable plaques, while yellow plaques are named unstable plaques

(Fig. 21-1). Yellow plaques have thin fibrous caps with a lipid-rich core, inadequate collagen content, and show an increased distensibility with compensatory enlargement (27,28). In contrast, white plaques have thick fibrous caps or are completely fibrous and show low distensibility and paradoxical shrinkage (27,28). Yellow plaques have been found more often in the setting of acute coronary syndromes compared to white (28–30), and in a prospective study, acute coronary syndromes occurred more often during the follow-up study period in patients with yellow plaques (31). These findings suggest a higher mechanical vulnerability of yellow plaques compared to white leading to acute coronary syndromes. Using intravascular ultrasound, Tanaka et al. (32) were able to demonstrate a higher occlusion rate of coronary arteries within minutes after successful coronary angioplasty in symptomatic echolucent plaques, thought to correlate to yellow plaques. With time, however, yellow plaques change into white plaques, a process that is thought to represent healing (33). Unfortunately, current

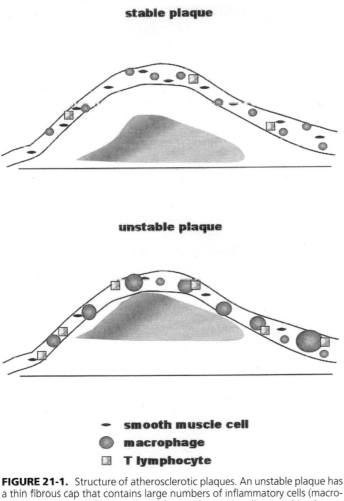

stable plaque

unstable plaque

- **smooth muscle cell**
- **macrophage**
- **T lymphocyte**

FIGURE 21-1. Structure of atherosclerotic plaques. An unstable plaque has a thin fibrous cap that contains large numbers of inflammatory cells (macrophages, T-cells) and few numbers of smooth muscle cells. Unstable plaques macroscopically appear yellow. A stable plaque has a thicker fibrous cap containing less inflammatory cells but larger numbers of smooth muscle cells. Stable plaques macroscopically appear white.

technology does not allow the *in vivo* examination of intracranial arteries by either angioscopy or intravascular ultrasound so that *in vivo* morphological data in these vessels are still lacking.

PATHOPHYSIOLOGY OF STROKE IN INTRACRANIAL ATHEROSCLEROSIS

Ischemic strokes in intracranial atherosclerosis can be caused by perfusion failure, local thrombosis at the site of the stenosis with arterioarterial thromboembolism, or occlusion at the origin of small penetrator's arteries. In the following sections, the different pathomechanisms of symptomatic intracranial atherosclerosis and their relevance to angioplasty are discussed.

Perfusion Failure

Depending on both stenosis severity and adequacy of collateral circulation, stenosis of cerebral arteries may lead to reduction of blood flow distal to it. In cerebral angiography, hemodynamic effects are usually demonstrated by delayed flow or border-zone shift. Examples of patients with intracranial stenoses and perfusion failure are demonstrated in Figs. 21-2, 21-3, and 21-4. The hemodynamic effects of cerebrovascular stenoses have been categorized into three stages [see Derdeyn et al. (34) for review]. Owing to good collateral circulation, a significant proportion of occlusive lesions have no effect on the distal circulation (stage 0: normal cerebral hemodynamics). However, when collateral circulation is inadequate, perfusion pressure distal to the lesion begins to fall. Because of an autoregulatory response, reflex vasodilatation occurs (stage 1 of hemodynamic compromise). In this stage, an increase in cerebral blood volume (CBV) and prolongation of mean transit time (MTT) are the result of autoregulatory vasodilatation, with cerebral blood flow (CBF) thus maintained. When autoregulatory vasodilatation is not adequate to maintain normal CBF, CBF begins to fall, and the brain increases the amount of extracted oxygen from the blood in order to maintain normal cerebral oxygen metabolism (stage 2 of hemodynamic compromise: misery perfusion). With further decrease in perfusion pressure above maximal oxygen extraction, disruption of oxygen metabolism leads to infarction of brain tissue. This concept evolves from several studies discussed below.

In one of the earliest studies, Naritomi et al. (35) demonstrated that the hemodynamic effect of MCA stenosis is usually present at a stenosis grade of 50% or higher and that the severity of perfusion deficit corresponded with the stenosis grade. This study involved a series of 36 patients examined by cerebral angiography and measurements of regional cerebral blood flow (rCBF) using ^{133}Xe inhalation. In the 16 patients with less than 50% MCA stenosis, no hemodynamic abnormality in angiographic and rCBF examinations was evident. In the nine patients with 50% to 74% MCA stenosis, angiography often revealed delayed filling of MCA branches, but with no significant rCBF reduction. All 25 patients with less than 75% MCA stenosis had small infarctions in the basal ganglia. In the 11 patients with 75% to 99% stenosis, a significant flow depression both in angiographical and rCBF examinations was observed, and three of them had large cerebral infarction in the watershed zone or the cerebral cortex (35).

In a small series of five patients with MCA occlusion and five patients with MCA-M1 stenosis (grade 50% to 83%) studied with positron emission tomography, Derdeyn et al. (36) suggested that MCA occlusion is associated with misery perfusion (stage 2) and MCA-M1 stenosis is not. Of the five patients with MCA occlusion, three had autoregulatory

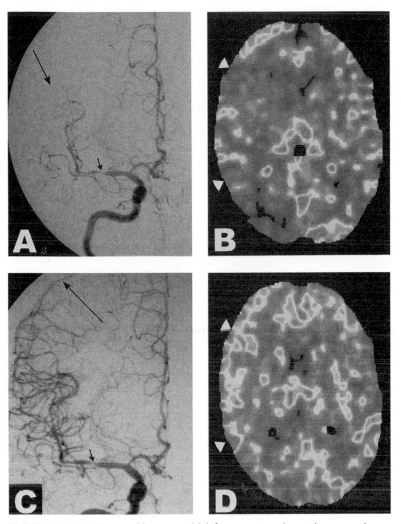

FIGURE 21-2. A 72-year-old woman with left upper extremity weakness, numbness, and intermittent limb shaking due to symptomatic right middle cerebral artery (MCA) stenosis failing medical therapy with aspirin, clopidogrel, and intravenous heparin. **A:** Right internal carotid arteriography in frontal projection during arterial phase demonstrates high-grade, focal stenosis of the right M1 segment (*short arrow*) and delayed filling of distal right MCA branch vessels (*long arrows*). **B:** Xenon computed tomography (CT) brain scan confirms asymmetric and reduced perfusion of the right MCA distribution (*white arrows*). **C:** Following angioplasty using a 1.5-mm-diameter coronary balloon (*short arrow*), the vessel diameter is only modestly increased although distal perfusion has increased markedly (*long arrows*). **D:** Repeat xenon CT perfusion study 24 hours following angioplasty demonstrates dramatically increased perfusion of the right MCA territory due to the small increase in cross-sectional diameter of the stenosis. (See also the color section following page 164 of this text.)

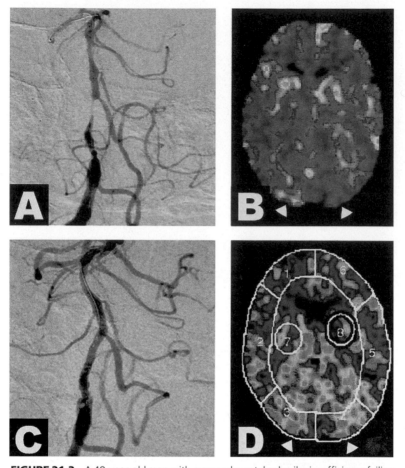

FIGURE 21-3. A 49-year-old man with crescendo vertebrobasilar insufficiency failing medical therapy with aspirin, clopidogrel, and intravenous heparin. **A**: Complete cerebral arteriography demonstrated high-grade focal stenosis of the intracranial right vertebral artery. The left vertebral artery was previously occluded, and there was no significant contribution to the posterior cerebral circulation by circle of Willis collaterals. **B**: Xenon computed tomography (CT) perfusion brain scan reveals diminished cortical perfusion in the posterior circulation (*white arrows*). **C**: Revascularization was performed under general anesthesia using a 2.5 × 9-mm metallic stent, which resulted in complete resolution of symptoms. **D**: Xenon CT perfusion scan within 24 hours of the procedure demonstrates hyperperfusion (increase in perfusion greater than 100%) in the posterior circulation (*white arrows*). This was managed by strict blood pressure control in the neurological intensive care unit until resolution. The patient recovered without complication. (See also the color section following page 164 of this text.)

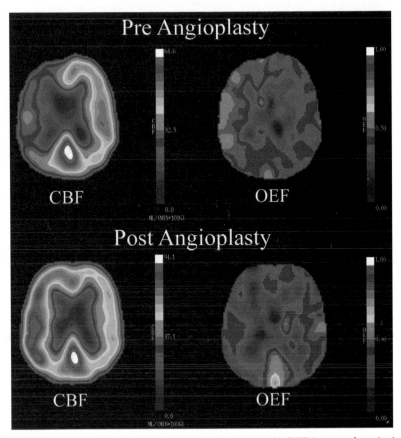

FIGURE 21-4. Quantitative positron-emission tomography (PET) images of cerebral blood flow (CBF, *left*) and oxygen extraction fraction (OEF, *right*). The top row of images (immediately before angioplasty) shows the reduction of CBF and compensatory increase in OEF in the right hemisphere distal to the stenosis. There are two basic compensatory responses of the cerebrovasculature to reduced perfusion pressure—autoregulatory vasodilation and increased oxygen extraction (134). These serve to maintain normal oxygen metabolism and neuronal function. When perfusion pressure drops below a critical level, the capacity for autoregulatory vasodilation is exceeded, and CBF will fall passively as a function of pressure. In this situation, OEF can increase from a baseline of 30% to a maximum of 80%. This phenomena has been called "misery perfusion" (135). The presence of increased OEF has been proven to be a powerful and independent predictor of subsequent stroke in patients with atherosclerotic occlusive cerebrovascular disease (34,39,136). The lower row of images acquired 36 hours after angioplasty shows the improvement in CBF and OEF. PET images courtesy of Colin P. Derdeyn, MD. (See also the color section following page 164 of this text.)

vasodilatation (stage 1) and four had increased oxygen extraction fraction distal to the lesion (stage 2). In contrast, four out of the five patients with focal MCA stenosis had normal hemodynamics (stage 0), and one patient had stage 1 hemodynamic status. In conclusion, Derdeyn et al. (36) suggested that stroke pathomechanism in MCA stenosis is probably thromboembolic rather than perfusion failure. A limitation of that study, however, is that the exact degree of MCA stenosis at the time of positron-emission tomography (PET) examination was unknown because angiography and PET were not performed on the same day in all patients (range 1–91 days). As has been demonstrated previously, MCA stenoses can be quite dynamic, with rapid regression and progression. In a subsequent paper, Derdeyn et al. (37) presented a patient with symptomatic 80% MCA-M1 stenosis who actually had misery perfusion (stage 2 of hemodynamic compromise) as detected by PET, immediately prior to angiography in the territory of the stenotic MCA. Successful angioplasty with a 40% residual MCA stenosis resulted in normalization of hemodynamic compromise as determined by PET at 36 hours postprocedure.

Studies with large sample sizes examining the relationship between different stages of perfusion failure and subsequent stroke in intracranial atherosclerosis are lacking. However, there is considerable evidence on the significance of stage 2 of hemodynamic compromise [increased oxygen extraction fraction (OEF)] as an independent stroke risk factor for ipsilateral stroke in atherosclerotic internal carotid occlusion. Increased OEF is associated with symptomatic carotid occlusion (38). Of 117 prospectively studied patients with carotid occlusion, 44 had increased OEF distal to the occluded carotid, and 73 had normal OEFs. Thirty-nine of the 81 patients with prior ipsilateral ischemic symptoms had high OEFs (42%), whereas only five of the 31 asymptomatic patients had high OEFs (16%, $p<0.001$). In a prospective, blinded, longitudinal cohort study by the same group, increased OEF was an independent risk factor for ipsilateral stroke (39). In this study, stroke occurred ipsilaterally in 11 of 39 patients with stage 2 hemodynamic failure due to internal carotid occlusion, and in only two of 42 patients without. Similar data on intracranial ICA stenoses are lacking, but data obtained from extracranial ICA occlusion might be extrapolated to intracranial carotid stenosis.

In summary, hemodynamic compromise as defined by neuroimaging seems to be an independent risk factor for ipsilateral stroke. The presence of a high-grade stenosis or even occlusion does not necessarily imply that there is actual perfusion failure. Patients with hemodynamic compromise due to intracranial atherosclerosis may represent a subgroup of patients for whom angioplasty may have the greatest chance of being proven effective.

Local Thrombosis at the Site of Stenosis

Findings of several autopsy studies suggest that thrombosis complicates intracranial athero-sclerosis associated with a preexisting stenosis (Fig. 21-5) (19,20,23–25). In some cases, intramural hemorrhage due to fibrinoid degeneration of the capillaries in the plaque could be responsible for cerebral arterial thrombosis (Fig. 21-5) (25,26).

In a careful autopsy study of the extracranial and intracranial vertebrobasilar systems, Castaigne et al. (19) were able to demonstrate that 38 of 40 primary thrombotic occlusions were related to stenotic atherosclerotic plaques. The degree of stenosis could be estimated in 35 lesions, and in 32 of these (94%), stenosis was tight (more than or equal to 75%). The same group previously published the association of local thrombosis with MCA stenosis in two out of 11 autopsy cases with MCA occlusion (23). Ogata et al. (25) could also demonstrate formation of nonocclusive mural and occlusive thrombi without plaque rupture in an autopsy series of eight patients. Thrombus formation in three of these cases was distal to the stenosis, and in one case a lamellated structure suggested stepwise progression with extension of the mural thrombus. These findings parallel those in coronary and extracranial carotid arteries and suggest plaque instability. However, in a recent autopsy series, Lammie et al. (22) found no direct evidence for plaque instability in 14 cases of intracranial ICA thrombosis. Of the 14 cases, three showed extracranial (carotid sinus), seven intracranial, and four both extracranial and intracranial carotid artery occlusion. In six of the seven occluded carotid sinuses, thrombus overlaid an ulcerated, unstable, atherosclerotic plaque. In one extracranial and all 11 intracranial occlusions, there was either no atheroma or a mildly stenotic, stable, fibrous plaque, and in these cases, the cause of occlusion was embolism

Mechanisms of Cerebral Artery Thrombosis

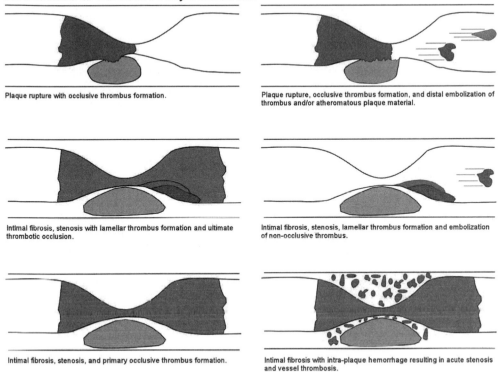

Plaque rupture with occlusive thrombus formation.

Plaque rupture, occlusive thrombus formation, and distal embolization of thrombus and/or atheromatous plaque material.

Intimal fibrosis, stenosis with lamellar thrombus formation and ultimate thrombotic occlusion.

Intimal fibrosis, stenosis, lamellar thrombus formation and embolization of non-occlusive thrombus.

Intimal fibrosis, stenosis, and primary occlusive thrombus formation.

Intimal fibrosis with intra-plaque hemorrhage resulting in acute stenosis and vessel thrombosis.

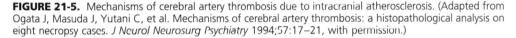

FIGURE 21-5. Mechanisms of cerebral artery thrombosis due to intracranial atherosclerosis. (Adapted from Ogata J, Masuda J, Yutani C, et al. Mechanisms of cerebral artery thrombosis: a histopathological analysis on eight necropsy cases. *J Neurol Neurosurg Psychiatry* 1994;57:17–21, with permission.)

(eight cases), giant-cell arteritis (one case), or was unknown (three cases). One limitation of this study is the study population: This included mainly Caucasians, in whom prevalence of intracranial atherosclerosis is lower compared to non-Caucasians (see introductory paragraph).

Local thrombus formation may result in distal arterioarterial embolism, as has been demonstrated in an autopsy case with MCA stenosis (24). In four of 16 patients with MCA stenosis studied by Hinton et al. (13), there was angiographic evidence suggesting peripheral embolism. Angiographic evidence for distal embolization was also found in four of 21 patients with MCA stenosis examined by Corston et al. (40). Wong et al. (41) identified microembolic signals using TCD monitoring in three (15%) of 20 patients with symptomatic MCA stenosis, compared with none of the 20 asymptomatic MCA stenosis patients. In a similar study, Segura et al. (3) detected microembolic signals distal to MCA stenoses in five (36%) of 14 symptomatic cases compared with none out of six asymptomatic cases. Detection of microembolic signals might therefore be a surrogate marker for plaque instability or local nonocclusive thrombus formation. Furthermore, detection of microemboli distal to stenotic intracranial vessels by TCD might be a surrogate marker for ischemic stroke distal to the stenosis. In vertebrobasilar disease, arterioarterial embolism is a well-established pathogenetic mechanism (42).

In the absence of perfusion failure, as discussed previously, these cases might primarily benefit from antithrombotic treatment and application of statins and angiotensin-converting enzyme (ACE) inhibitors to prevent local thrombus formation and to promote stabilization or even regression of the stenotic plaque.

Occlusion of Small Penetrating Arteries at the Site of Stenosis

The stenotic atheromatous plaque might include the origin of small arteries. Small arteries are specifically found in the proximal and distal MCA (lenticulostriate arteries), PCA (thalamogeniculate branches), as well as in the basilar artery (median perforating and short or long circumferential arteries). Stenosis or occlusion of the origin of these small arteries due to focal atherosclerosis may therefore lead to infarctions in the deep structures of the cerebral hemispheres or brainstem (43,44).

C. Miller Fisher (45) and Fisher and Caplan (46) demonstrated the occlusion of small arteries of the basilar artery in three autopsied patients with infarctions of the pons. The first patient suffered from a small infarct in the right basis pontis (46). The artery supplying that territory was a small 0.5-mm-diameter circumferential branch originating from the posterior aspect of the basilar artery at the level of the junction of the vertebral arteries. The origin of the small artery was within an atherosclerotic plaque consisting mostly of macrophages, and a mixture of macrophages, connective tissue, and some red blood cells obstructed the lumen. The second patient suffered an infarction of the left basis pontis. The small artery supplying the infarcted area arose from the posterior aspect of the proximal basilar artery, and its origin was through a large atheromatous plaque, which narrowed the intramural part of the artery and extended into its most proximal part (46). The third patient had a bilateral midline infarction of the basis pontis, which resulted from occlusion of a small branch of the lower basilar artery (45). This small branch originated through a fibrous atheromatous plaque of the basilar artery that was 2 mm thick, and a small local dissection was present. The occlusion of that branch was 1 mm from its origin from the basilar artery. Despite this careful analysis, however, it remained unclear how thrombotic occlusion of the small penetrators finally resulted. Fisher suggested that the small artery either had become severely narrowed by a lipid-rich atheroma in which a local hemorrhage had occurred or, alternatively, that trauma with subsequent microdissection had damaged the intramural part of the vessel. Clinical studies have suggested that occlusion of perforating arteries arising from a stenotic basilar artery might be a frequent finding. Bogousslavsky et al. (47) demonstrated that 15 out of 23 patients (65%) with basilar artery stenosis by MRA had paramedian infarcts of the brainstem.

In an autopsy series of 11 patients with thrombotic MCA occlusion, one patient had occlusion of the mouth of a basal perforating branch of the MCA. The authors suggested that the occlusion resulted from the development of an atherosclerotic stenosis reducing the MCA lumen by about 5% (23). Subsequent clinical studies have confirmed the association of deep MCA infarctions with stenosis of the M1 and M2 segments. In the Extracranial-Intracranial (EC-IC) Bypass Study, 166 patients had visible infarctions in the appropriate MCA territory on the initial computed tomography (CT) scan. This infarct was confined to deep structures (lenticulocapsular, corona radiata) in 39% of the patients with MCA stenosis and in 25% of patients with MCA occlusion (48). In a retrospective series of 22 patients with ultrasonographic or angiographic evidence of isolated MCA stenosis, Lyrer et al. (49) found ten patients (46%) with deep infarcts in the basal ganglia, and six patients (27%) had striatocapsular infarctions of various sizes. In a recent retrospective study of 102 consecutive Korean patients with small striatocapsular infarctions, Bang et al. described a high prevalence of MCA stenosis of at least 50% diagnosed by MRA or angiography with 50% to 79% stenosis in 16 of the patients and at least 70% stenosis in 21.

The main point of these studies is that stenotic atheromatous plaques in large intracranial arteries might cause symptomatic stenosis or occlusion of small penetrating arteries. Careful correlation of the ischemic clinical syndrome with neuroimaging is necessary in these cases because angioplasty of the stenotic plaque may result in complete obstruction and subsequent ischemic stroke in the territory of the penetrators, resulting in an adverse outcome of the procedure.

PROGNOSIS OF PATIENTS WITH INTRACRANIAL ATHEROSCLEROSIS

The prognosis after stroke associated with intracranial stenosis seems to be dependent on location and extent of intracranial atherosclerosis. Most of our knowledge about prognosis in intracranial atherosclerosis is based on retrospective series, reviewed in the following section.

Chimowitz et al. (50) published the largest series of patients with angiographically proven intracranial stenosis of at least 50%. This retrospective, multicenter study compared major vascular outcomes (vascular death and stroke) in 88 patients treated with warfarin and 63 patients treated with aspirin. All patients were symptomatic; 62 patients (41%) presented with TIA and 89 patients (56%) with stroke. In 68 patients (45%), the stenoses were located in the posterior cerebral circulation (vertebrobasilar and PCA) and in 83 patients (55%) in the anterior cerebral circulation (ICA, MCA, and ACA). At the end of follow-up, 40 patients (26%) had reached an end point, four patients (3%) died of nonvascular causes, and two patients (1%) died of hemorrhage. Of the 40 patients reaching an endpoint, 14 patients (9%) had a stroke in the territory of the stenotic artery, seven patients (5%) had a stroke in a site distant from the stenotic artery, and 19 patients (13%) either had a myocardial infarction or sudden death. Chimowitz et al. provided no data on mean annual death or stroke rates for the whole study population. However, the rates of major vascular events were 18.1 per 100 patient-years of follow-up in the aspirin group (stroke rate, 10.4 per 100 patient-years; myocardial infarction or sudden death rate, 7.7 per 100 patient-years) and were statistically higher when compared with 8.4 per 100 patient-years of follow-up in the warfarin group (stroke rate, 3.6 per 100 patient-years; myocardial infarction or sudden death rate, 4.8 per 100 patient-years). Recurrent stroke rates seem to be associated with the stenosis grade. Of the 84 patients with 50% to 79% stenosis, five patients (6%) had a recurrent stroke in the territory of the stenotic artery. Of the 67 patients with 80% to 99% stenosis, nine patients (13%) suffered a recurrent stroke in the territory of the stenotic artery.

In a recent retrospective study of 52 patients with symptomatic intracranial atherosclerosis, 29 patients (56%) failed antithrombotic therapy (antiplatelet agents in 55%, warfarin in 31%, or heparin in 14%) (51). The median time to recurrent TIA, stroke, or death was only 36 days [95% confidence interval (CI) 13–59]. Among patients who failed antithrombotic therapy, the subsequent rate of stroke or death was extremely high (45% per year). In a Cox regression model, older age was an independent predictor of failure of antithrombotic therapy, and warfarin use was associated with a decrease in risk (51). This study, therefore, suggests that patients with symptomatic intracranial atherosclerosis are at a high risk for recurrent stroke or death. However, the results of that study suggesting early and high rates of medical failure contradict results of older studies on recurrent stroke and death, summarized in the following sections.

PROGNOSIS OF PATIENTS WITH INTRACRANIAL CAROTID SIPHON STENOSIS

A summary of published data on mean annual death and stroke rates of patients with carotid siphon stenosis is presented in Table 21-1. Generally, annual mortality rates range from 4.7% to 17.2% and annual ipsilateral stroke rates from 3.1 to 7.6 (Table 21-1).

Marzewksi et al. (52) published the first detailed retrospective series of patients with angiographically proven ICA stenosis of 50% or more. Forty-six of the 66 patients (70%) presented with ischemic symptoms. Only 27 patients (41%) presented initially with ischemic events ipsilateral to the ICA stenosis; 16 patients (24%) had a tandem ICA stenosis, and 11 patients (16.7%) had an intracranial ICA stenosis as the only apparent cause for their ischemic symptoms. During an average follow-up period of 3.9 years, eight patients (12.1%) suffered an isolated TIA in the ICA territory, and ten patients (15%) suffered a stroke. The stroke was ipsilateral to the siphon stenosis in eight patients (12%). Six of these eight patients had a tandem stenosis on the initial angiogram. Thirty-three patients (50%) died during follow-up. The cause of death was due to cardiac disease in 18 patients, and there were no stroke-related deaths. The annual death rate was 12.8% per year, and the ipsilateral annual stroke rate was 3.1% per year (Table 21-1) (52).

Another retrospective series of 58 patients with angiographically proven intracranial internal artery stenosis of 30% or more, published by Craig et al. (5), comprising 47 (81%) symptomatic and 11 (19%) asymptomatic patients, reports an annual ipsilateral stroke rate of 7.6% per year and an annual mortality rate of 17.2% per year. Overall, at the end of the mean follow-up time of 30 months, only 19 of the 58 patients (33%) were alive or free from subsequent cerebrovascular events. Twenty-five of the patients (43%) suffered a TIA or stroke during follow-up. Among those, 17 (29%) patients suffered an ischemic stroke; in 11 patients, the stroke was distal to the ICA stenosis. Twenty-one of the 47 symptomatic patients (45%) suffered a cerebrovascular event as compared to four of the 11 asymptomatic patients (36%) in the follow-up period. None of six patients with tandem ICA lesions suffered a stroke during follow-up. A total of 25 patients (43%) died during follow-up: Eleven of the deaths (44%) were due to cardiac disease and nine were due to stroke (36%). There were no differences between death rates in symptomatic and asymptomatic patients (42% versus 45%, respectively) (5).

In a retrospective series of 15 patients with angiographically-proven carotid siphon stenosis of 50% or more followed for an average of 51 months, Wechsler et al. (53) report an annual mortality rate of 4.7% per year and annual ipsilateral stroke rate of 3.1% per year (Table 21-1). Twelve patients (80%) were symptomatic and three (20%) were asymptomatic. During a mean follow-up time of 51 months, four of the 12 symptomatic patients (25%) and none of the asymptomatic patients suffered a stroke. Three of the four strokes occurred ipsilateral to the carotid stenosis, and the last case died from fatal basilar thrombosis. A total of three patients (20%) died during follow-up: two of the deaths were due to presumed myocardial infarction and one was due to stroke. One main finding of the study was that initial clinical presentation correlated with the presence of hemodynamically significant stenosis. Five of the seven patients with TIAs at presentation had evidence of impaired flow on angiography. The TIAs were mostly multiple and stereotyped. Unlike the TIA group, only one of the five patients with stroke at presentation had evidence of impaired flow on angiography and in only one patient was the stroke preceded by a TIA. The authors suggested that strokes were due to embolism distal to the stenosis, whereas TIAs were due to slow flow.

In a series of 22 patients with siphon stenosis of 30% or more followed for an average

TABLE 21-1. ANNUAL DEATH AND STROKE RATES IN PATIENTS WITH INTRACRANIAL CAROTID STENOSIS

Author, Year	Study Type	Study Period	Diagnosis and Degree of Stenosis	No. of Patients	Follow-up (Range)	Mean Annual Death Rate	Mean Annual Stroke Rate in Any Vascular Territory[a]	Mean Annual Stroke Rate in the Territory of the Stenotic Artery
Marzewski et al., 1982 (52)	Retrospective	1966–1977; London, Ontario: 1972–1980	Cerebral angiography, ≥50%	66	47 mo (0–79)	12.8%	3.9%	3.1%
Craig et al., 1982 (5)	Retrospective	VA hospital; Memphis, Tennessee: 1975–1981	Cerebral angiography, ≥30%	58	30 mo (2–78)	17.2%	11.7%	7.6%
Borozan et al., 1984 (55)	Retrospective	1978–1983	Cerebral angiography, ≥20%	93	22.5 mo (1–62)	10.3%	5.1%	5.1%
Wechsler et al., 1986 (53)	Retrospective	1980–1985	Cerebral angiography, ≥50%	15	51 mo (4–123)	4.7%	6.5%	3.1%
Bogousslavsky 1987 (54)	NN	NN	Cerebral angiography, ≥30%	22	40.4 mo	9.5%	NN	8.1%

[a] Per 100 person-years.

of 40.4 months, Bogousslavsky (54) reported an annual death rate of 9.5% per year and an annual ipsilateral stroke rate of 8.1% per year. The cause of death was cardiac in six patients and stroke in one patient.

Borozan et al. (55) identified 93 patients with isolated carotid siphon stenosis among 885 consecutive patients with cerebral angiograms, of whom 71 had unilateral and 22 bilateral disease. During a mean follow-up time of 22.5 months, the calculated annual ipsilateral stroke rate was 5.1% per year for both symptomatic and asymptomatic patients combined. Sixteen of the 71 asymptomatic patients died (22.5%) during the follow-up period. The causes of death in the asymptomatic patients were myocardial infarction (three patients), stroke (three patients), carcinoma (three patients), other causes (three patients), and unknown (four patients). In two of the three symptomatic patients who suffered a fatal stroke, the event occurred ipsilateral to the siphon stenosis, and in the last patient, the stroke location was unknown. Five of the 22 symptomatic patients died during follow-up. The causes of death in the symptomatic patients were due to myocardial infarction (three patients), stroke (one patient), and carcinoma (one patient). Borozan et al. (55) did not report the total annual death rate. However, taking the annual death rate due to myocardial infarction of 3.0% per year given by the authors and extrapolating that number to all causes of death, the annual death rate for the cohort is 10.3% per year.

The only prospective study in patients with carotid siphon stenosis comes from the EC-IC Bypass Study Group (56). One of the subgroups enrolled in this study was composed of patients with stenosis of the ICA at or above the C-2 vertebral body, and it is likely that most of these patients actually had a carotid siphon stenosis. Twenty-six of 72 medically treated patients (36%) with ICA stenosis more than 70% at or distal to C-2 had a nonfatal or fatal stroke in any vascular distribution; data on ipsilateral strokes were not provided. The exact follow-up period for this subgroup of patients was not specified, but the mean follow-up for all patients included in the study was 55.8 months.

Besides the retrospective design of most of the published series of patients with carotid siphon stenosis, there are several other limitations making a definite conclusion difficult regarding short-term and long-term prognosis. The limitations are as follows:

- The cohorts are highly selected because patients collected had cerebral angiography as a main entry criterion into the studies (5,52–55). Most stroke patients are not evaluated with cerebral angiography.
- Some series included carotid stenoses of different grades, with ranges as low as 20% (5,52–55).
- The patient populations are heterogeneous, consisting of patients with variable proportions of unilateral versus bilateral intracranial carotid stenosis and also patients with intracranial and extracranial ICA tandem stenosis (5,52).
- The severity of ipsilateral strokes due to carotid siphon stenosis is not clearly described in all cases (5,52).
- Often, no hemodynamic parameters, like delayed flow distal to the stenosis, shift of the borderzone region, or collateral flow, are presented (5,52).

PROGNOSIS OF PATIENTS WITH STENOSIS OF THE MIDDLE CEREBRAL ARTERY

Retrospective studies with small numbers of patients suggested that the long-term risk of stroke or death was low in patients with stenosis of the MCA (13,40,57). In the retrospective study of 16 patients by Hinton et al. (13) with angiographically proven MCA stenosis of 45% or more, the initial presentation was TIA in 15 patients and minor stroke in 11 patients. In all but two patients, angiography demonstrated hemodynamic effects, evidenced by border zone shift or delayed flow. During a follow-up between 1 and 72 months, only two of the 16 patients with angiographically proven MCA stenosis developed a severe stroke; this occurred in both patients prior to initiating treatment soon after the diagnosis of the MCA stenosis (13).

In a retrospective series of 13 patients with an angiographically proven MCA stenosis of 34% or more, Feldmeyer et al. (57) report a mean annual death rate of 4.3% and mean annual stroke rate of 1.5% (Table 21-2). Two of the 13 patients were thought to have MCA stenosis due to fibromuscular dysplasia or due to radiation angiopathy, and, therefore, these cases are atypical for intracranial atherosclerosis. In ten patients (77%), there was hemodynamic significance as assessed by angiography, and in four patients (31%), there was suggestion of a mural thrombus. In nine patients (70%), the MCA stenoses were associated with additional stenoses in the proximal or distal ICA. Overall, three (23%) of the 13 patients died during a mean follow-up of 63.6 months. The causes of death were presumed basilar thrombosis (n = 1), carcinoma (n = 1), and unknown (n = 1). Two patients (15%) suffered a recurrent stroke: one patient a fatal basilar stroke, and the second patient presumably an MCA infarct. No clear statement is made if the MCA infarct developed ipsilateral to the MCA stenosis.

Corston et al. (40) identified 21 patients with angiographically proven MCA stenosis; 19 had stenosis of the M1 segment and two of more distal branches. Fourteen patients (67%) presented with stroke and seven patients (33%) with TIA alone. Eight of the 14 patients with stroke at presentation had prior TIA. Angiography demonstrated hemodynamic significance in six patients (29%), as shown by border zone shift or delayed flow. During a mean follow-up period of 6.5 years (range 4 months to 25 years), six patients (29%) suffered a stroke; no sufficient data relating the location of the strokes to the site of stenosis are provided. Ten patients died during follow-up. The cause of death was recurrent stroke in four patients (in three ipsilateral to the stenosis), myocardial infarction in two patients, cancer in three patients, and unknown in one patient.

The EC-IC Bypass Study is the only prospective study on the long-term outcome of patients with angiographically proven atherosclerotic MCA disease (48,56). In the EC-IC Bypass Study, 85 patients with MCA stenosis were treated medically [management of risk factors and antithrombotic therapy with aspirin (the majority) or warfarin]. The stenosis was graded as moderate if less than 70% and as severe if 70% or more. All of these patients had a TIA or nondisabling stroke in the distribution of the diseased MCA within 3 months of study entry, and none had a cardiac source of embolus or severe extracranial carotid stenosis. In the 85 patients with MCA stenosis followed for a mean of 43.3 months, 18 patients (21%) had a stroke and ten patients (12%) died (three from stroke, two from coronary artery disease, and five from other causes). The annual mortality rate was 3.3% per year. The mean annual stroke in any vascular territory was 5.9%, and the mean annual of ipsilateral stroke was 4.6% per year. Because some patients suffered more than one stroke, the rate of stroke in any vascular territory was 9.5% per patient-year, and the rate of ipsilateral stroke was 7.8% per patient-year. Seven of the 18 patients with a stroke experienced warning TIAs. Seventy-one percent of patients with moderate MCA stenosis experienced warning TIAs compared to 18% with severe MCA stenosis. Eighty-three percent of all strokes occurred ipsilateraly to the MCA stenosis. There was no apparent difference in the rate of stroke or death in patients with less than 70% stenosis versus patients with more than 70% stenosis of the MCA (48).

TABLE 21-2. ANNUAL DEATH AND STROKE RATES IN PATIENTS WITH MIDDLE CEREBRAL ARTERY STENOSIS

Author, Year	Study Type	Study Period	Diagnosis and Degree of Stenosis	No. of Patients	Follow-up	Mean Annual Death Rate	Mean Annual Stroke Rate in any Vascular Territory[a]	Mean Annual Stroke Rate in the Territory of the Stenotic Artery
Corston et al., 1984 (40)	Retrospective	1957–1982	Cerebral angiography ≥33%	21	78.5 mo	7.1%	4.2%	NS
Feldmeyer et al., 1983 (57)	Retrospective	1970–1981	Cerebral angiography ≥34%	13	63.6 mo	4.3%	2.8%	NS
Bougousslavsky et al., 1986 (48)	Prospective	08/1977–09/1982	Cerebral angiography	85	43.3 mo	3.3%	5.9%	4.7%

[a] Per 100 person-years.
NS, not specified.

In summary, there are limited data on the natural history of MCA stenosis. The reported mean annual death rate is in the range of 3.3% to 7.7% and the mean annual stroke rate in any territory in the range of 2.8% to 4.2% (Table 21-2). Only the EC-IC Bypass Study reports an annual stroke rate for ipsilateral stroke, which is 4.7%. These rates seem to be lower compared to those for intracranial ICA stenosis.

PROGNOSIS OF PATIENTS WITH INTRACRANIAL STENOSIS OF THE VERTEBROBASILAR TERRITORY

As is true for carotid siphon and MCA stenosis, there are limited studies on long-term outcome for intracranial posterior circulation atherosclerosis. Most published studies are retrospective or use noninvasive techniques for the diagnosis of posterior circulation occlusive disease.

Moufarrij et al. (58) retrospectively studied 44 patients with angiographically proven stenosis in the distal vertebral or basilar arteries of 50% or more; two of the patients had an extracranial distal vertebral artery stenosis between C-2 and the foramen magnum. A total of 17 patients (38%) had stenotic lesions in two or more sites of the distal vertebrobasilar vascular territory. During a mean follow-up period of 6.1 years, eight patients died and five had a nonfatal stroke (Table 21-3). The causes of death were stroke in three patients (two patients in the brainstem), cardiac in two patients, and other causes in three patients. The location of the stroke was in the vertebrobasilar territory in five of the eight patients (63%) with an infarct during follow-up (four brainstem, one occipital lobe). The period between angiography and stroke varied between 2 days and 6 years. However, in seven patients, the stroke occurred within 2 years after angiography.

In the retrospective study by Pessin et al. (59) of nine patients with angiographically proven stenosis of the mid-distal basilar artery 40% or more, eight patients had a single stenosis and one patient had a tandem stenosis. Anterograde flow was observed in all patients, and only one patient demonstrated a slow anterograde filling through a 90% stenosis. During a mean follow-up of 21 months, only one patient suffered from a recurrent basilar artery stroke with fatal outcome after 2 years. A total of three patients died during follow-up. The cause of death was alcohol abuse in one patient, basilar artery stroke in one patient, and death due to the original stroke leading to the basilar artery stenosis in one patient.

Pessin t al. (60) also published a paper of six patients with stenosis in the posterior cerebral artery of 50% to 80%; five patients had unilateral and one patient had bilateral disease. Angiography demonstrated no hemodynamic abnormalities in all patients, like slow anterograde filling through the stenosis. During a mean follow-up of 84 months, no patient developed an infarction in the ipsilateral territory of the PCA. One patient suffered a large MCA infarction. Three patients died. The cause of death was fatal MCA stroke in one patient, traumatic brain hemorrhage in one patient, and unknown in one patient.

The Warfarin-Aspirin Symptomatic Intracranial Disease Study (WASID) provides the largest retrospective series on outcome in 68 patients with angiographically proven stenosis of 50% or more in vertebral or basilar arteries (61). Thirteen patients (20%) had more than one stenotic lesion in the vertebrobasilar territory. During a median follow-up of 13.8 months, 15 patients (22%) had an ischemic stroke; in ten patients (15%), the stroke was in the same territory of the stenotic vessel. Six patients (9%) had a nonfatal myocardial infarction. Seven patients died; the cause of death was fatal stroke in four patients and fatal myocardial infarction or sudden death in three patients. The rates per 100 person-years of follow-up for ischemic stroke in any vascular territory was 13.1% and for death 6.1% (Table

TABLE 21-3. PROGNOSIS OF INTRACRANIAL ATHEROSCLEROSIS: POSTERIOR CIRCULATION

Author, Year	Study Type	Study Period	Diagnosis of Stenosis	Vessels Analyzed	N	Follow-up (Mean)	Death Rate[a]	Stroke Rate in any Vascular Territory[a]	Stroke Rate in the Territory of the Stenotic Artery[a]
Moufarrij et al., 1986 (58)	Retrospective, single-center, consecutive cases	1974–1984	Conventional angiography, 50% to 99% stenosis	VA, BA	44	6.1 yr	7.0%[b]	7.0%	4.3%
Pessin et al., 1987 (59)	Retrospective, single-center, consecutive cases	NS	Conventional angiography, 40%–90%	Mid-distal BA	9	21 mo	9.7%[c]	4.8%[d]	4.8%[d]
Pessin et al, 1987 (60)	Retrospective, single center, consecutive cases	1978–1985	Conventional angiography 40%–90%	PCA	6	14 mo	7.1%	2.4%	0%
WASID, 1998 (61)	Retrospective, multicenter, consecutive cases	1985–1991	Conventional angiography, 50%–99% stenosis	VA, BA, PCA	68	13.8 mo	6.1%	13.1%	8.7%

[a] Per 100 person-years.

[b] Total deaths: n = 8 (fatal stroke: n = 3, 2 of them in brainstem; cardiac death: n = 2; other or unclear cause of death: n = 3).

[c] Total deaths: n = 2 (fatal basilar stroke: n = 1; alcohol abuse: n = 1), rate based on inference of 20.7 person-years of follow-up calculated from data presented in Table 1 of reference.

[d] One patient developed a fatal basilar artery stroke. One other patient not included in this calculation died from his original basilar stroke; total deaths: n = 7 (fatal strokes n = 4; fatal myocardial infarction or sudden death: n = 3), rate based on inference of 115 person-years follow-up calculated from the reported number in the reference.

NS, not specified; VA, vertebral artery; BA, basilar artery; PCA, posterior cerebral artery.

21-3). A main finding of that study is the variation of stroke rates in the different stenotic arteries. The stroke rate in the territory of the stenotic artery per 100 person-years was 7.8 for vertebral artery stenosis, 10.7 for basilar artery stenosis, and 6.0 for PCA/posterior inferior communicating artery (PICA) stenosis.

In summary, there are limited data on the natural history of intracranial vertebrobasilar artery stenosis. The reported mean annual death rate is in the range of 6.1 to 9.7 per 100 person-years, the mean annual stroke rate in any territory is in the range of 2.4 to 13.1 per 100 person-years, and the mean annual stroke rate in the territory of the stenotic artery is in the range of 0 to 8.7 per 100 person-years (Table 21-3).

IDENTIFYING THE SYMPTOMATIC PATIENT WITH INTRACRANIAL ATHEROSCLEROSIS

At the present time, angioplasty and stenting is usually performed for patients with symptomatic intracranial stenoses. A detailed description of the different stroke syndromes is beyond the scope of this review, and the interested reader can refer to standard textbooks on stroke and stroke syndromes (1,62). However, there are some general recommendations. An experienced stroke neurologist should evaluate all patients prior to any angioplasty to correlate the patient's symptoms and clinical findings with the presumed symptomatic vessel and to exclude other potential diagnoses with alternative treatment options, i.e., cerebral vasculitis. Part of this evaluation should include type and duration of medical therapy and adjusting of medical treatment as necessary.

As already outlined above, the clinical symptoms of intracranial stenosis may be due to perfusion failure or arterioarterial embolism. Perfusion failure manifests clinically by the presence of neurological symptoms attributable to the stenotic vessel when the patient changes body position, like an orthostatic reaction (Fig. 21-6). A classical presentation of perfusion failure is the so-called orthostatic limb shaking from hypoperfusion in the carotid territory (63–65). Symptomatology in arterioarterial embolism distal to a stenosis depends on the vascular territory involved. The presence of ischemic lesions in the border zone territories of major cerebral arteries suggests perfusion failure. In hemispheric disease due to MCA stenosis, this may be visible as nonconfluent or confluent in the ipsilateral supraventricular or paraventricular white matter (66). Careful analysis of the clinical syndrome and the results of neuroimaging should be performed to identify patients with perfusion failure due to proximal stenosis and to differentiate them from symptomatic penetrating artery disease at the site of the stenosis as the cause of ischemia, because patients with the latter condition might not benefit from angioplasty and stenting. Also, an angiographically visible intracranial stenosis might not be hemodynamically significant, and in these cases, angioplasty might be of no value.

The usual vascular workup of stroke patients includes TCD or duplex sonography, CT angiography, or magnetic resonance imaging (MRI) with MRA. Intracranial stenoses in the arteries accessible to angioplasty and stenting can be easily identified with any of those studies. In individual cases, verification of the findings of the noninvasive studies with conventional cerebral angiography might be necessary. Impaired cerebrovascular reserve as an indicator for perfusion failure distal to the stenosis is diagnosed by several methods, each of them having its own advantages and disadvantages [see Derdeyn et al. (34) for review]. CBF can be evaluated at baseline and after a cerebral vasodilatatory stimulus, like hypercapnia, or acetazolamide. In the normal situation, each of those stimuli results in an increase of CBF. If the CBF response is muted or absent, preexisting cerebral vasodilatation due to

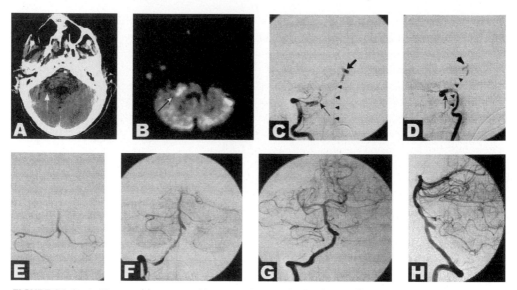

FIGURE 21-6. A 68-year-old woman with progressive vertebrobasilar insufficiency despite maximal medical therapy developed postural syncope. She was unable to rise from a horizontal position without fainting. **A**: Non-enhanced computed tomography (CT) brain scan. **B**: Diffusion-weighted magnetic resonance imaging (MRI) demonstrates acute infarction in the right middle cerebellar peduncle (*arrows*). **C** and **D**: Complete cerebral arteriography including right vertebral arteriography in frontal and lateral projections demonstrates complete occlusion of the vertebral arteries (*thin arrow*) and reconstitution of the proximal basilar artery (*thick arrow*) via retrograde filling of the anterior spinal artery (*arrowheads*). The occlusion remained unchanged despite attempted thrombolysis using a total of 15 mg intraarterial recombinant tissue-type plasminogen activator (rt-PA). **E**: Under general anesthesia, a microcatheter and 0.014-inch microguide wire were used to gently traverse the occluded segment. Arteriography through the microcatheter confirms patency of the basilar artery beyond the occlusion and intraluminal position of the microcatheter. **F**: Following angioplasty using a 3.0 mm balloon, the vertebral artery is patent but markedly irregular. **G** and **H**: A 3.5 × 15-mm stent was used to improve luminal diameter and maintain vessel patency. Stent placement was complicated by dislodgement of organized thrombus or plaque that initially occluded the basilar artery terminus. The embolus could not be retrieved with the retrieval devices available at the time. The embolus was forced distally into the right posterior cerebral artery beyond important thalamic and brainstem perforators. The patient suffered a small periventricular infarct in the right occipital lobe but did not lose vision.

reduced cerebral perfusion pressure is assumed. Measurements of CBF can be made by several methods, including ^{133}Xe by inhalation or intravenous injection, single photon emission computed tomography (SPECT), stable xenon CT (Xe-CT), PET, and CT and MRI-perfusion studies after the injection of an adequate contrast medium (34,67–71). The changes in flow velocity as determined by TCD and CO_2 inhalation as compared to baseline also serve to estimate reduced poststenotic vasoreactivity (72–74). However, for technical reasons, all of these techniques allow only the diagnosis of stage 1 of hemodynamic compromise (see section 4.1). At the present time, the diagnosis of stage 2 of hemodynamic compromise (increased OEF) is only possible with PET using ^{15}O labeled radiotracers (75). Unfortunately, PET is expensive and not readily available in most institutions. To what extent the information of these studies might be helpful for the indication and timing to perform an angioplasty remains to be established in future studies.

MEDICAL TREATMENT OF INTRACRANIAL ATHEROSCLEROSIS

The medical treatment of intracranial atherosclerosis is similar to the treatment of atherosclerosis in other vascular territories and includes the control of vascular risk factors and the prescription of antithrombotics (platelet-active drugs or warfarin), statins, and ACE inhibitors. Patients are usually referred for elective intracranial angioplasty if they have failed "maximal medical" therapy. However, the term "maximal medical" therapy is not clearly defined. In most instances, failure of maximal medical therapy is defined as TIA or recurrent ischemic stroke while on therapeutic doses of aspirin (more than or equal to 81 mg per day), ticlopidine (500 mg per day), clopidogrel (75 mg per day), warfarin [international normalized ratio (INR) more than or equal to 2.0], or intravenous heparin (prolongation of partial thromboplastin time more than 1.2 times baseline value) (50,51). Symptomatic patients on platelet-active drugs are often switched to anticoagulants, i.e., warfarin or heparin. Retrospective studies have suggested that warfarin compared to aspirin had a more favorable risk/benefit ratio for the prevention of major vascular events in patients with symptomatic intracranial large artery disease (50,51). In the prospective, randomized, placebo-controlled Warfarin-Aspirin Recurrent Stroke Study (WARSS), warfarin had no benefit over aspirin for secondary prevention in the subgroup of patients with large artery thrombotic stroke (stenosis or occlusion) (76). However, that study was not specifically designed for patients with intracranial atherosclerosis.

At the present time, two randomized trials are specifically evaluating different antithrombotic treatments for secondary stroke prevention in intracranial atherosclerosis. The Warfarin-Aspirin Symptomatic Intracranial Disease (WASID) trial is a randomized, double-blind, clinical trial in which 806 patients with TIA or minor stroke that is related to an angiographically proven stenosis (50% to 99%) of a major intracranial artery are randomized to warfarin sodium (INR 2.3) or aspirin (1300 mg per day). The main aim of the study is to determine whether warfarin is superior to aspirin for preventing ischemic stroke or death in those patients (77). The Aspirin Versus Anticoagulants in Symptomatic Intracranial Stenosis (AVASIS) study is a randomized, multicenter, open trial designed to compare the efficacy and safety of aspirin (300 mg per day) and coumarin (INR 2–3) in the secondary prevention of ischemic stroke, other vascular events, and major hemorrhagic complications among patients with TIA and/or cerebral infarction attributable to MCA stenosis (77).

SYMPTOMATIC INTRACRANIAL STENOSIS: SURGICAL OPTIONS

Conventional Surgical Revascularization with Craniotomy

EC-IC bypass has largely been discredited as a valid therapeutic option for symptomatic intracranial stenosis (56,78). The EC-IC Bypass Study Group performed a randomized, controlled trial evaluating the efficacy of surgical revascularization for a variety of indications. In general, the technical success was variable by operator and failed to demonstrate improvement in patient outcomes. Particularly in the subgroup with MCA stenosis, surgical bypass from the superficial temporal artery to the distal MCA branches (M2-M4) met with the most disastrous results. Patients with severe MCA stenoses treated with EC-IC bypass had the worst outcomes as a result of basal ganglia and internal capsule infarction from obliteration of lenticulostriate perforators in proximity to the stenosis (79,80). The apparent hemodynamic mechanism is removal of the pressure gradient responsible for continued anterograde blood flow across the stenosis, causing thrombosis of the MCA from the stenotic segment to the site of the surgical anastomosis. Perforating end-arteries, including the lateral lenticulostriate branches, occlude without likelihood of adequate collateral blood flow. Similarly, surgical series reporting bypass procedures for symptomatic vertebrobasilar stenosis have met with limited success (81,82).

Encephaloduro arterio-synangiosis (EDAS) was developed as a limited craniotomy to treat symptomatic cerebral stenosis, particularly due to moyamoya disease and syndrome (83), a cryptogenic condition resulting in progressive distal ICA and MCA stenosis, and occlusion that most often affects children of Asian descent. The result is an arteriographic pattern of asymmetric obliterative vasculitis with lenticulostriate collateralization likened to a "puff of [cigarette] smoke" in a darkened room. Adults and other ethnic groups are not immune. The natural history is one of progressive perfusion failure with neurological deficit and dementia.

EDAS was proposed when it was observed that conventional surgical bypass could cause a rapid progression of disease. Even in a contralateral hemisphere that had been relatively less symptomatic or asymptomatic hours to days before treatment, it was observed that a surgical bypass procedure on one side could cause sudden stenosis and infarction in the other. A less invasive procedure without transgression of the dural membranes limited this rapid progression. In the classical EDAS procedure, the vascular pedicle of the temporal muscle is placed in proximity to the dura mater through a craniectomy. The ischemic hemisphere then induces the temporalis pedicle to provide exuberant transdural collateral vessels over a 6-week interval, demonstrable at arteriography and perfusion studies, with concomitant neurological stabilization.

EDAS has been performed with limited success in adults with atherosclerotic cerebrovascular stenosis or occlusion. It has been observed in adults that the EDAS procedure has a limited ability to mitigate the inexorable neurological decline associated with atherosclerotic disease, likely due to poor collateral formation. Furthermore, collateral perfusion cannot address thrombosis at the site of an anatomic stenosis. At our institution, EDAS is performed in patients in whom an endovascular procedure and anticoagulant therapy are contraindicated or in patients refusing endovascular revascularization.

Endovascular Revascularization

During the last decade, dramatic improvements in microcatheter technology have allowed for innovative endovascular neurovascular procedures and popularization of existing technology. The successful use of balloon angioplasty for the treatment of intracranial atherosclerosis has been reported by an increasing number of medical centers, predominantly academic centers and high-volume medical centers with significant neurovascular expertise. Results to date are encouraging, yet the procedure is technically demanding at many levels and carries substantial risk. In general, most practitioners reserve endovascular revascularization for patients who are refractory to maximal medical therapy.

Not all patients with cerebrovascular stenoses are equivalent: Careful neurological and imaging assessments are mandatory for planning a successful individualized treatment strategy. Moreover, treatment requires a multidisciplinary approach, as weakness in any link of the chain can have devastating consequences. An important theme of this monograph is the customized approach needed to address each patient. No single operator works in a vacuum. Technically successful revascularization of cerebrovascular stenosis is only one step to achievement of acceptable treatment outcomes.

Mori et al. (84,85) developed an arteriographic classification system to predict the outcome of cerebral revascularization with primary angioplasty alone. Lesions were categorized at high-resolution digital subtraction arteriography by length and geometry:

Type A: short (less than or equal to 5 mm in length); concentric or moderately eccentric; nonocclusive

Type B: tubular (5–10 mm in length); extremely eccentric; moderately angulated (curved)

TABLE 21-4. TREATMENT SUCCESS AND RESTENOSIS ACCORDING TO TYPE OF INTRACRANIAL ATHEROSCLEROSIS

Mori Type, Cerebral Stenosis	A	B	C
Treatment success, %	92	86	33
One-year critical restenosis, %	0	33	100

Adapted from Mori T, Fukuoka M, Kazita K, et al. Follow-up study after percutaneous transluminal cerebral balloon angioplasty. *AJNR Am J Neuroradiol* 1998;19:1525–1533.

Type C: diffuse (more than 10 mm in length); extremely angulated (more than 90 degrees); very tortuous proximal segment

Clinical outcomes are summarized in Table 21-4 (84). The more complex the target lesion, the less satisfactory immediate and long-term outcomes become using the currently available devices. As we will discuss, the use of currently available stent technology resolves certain limitations inherent to angioplasty alone.

Nahser et al. (86) reported resolution of symptoms in 100% of patients treated with balloon angioplasty for posterior circulation stenoses. Improvements in luminal diameter (less than 50% residual stenosis) and flow depicted on angiography following angioplasty have also been documented (87). In the largest series of intracranial angioplasty to date, Mori et al. (84) treated 42 patients with symptomatic intracranial stenoses of more than 70% or occlusion failing maximal medical therapy, with a 76% technical success rate and 5% (two) major complications.

Specific risks of balloon angioplasty include thromboembolism, vascular dissection with acute or delayed occlusion, pseudoaneurysm formation, vessel rupture, and occlusion of small perforators (88). The rate of procedure-related stroke has varied from 8% to 50% (89–91). Vascular dissection has been observed in up to 38% of angioplasty cases performed for subarachnoid hemorrhage-induced vasospasm (92).

In a series of 23 patients undergoing intracranial angioplasty by Marks et al. (93), the annual rate for strokes in the territory of angioplasty was reduced to 3.2% during the mean follow-up period of 35.4 months.

Stent-assisted Angioplasty

Immediate complications of balloon angioplasty include plaque/vessel recoil, vessel dissection, acute closure, perforation, and rupture. Stent-assisted angioplasty in the peripheral, extracranial cerebral, and coronary circulation has been shown to have a superior safety profile and efficacy compared with balloon angioplasty alone (94–98). Stents limit vessel wall recoil and the extent of iatrogenic dissection by compressing the intimal flap (99).

The feasibility of stent-assisted angioplasty of the intracranial circulation was, until recently, limited by the inability of available stents to negotiate the tortuosity of intracranial vessels. Newer coronary stents are lighter and more flexible than their predecessors, providing the required performance for intracranial navigation. Moreover, thin struts that are widely spaced may have a theoretical advantage in preserving side branches such as perforating arteries. The successful use of coronary stents including the GRII (Cook, Bloomington, IN)(100,101), Multilink Duet (Guidant, Santa Clara, CA) (99,102–104), and GFX I and II (Medtronic/AVE, Santa Rosa, CA) (99,103–106) for treatment of intracranial stenoses has been reported. Most applications have related to the vertebrobasilar system (99,101,103,104) with limited reports of their use in the MCA (102) and intracranial internal carotid (100,104). Investigations utilizing the INX stent (Medtronic/AVE, Santa Rosa, CA), the first stent designed primarily for neurovascular use, are ongoing. However, most work has focused on its application in stent-supported coil embolization for wide-necked aneurysms rather than intracranial stenoses.

Mori et al. (104), primarily utilizing the GFX stent in ten patients with 12 intracranial stenoses, reported a technical success rate of 83%. None of the procedures was complicated, and the restenosis rate at 3 months for Type B and Type C lesions was 0%. In a series of 12 patients who underwent stent-assisted angioplasty for symptomatic basilar artery stenoses, ten patients (83%) were asymptomatic after a mean follow-up period of 5.5 months (102).

TECHNICAL CONSIDERATIONS

Patient Selection

Informed consent must include a discussion of the experimental nature of the procedure and the "off-label" use of equipment approved by the Food and Drug Administration for other applications. The technical risk of vessel occlusion is in the range of 10% for anterior circulation lesions and 20% for the posterior circulation (107). Patient selection is a major factor in determining patient outcomes. As the anatomic configuration of the lesion can affect technical outcome, the patient's neurological and hemodynamic status certainly affects functional outcome. Although patients failing maximal medical therapy with anticoagulant and antiaggregate therapy comprise the treatment group for this procedure, patients with acute stroke and cerebral perfusion failure are at extremely high risk for perioperative complication, approaching 50%. In this high-risk group, satisfactory functional outcomes can be achieved only with medical management to complement the revascularization procedure.

Patient Preparation

MRI with diffusion-weighted imaging is currently the optimal pretreatment imaging study to evaluate for acute cerebral infarction. Historically, the nonenhanced CT brain scan has been the screening tool used in major stroke therapy trials and is the most well-validated test to predict the risk of treatment in the presence of a recent cerebral infarction. Because fibrinolytic therapy may be required to treat the intraprocedural complications of cerebral revascularization, recent infarction remains a relative contraindication to angioplasty. Prior to the use of small diameter stents (2.5 to 4 mm), antiaggregate therapy with strong antiplatelet medications may exacerbate the effects of intraoperative anticoagulations. For all the reasons described, a 6-week waiting period following cerebral infarction before proceeding with angioplasty has been suggested (107). This must be weighed against the risk of recurrent or progressive infarction if early revascularization is not achieved.

Premedication

Because the target population for treatment has failed maximal medical therapy, most patients are already on an antiplatelet regimen of aspirin and clopidogrel, dipyridamole, ticlopidine, or other combination therapy. Aspirin is a weak antiplatelet agent, but the benefits of its administration have been demonstrated (76). Aspirin therapy should be initiated at least 3 days before the procedure and continued indefinitely.

Antiplatelet agents, typically clopidogrel or ticlopidine in addition to aspirin, are routinely administered 1 to 3 days before the procedure. Some operators also administer abciximab as a 0.25 mg per kg intravenous bolus before stent deployment, which is continued at a rate of 10 mcg per minute for 12 hours. Others prefer to use dextran 40 (10% weight/volume low-molecular-weight dextran) (104,106). Intraarterial injection of isosorbide dinitrate via the guide catheter may help limit vasospasm. Preoperative administration of 10 mg intravenous dexamethasone and antibiotics have also been proposed (105).

Heparin is given to achieve an ACT of 250 to 300 seconds throughout the procedure. An appropriate guide catheter is placed into the cervical ICA or vertebral artery via a standard transfemoral approach. Biplane digital roadmaps are obtained and the lesion traversed with a floppy-tipped guide wire. A microcatheter is then advanced across the lesion and a small volume of contrast injected to confirm an intraluminal position. An exchange-length floppy-tipped hydrophilic guide wire is positioned with its tip sufficiently distal to the lesion to provide sufficient support for the stent. This usually requires the tip to be in the insular (M2) branches of the MCA for MCA stenoses (102), P2 segments of the PCA for basilar artery stenoses (103), or M1 segment of the MCA for distal ICA stenoses (100).

Combination therapy with other antiaggregate therapy has been demonstrated in the coronary and neurological literature to help prevent early restenosis (108–110); its use has been extrapolated to the revascularization of neurovascular disease. Some operators administer low-molecular-weight dextran 40 as an intravenous infusion (20 to 40 mL per hour) the day before treatment, continued to the day after treatment (88,106). Oral nimodipine, a calcium channel blocker (60 mg every 4 hours), beginning 12 hours prior to the procedure and continuing 24 hours after the procedure may provide a neuroprotective effect (87). The benefits of nimodipine were previously demonstrated in the treatment of hemorrhagic stroke (111).

Intraprocedural use of heparin, given as an intravenous bolus, is commonly used in neurovascular procedures, although there is little consensus on the loading dose or rate of infusion. We prefer a loading dose given as a bolus as 70 units per kg followed by an infusion of 1000 U per hour to achieve an ACT of 2.5 to 3.0 times baseline. Some operators routinely administer abciximab (ReoPro, Eli Lilly and Co., Indianapolis, IN) as a 0.25 mg per kg intravenous bolus immediately before angioplasty and continue an infusion of 10 mcg per minute for 12 hours. In general, strong intravenous antiaggregating agents are not well characterized in the neurovascular literature. ReoPro is the only agent in which any substantial neurovascular experience has been obtained. Nevertheless, anecdotal complication rates in neurovascular revascularization applications have far exceeded those reported in the coronary literature, likely due to differences in the perfusion status of the brain between the two applications. If the use of ReoPro is warranted, then most operators will opt for less anticoagulant effect with an ACT 2.0 to 2.5 times baseline value.

A slow infusion of isosorbide dinitrate through the guide catheter (88) or application of two inches of nitroglycerin paste (107) can be used to minimize iatrogenic vasospasm. The direct vasodilatory (112) and cerebral protection effects (113) of intraarterial verapamil are under investigation.

Anesthesia

A complete discussion of the anesthetic considerations in the treatment of the neurologically symptomatic patient is beyond the scope of this text. For a more complete discussion, please refer to one of many authorities on this subject (114). In general, the anesthesiologist should be consulted in advance of the procedure and sensitized to the goals of the procedure. The neurologically impaired patient will poorly tolerate periods of relative hypotension such as those that frequently occur after induction. The anesthesiologist should have a full complement of equipment during the procedure, not the subset that is often provided for "off-site" or outside the conventional operating room cases.

These procedures have been performed successfully under general anesthesia (99,105) or local anesthesia (102–104,106). Basilar artery lesions should be treated under general anesthesia, as occlusion of the artery during balloon inflation can result in loss of consciousness and apnea. In a series of 12 patients stented under local anesthesia, three (25%) complained of severe headache at the time of stent deployment, which subsided rapidly following balloon deflation (102).

Most operators prefer to perform the procedure with the patient under general anesthesia to maximize safety and reduce procedure time (86,88,89). Four-vessel cerebral angiography is mandatory to determine the optimal working projection, assess collateral blood supply to the territory at risk, identify tandem lesions, characterize the length and geometry of the stenotic area, and guide further therapy if the revascularization procedure were to fail. Accurate and precise measurement of the stenosis, its length, and normal vessel caliber adjacent to the stenosis is used to select appropriate balloon length and diameter. Patient motion artifact limits resolution, may require repeat angiographic sequences, and increases contrast load. The injured brain can be intolerant of smaller doses of iodinated contrast than the uninjured brain. Contrast dose should be limited to 6 mg per kg even with good renal function.

Guide Catheter

Adequate support for the microcatheter–guide wire assembly and the ability to inject contrast injection around the balloon catheter for evaluation of angioplasty result and for digital roadmapping is essential. Small bore (5–6 French) guiding catheters may appear favorable relative to the size of the cervical vessels, especially the vertebral artery. Larger catheters (7–8 French), when safely placed directly or using exchange technique with a 300-cm, 0.035-inch to 0.038-inch guide wire, can provide a firmer platform when needed.

The rapid-delivery, or "monorail," systems now popular in cardiology catheterization labs because of ease of single operator use are distinctly suboptimal for intracranial navigation and revascularization procedures for three important reasons. The greater tortuosity of intracranial vessels and the longer distance from the orifice of the guiding catheter to the target lesion by comparison with coronary procedures leads to a "bow-string" effect, as additional forward pressure is required to advance the microcatheter device over the guide wire.

Secondly, balloon dilatation catheters and balloon-mounted stents developed for coronary application remain excessively rigid for cerebral application. Tremendous research efforts are underway to design more malleable devices for intracranial navigation. To advance the available devices, significant forward pressure is often necessary.

Thirdly, softer guide wires are required for intracranial application than coronary application. The cerebral vessels are comparatively stationary and suspended in cerebrospinal fluid. Innumerable small perforating vessels [many less than 250 microns in diameter and invisible even on high resolution digital subtraction angiography (DSA) equipment] arise from the larger cerebral arteries. Even with soft microcatheters and guide wires designed for cerebral application, deformation of cerebral branches can easily avulse these small branches.

Concurrent with the administration of strong anticoagulant and antiaggregate drugs, perforator branch injury can lead to catastrophic intracranial hemorrhage. By analogy, intracranial navigation for treatment of arteriovenous malformations is complicated by perforator branch injury and hemorrhage in up to 5% of procedures owing to use of over-the-wire catheters. Consequently, many interventional neuroradiologists prefer the use of soft flow-directed catheters for distal catheterization of tortuous vessels to these lesions. Unfortunately, the flow-directed systems available to treat vascular malformations are not applicable to treatment of cerebrovascular stenosis.

The microcatheter–guide wire assembly is passed through a rotating hemostatic valve into the guide catheter. Anterograde flow must be preserved in the cervical artery in which the guiding catheter lies. Continuous forward flushing of the guiding catheter with heparinized saline (3 units heparin/cc normal saline at 1 to 2 cc per second) must be maintained. Digital roadmap images should be obtained in two projections determined by previously acquired arteriographic sequences to advance the microcatheter assembly to the skull base. Trauma to the endothelium of the cervical vessels may lead to excessive platelet activation and suboptimal technical results.

Lesion Navigation and Angioplasty

Once the microcatheter assembly has been passed in proximity to the intracranial vessels, a second set of high-resolution, high-magnification (4.5 to 5 cm field of view) roadmap images are obtained in two planes by injection through the guiding catheter. Coordination with the attending neuroanesthesiologist is imperative to maintain cerebral perfusion prior to revascularization and to provide additional cerebral protection, if appropriate. Burst-suppression doses of etomidate (0.3 to 0.6 mg per kg) may help to protect the brain from further ischemia during the brief time that the treatment device traverses the stenosis. For high-grade or tortuous stenosis, flow arrest is not uncommon. Prior preparation and rapid execution of the treatment plan are a necessity to best ensure satisfactory outcomes.

Although it is often tempting to use the treatment device (balloon catheter or balloon-mounted stent) and microguide wire to cross primarily and revascularize the stenosis, use of a microcatheter and soft microguide wire to cross the stenosis initially is technically superior. It is relatively rare that soft, steady forward pressure on currently available low-profile balloons and stent catheters will not cross an intracranial stenosis using over-the-wire technique. Predilatation with a small, noncompliant balloon (1.5 to 2.0 mm) is seldom necessary. However, the risk of dissection and subintimal passage of the microguide wire in the cerebral circulation is significant. Little effort is required to dissect the delicate cerebral vessels. Operator error leading to subintimal dilatation or stent deployment in the cerebral circulation is generally unsalvageable.

Typically, a low-profile, semicompliant balloon such as the Valor (Cordis, Miami Lakes, FL) is used with the Transend EX or Platinum Tip (BSC/SciMed, Maple Grove, MN) guide wire.

If superimposed thrombus is thought to be contributing to the degree of stenosis and recent infarction has been excluded, superselective infusion of 1 to 5 mg recombinant tissue-type plasminogen activator (rt-PA) or 125,000 IU urokinase may reveal the true extent of the underlying lesion (107). However, this practice is highly controversial, as the available thrombolytic agents have procoagulant properties mediated through release of clot-bound thrombin and/or platelet activation (105). In addition, acute cerebral ischemia leads to poorly characterized vascular permeability due to increased production of metallo-proteinases (115–117) and endothelial injury (118), predisposing to catastrophic hemorrhage following the administration of thrombolytic agents. For the same reasons that administration of thrombolytic agents outside of the treatment "window" for acute cerebral stroke leads to excessive risk of cerebral hemorrhage (119–122), administration of thrombolytic agents during cerebral revascularization in the symptomatic patient must be approached with extreme caution.

With a microcatheter designed for neurological application the lesion is carefully traversed under high-resolution roadmapping. To cross the lesion initially, a gentle curve on a soft-tip microguide wire is preferable, allows greatest directional control, and may be least likely to dislodge plaque or thrombus. Once across, the guide wire is gently removed. Under a blank roadmap image, injection of a small amount of contrast (0.1 to 0.2 cc) is used to confirm intraluminal position of the microcatheter. An arteriographic sequence is useful to document appropriate position of the microcatheter across the stenosis, within the true lumen of the target vessel distal to the stenosis, and to assess for flow arrest.

An exchange-length, soft-type microwire is prepared with the J-curve on the distal tip of the guide wire. Under high-resolution roadmapping, the exchange length microwire is passed into the vessel distal to the stenosis. The wire tip must be kept within the field of view throughout the procedure. Failure to maintain visualization of the wire tip is poor technique and may predispose to vessel perforation during the exchange process. Distal placement of the wire allows greater distribution of radial forces during passage of the treatment device and places a more structurally rigid segment of the wire across the site of stenosis. These factors must be balanced against the risk of vessel distortion, perforator avulsion, and wall penetration. Careful assessment is made regarding the ease of wire advancement and the preferred path of the guide wire in relation to the roadmap and other radiographic landmarks to ensure an intraluminal position.

Primary stenting without predilatation may be feasible depending on lesion severity and morphology. Undersizing of the stent and angioplasty balloon if the lesion requires predilation is recommended to minimize intimal trauma. Intimal damage is related to immediate occlusion and delayed restenosis as previously discussed. This has particular implications in the current setting, as reangioplasty of a stented lesion may be difficult if not impossible. Stent length should be selected to allow 2 mm of stent to protrude beyond each end of the stenosis.

The stent is then positioned across the lesion and deployed using an insufflation device. Postprocedural angiography is performed after the balloon is carefully withdrawn from the stent to define any residual stenosis and exclude branch occlusions.

A screw-type inflation device is used to slowly and accurately distend the balloon over several minutes. Manual inflation using a 1-cc syringe alone is used with compliant balloons for treatment of vasospasm associated with hemorrhagic stroke. This technique is discouraged when using less compliant balloons for treatment of intracranial atherosclerosis where fine pressure and temporal control are necessary. Gradually incremented inflations are continued in 0.5-atmosphere (atm) steps with a pause between each stage until a maximum pressure of 6 to 7 atm is reached. Connors (107) has reported immediate technical improvement and reduced short-term and mid-term restenosis when slow inflation of the device is performed. Again, flow arrest is present throughout device inflation. The duration that flow arrest will be tolerated by the involved vascular distribution varies on an individual basis according to cerebral metabolic status, presence of prior parenchymal injury, and the degree of collateral cerebral blood flow. In many cases, tolerance of prolonged flow arrest is not well characterized before the treatment procedure.

Angiography is obtained with the deflated balloon in position across the site of stenosis by injection of contrast through the guide catheter. If required, the balloon can be withdrawn from the angioplasty site, leaving the wire in place to reveal the true angiographic result. With primary angioplasty, modest restoration of luminal diameter is acceptable and to be expected given deliberate undersizing of the balloon. Increasing luminal diameter has an exponential effect (proportional to the fourth power of the radius) on flow rate, which is likely to be adequate even with modest improvement in the angiographic appearance. Primary placement of an appropriately sized stent device will immediately result in normal, or near normal, vessel caliber. "Undersizing," the purposeful selection of a balloon at least 0.5 mm smaller in diameter than the normal vessel surrounding the stenosis, is recommended (48,89) owing to the fragility of intracranial vessels that possess a thin muscularis and adventitia. Although this does not restore the lumen to its native diameter, the risk of vessel dissection and rupture, which is greater with eccentric lesions, is reduced to an acceptable level. Furthermore, restenosis is believed to be proportional to the degree of intimal damage produced (123) and the rate at which dilatation is performed (107). At least 2 mm of the stent must extend beyond the proximal and distal margins of the stenosis for stable positioning and limitation of the risk of dissection. In either case, the microguide wire must be left in position across the stenosis until it is determined that hyperacute or acute vessel thrombosis will not occur. For this reason and any rescue procedure that may be required, an exchange-length microguide wire is a technical necessity.

Once the guide wire has been removed, attempts at recrossing the recent angioplasty site with a guide wire should be resisted, as selection of a false lumen may occur. Similarly, the smallest of stent devices may be displaced. Further dilatation, if required, may be performed at the 3-month follow-up, by which time the vessel has healed.

Reactive vasospasm at the angioplasty site can be aggressively treated with papaverine (3 mg per cc, maximum dose 150 mg per major vascular territory), nitroglycerin (10 to 25 micrograms per cc, maximum dose unknown), or verapamil (1 mg per cc, maximum dose not known, likely 8 mg per major vessel distribution). If refractory to medical therapy, a compliant balloon catheter designed for dilatation of cerebral vasospasm (Sentry, BSCI/ Target Therapeutics, Fremont, CA; Commodore, Cordis Neurovascular, Miami Lakes, FL) may be used.

Observation of the angioplasty site by performing intermittent angiography for an hour following the procedure is important, unless contraindicated. Exposure of subendothelial layers can stimulate "malignant" activation of the coagulation cascade with platelet adhesion and activation of complement and intrinsic clotting cascade. If thrombus is detected, infusion of fibrinolytics typically clears the fresh "red" thrombus easily. Similarly, the glycoprotein IIB/IIIA inhibitors will also rapidly clear acute "white" thrombus formation. Either agent may be used for emergency salvage in presence of impending or acute occlusion despite certain risk of cerebral hemorrhage.

Postprocedure Management

It is often advantageous to extubate the patient in the neuroangiography suite and perform clinical assessment prior to transfer to the neurological intensive care unit. In certain situations, it may be advantageous to arouse the patient from general anesthesia in the intensive care unit if blood pressure instability mitigates toward continuous physiological monitoring. The patient transport process often exposes weaknesses in the ability to perform intensive pressure modulation often seen in the patient population requiring these procedures.

After revascularization and catheter removal, blood pressure must be reduced 25% to 30% in an effort to prevent hyperperfusion hemorrhage that may complicate up to 5% of technically successful procedures (124). Posttreatment perfusion studies such as TCD with evaluation of pulsatility index (125,126), Xenon CT (127), or other perfusion studies, such as SPECT and MRI (128,129), may help to guide blood pressure modulation in an effort to prevent the sequela of hyperperfusion (124). If not contraindicated for cardiopulmonary factors, antihypertensive agents such as metoprolol are optimal owing to alpha-receptor and beta-receptor blockage with reduction in pressure and pulsatility. Heparin is continued for 24 to 48 hours to maintain a partial thromboplastin time (APTT) of 60 to 80 seconds. Some operators add ticlopidine or clopidogrel to the antiplatelet regimen for 2 to 4 weeks (86,107). We prefer administration of enteric-coated aspirin and clopidogrel for 6 weeks from the date of the procedure if not otherwise contraindicated, with aspirin administered indefinitely thereafter.

Acute and subacute stent thrombosis may result from platelet aggregation on stent struts and damaged intima. Continuation of an antiplatelet regimen consisting of aspirin and clopidogrel or ticlopidine with or without abciximab minimizes the incidence of this complication (99). Some authors state that heparin can be discontinued, as persistent anticoagulation is unnecessary owing to the mechanism of early stent occlusion and superior restoration of luminal diameter compared with angioplasty alone (103,105). Unless an intravenous glycoprotein IIB/IIIA inhibitor has been given, we prefer administration of heparin for 1 to 3 days.

FOLLOW-UP

Subacute to late restenosis is related to intimal hyperplasia (cellular proliferation) and vascular remodeling. MRI with MRA is useful for noninvasive surveillance (86,87), but not all stenoses are detected with these modalities, and measurements of stenosis severity can be inaccurate. The role of CT angiography to accurately depict restenosis is uncertain but likely limited by beam-hardening artifact. Some authors advocate rigorous angiographic follow-up beginning at 3 months (88,107,130) given the 33% and 100% incidence of restenosis for Type B and Type C lesions, respectively, at 1 year (130). It is recommended that conventional angiographic follow-up be obtained initially at 3 months, at which stage additional endovascular treatment can be undertaken if required (107). Depending on patient age, medical condition, and other angiographic risk factors, the value of aggressive arteriographic surveillance must be weighed against the potential complications (131–133).

CONCLUSION

The poor prognosis of patients with symptomatic intracranial atherosclerotic stenoses despite best medical management has defined a new role for endovascular revascularization of the intracranial circulation. However, the procedure is associated with a morbidity and mortality rate of 10% to 20%, and restenosis remains problematic. Undersizing of the balloon is recommended to minimize complications. Stent-assisted angioplasty is now feasible, with recent coronary stent technology allowing improved restoration of vessel diameter while reducing the incidence of local complications. Restenosis after stenting appears to be less problematic at early follow-up compared with angioplasty alone, but the long-term patency of intracranial stenting has yet to be determined. A multidisciplinary approach to patients with symptomatic intracranial atherosclerosis is imperative to achieve appropriate outcomes across the spectrum of disease.

REFERENCES

1. *Stroke. Pathophysiology, diagnosis, and management*, 3rd ed. New York: Churchill Livingstone, 1998.
2. Sacco RL, Kargman DE, Gu Q, et al. Race-ethnicity and determinants of intracranial atherosclerotic cerebral infarction. The Northern Manhattan Stroke Study. *Stroke* 1995;26:14–20.
3. Segura T, Serena J, Castellanos M, et al. Embolism in acute middle cerebral artery stenosis. *Neurology* 2001;56:497–501.
4. Wityk RJ, Lehman D, Klag M, et al. Race and sex differences in the distribution of cerebral atherosclerosis. *Stroke* 1996;27:1974–1980.
5. Craig DR, Meguro K, Watridge C, et al. Intracranial internal carotid artery stenosis. *Stroke* 1982; 13:825–828.
6. Fisher CM, Gore I, Okabe N, et al. Atherosclerosis of the carotid and vertebral arteries: extracranial and intracranial. *J Neuropathol Exp Neurol* 1965;24:455–476.
7. Inzitari D, Hachinski VC, Taylor DW, et al. Racial differences in the anterior circulation in cerebrovascular disease. How much can be explained by risk factors? *Arch Neurol* 1990;47:1080–1084.
8. Resch JA, Okabe N, Loewenson RB, et al. Pattern of vessel involvement in cerebral atherosclerosis. A comparative study between a Japanese and Minnesota population. *J Atheroscler Res* 1969;9:239–250.
9. Wong KS, Huang YN, Gao S, et al. Intracranial stenosis in Chinese patients with acute stroke. *Neurology* 1998;50:812–813.
10. Caplan LR, Gorelick PB, Hier DB. Race, sex and occlusive cerebrovascular disease: a review. *Stroke* 1986;17:648–655.
11. Ingal TJ, Horner D, Baker HI, Jr, et al. Predictors of intracranial carotid atherosclerosis: duration of cigarette smoking and hypertension are more powerful than serum lipid levels. *Arch Neurol* 1991; 48:687–691.
12. Allcock JM. Occlusion of the middle cerebral artery: serial angiography as a guide to conservative therapy. *J Neurosurg* 1967;27:353–363.
13. Hinton RC, Mohr JP, Ackerman RH, et al. Symptomatic middle cerebral artery stenosis. *Ann Neurol* 1979;5:152–157.
14. Lascelles RG, Burrows EH. Occlusion of the middle cerebral artery. *Brain* 1965;88:85–96.
15. Akins PT, Pilgram TK, Cross DT III, et al. Natural history of stenosis from intracranial atherosclerosis by serial angiography. *Stroke* 1998;29:433–438.
16. Schwarze JJ, Babikian V, DeWitt LD, et al. Longitudinal monitoring of intracranial arterial stenoses with transcranial Doppler ultrasonography. *J Neuroimaging* 1994;4:182–187.
17. Wong KS, Li H, Lam WW, et al. Progression of middle cerebral artery occlusive disease and its relationship with further vascular events after stroke. *Stroke* 2002;33:532–536.
18. Castaigne P, Lhermitte F, Gautier JC, et al. Internal carotid artery occlusion. A study of 61 instances in 50 patients with post-mortem data. *Brain* 1970;93:231–258.
19. Castaigne P, Lhermitte F, Gautier JC, et al. Arterial occlusions in the vertebro-basilar system. A study of 44 patients with post-mortem data. *Brain* 1973;96:133–154.
20. Constantinides P. Pathogenesis of cerebral artery thrombosis in man. *Arch Pathol* 1967;83:422–428.
21. Fisher CM. Cerebral arterial occlusion–remarks on pathology, pathophysiology, and diagnosis. *Clin Neurosurg* 1963;9:88–105.
22. Lammie GA, Sandercock PA, Dennis MS. Recently occluded intracranial and extracranial carotid arteries. Relevance of the unstable atherosclerotic plaque. *Stroke* 1999;30:1319–1325.
23. Lhermitte F, Gautier JC, Derouesne C. Nature of occlusions of the middle cerebral artery. *Neurology* 1970;20:82–88.
24. Masuda J, Ogata J, Yutani C, et al. Artery-to-artery embolism from a thrombus formed in stenotic middle cerebral artery. Report of an autopsy case. *Stroke* 1987;18:680–684.
25. Ogata J, Masuda J, Yutani C, et al. Mechanisms of cerebral artery thrombosis: a histopathological analysis on eight necropsy cases. *J Neurol Neurosurg Psychiatry* 1994;57:17–21.
26. Sadoshima S, Fukushima T, Tanaka K. Cerebral artery thrombosis and intramural hemorrhage. *Stroke* 1979;10:411–414.
27. Takano M, Mizuno K, Okamatsu K, et al. Mechanical and structural characteristics of vulnerable plaques: analysis by coronary angioscopy and intravascular ultrasound. *J Am Coll Cardiol* 2001;38: 99–104.
28. Thieme T, Wernecke KD, Meyer R, et al. Angioscopic evaluation of atherosclerotic plaques: validation by histomorphologic analysis and association with stable and unstable coronary syndromes. *J Am Coll Cardiol* 1996;28:1–6.

29. Mizuno K, Miyamoto A, Satomura K, et al. Angioscopic coronary macromorphology in patients with acute coronary disorders. *Lancet* 1991;337:809–812.

30. Ramee SR, White CJ, Collins TJ, et al. Percutaneous angioscopy during coronary angioplasty using a steerable microangioscope. *J Am Coll Cardiol* 1991;17:100–105.

31. Uchida Y, Nakamura F, Tomaru T, et al. Prediction of acute coronary syndromes by percutaneous coronary angioscopy in patients with stable angina. *Am Heart J* 1995;130:195–203.

32. Tanaka A, Kawarabayashi T, Taguchi H, et al. Use of preintervention intravascular ultrasound in patients with acute myocardial infarction. *Am J Cardiol* 2002;89:257–261.

33. Ueda Y, Asakura M, Yamaguchi O, et al. The healing process of infarct-related plaques. Insights from 18 months of serial angioscopic follow-up. *J Am Coll Cardiol* 2001;38:1916–1922.

34. Derdeyn CP, Grubb RL Jr, Powers WJ. Cerebral hemodynamic impairment: methods of measurement and association with stroke risk. *Neurology* 1999;53:251–259.

35. Naritomi H, Sawada T, Kuriyama Y, et al. Effect of chronic middle cerebral artery stenosis on the local cerebral hemodynamics. *Stroke* 1985;16:214–219.

36. Derdeyn CP, Powers WJ, Grubb RL Jr. Hemodynamic effects of middle cerebral artery stenosis and occlusion. *AJNR Am J Neuroradiol* 1998;19:1463–1469.

37. Derdeyn CP, Videen TO, Fritsch SM, et al. Compensatory mechanisms for chronic cerebral hypoperfusion in patients with carotid occlusion. *Stroke* 1999;30:1019–1024.

38. Derdeyn CP, Yundt KD, Videen TO, et al. Increased oxygen extraction fraction is associated with prior ischemic events in patients with carotid occlusion. *Stroke* 1998;29:754–758.

39. Grubb RL Jr, Derdeyn CP, Fritsch SM, et al. Importance of hemodynamic factors in the prognosis of symptomatic carotid occlusion. *JAMA* 1998;280:1055–1060.

40. Corston RN, Kendall BE, Marshall J. Prognosis in middle cerebral artery stenosis. *Stroke* 1984;15:237–241.

41. Wong KS, Gao S, Lam WW, et al. A pilot study of microembolic signals in patients with middle cerebral artery stenosis. *J Neuroimaging* 2001;11:137–140.

42. Koroshetz WJ, Ropper AH. Artery-to-artery embolism causing stroke in the posterior circulation. *Neurology* 1987;37:292–295.

43. Caplan LR. Intracranial branch atheromatous disease: a neglected, understudied, and underused concept. *Neurology* 1989;39:1246–1250.

44. Fisher CM. Lacunar strokes and infarcts: a review. *Neurology* 1982;32:871–876.

45. Fisher CM. Bilateral occlusion of basilar artery branches. *J Neurol Neurosurg Psychiatry* 1977;40:1182–1189.

46. Fisher CM, Caplan LR. Basilar artery branch occlusion: a cause of pontine infarction. *Neurology* 1971;21:900–905.

47. Bogousslavsky J, Regli F, Maeder P, et al. The etiology of posterior circulation infarcts: a prospective study using magnetic resonance imaging and magnetic resonance angiography. *Neurology* 1993;43:1528–1533.

48. Bogousslavsky J, Barnett HJ, Fox AJ, et al. Atherosclerotic disease of the middle cerebral artery. *Stroke* 1986;17:1112–1120.

49. Lyrer PA, Engelter S, Radu EW, et al. Cerebral infarcts related to isolated middle cerebral artery stenosis. *Stroke* 1997;28:1022–1027.

50. Chimowitz MI, Kokkinos J, Strong J, et al. The Warfarin-Aspirin Symptomatic Intracranial Disease Study. *Neurology* 1995;45:1488–1493.

51. Thijs VN, Albers GW. Symptomatic intracranial atherosclerosis: outcome of patients who fail antithrombotic therapy. *Neurology* 2000;55:490–497.

52. Marzewski DJ, Furlan AJ, St Louis P, et al. Intracranial internal carotid artery stenosis: longterm prognosis. *Stroke* 1982;13:821–824.

53. Wechsler LR, Kistler JP, Davis KR, et al. The prognosis of carotid siphon stenosis. *Stroke* 1986;17:714–718.

54. Bogousslavsky J. Prognosis of carotid siphon stenosis. *Stroke* 1987;18:537.

55. Borozan PG, Schuler JJ, LaRosa MP, et al. The natural history of isolated carotid siphon stenosis. *J Vasc Surg* 1984;1:744–749.

56. Failure of extracranial-intracranial arterial bypass to reduce the risk of ischemic stroke. Results of an international randomized trial. The EC/IC Bypass Study Group. *N Engl J Med* 1985;313:1191–1200.

57. Feldmeyer JJ, Merendaz C, Regli F. [Symptomatic stenoses of the middle cerebral artery]. *Rev Neurol (Paris)* 1983;139:725–736.

58. Moufarrij NA, Little JR, Furlan AJ, et al. Basilar and distal vertebral artery stenosis: long-term follow-up. *Stroke* 1986;17:938–942.

59. Pessin MS, Gorelick PB, Kwan ES, et al. Basilar artery stenosis: middle and distal segments. *Neurology* 1987;37:1742–1746.
60. Pessin MS, Kwan ES, DeWitt LD, et al. Posterior cerebral artery stenosis. *Ann Neurol* 1987;21: 85–89.
61. Prognosis of patients with symptomatic vertebral or basilar artery stenosis. The Warfarin-Aspirin Symptomatic Intracranial Disease (WASID) Study Group. *Stroke* 1998;29:1389–1392.
62. *Stroke syndromes*, 2nd ed. New York: Cambridge University Press, 2001.
63. Tatemichi TK, Young WL, Prohovnik I, et al. Perfusion insufficiency in limb-shaking transient ischemic attacks. *Stroke* 1990;21:341–347.
64. Yanagihara T, Piepgras DG, Klass DW. Repetitive involuntary movement associated with episodic cerebral ischemia. *Ann Neurol* 1985;18:244–250.
65. Zaidat OO, Werz MA, Landis DM, et al. Orthostatic limb shaking from carotid hypoperfusion. *Neurology* 1999;53:650–651.
66. Mull M, Schwarz M, Thron A. Cerebral hemispheric low-flow infarcts in arterial occlusive disease. Lesion patterns and angiomorphological conditions. *Stroke* 1997;28:118–123.
67. Furukawa M, Kashiwagi S, Matsunaga N, et al. Evaluation of cerebral perfusion parameters measured by perfusion CT in chronic cerebral ischemia: comparison with xenon CT. *J Comput Assist Tomogr* 2002;26:272–278.
68. Kikuchi K, Murase K, Miki H, et al. Measurement of cerebral hemodynamics with perfusion-weighted MR imaging: comparison with pre- and post-acetazolamide 133Xe-SPECT in occlusive carotid disease. *AJNR Am J Neuroradiol* 2001;22:248–254.
69. Kim JH, Lee SJ, Shin T, et al. Correlative assessment of hemodynamic parameters obtained with T2*- weighted perfusion MR imaging and SPECT in symptomatic carotid artery occlusion. *AJNR Am J Neuroradiol* 2000;21:1450–1456.
70. Lythgoe DJ, Ostergaard L, William SC, et al. Quantitative perfusion imaging in carotid artery stenosis using dynamic susceptibility contrast-enhanced magnetic resonance imaging. *Magn Reson Imaging* 2000;18:1–11.
71. Ozgur HT, Kent WT, Masaryk A, et al. Correlation of cerebrovascular reserve as measured by acetazolamide-challenged SPECT with angiographic flow patterns and intra- or extracranial arterial stenosis. *AJNR Am J Neuroradiol* 2001;22:928–936.
72. Cigada M, Marzorati S, Tredici S, et al. Cerebral CO_2 vasoreactivity evaluation by transcranial Doppler ultrasound technique: a standardized methodology. *Intensive Care Med* 2000;26:729–732.
73. Kleiser B, Widder B. Course of carotid artery occlusions with impaired cerebrovascular reactivity. *Stroke* 1992;23:171–174.
74. Silvestrini M, Vernieri F, Pasqualetti P, et al. Impaired cerebral vasoreactivity and risk of stroke in patients with asymptomatic carotid artery stenosis. *JAMA* 2000;283:2122–2127.
75. Mintun MA, Raichle ME, Martin WR, et al. Brain oxygen utilization measured with O-15 radiotracers and positron emission tomography. *J Nucl Med* 1984;25:177–187.
76. Mohr JP, Thompson JL, Lazar RM, et al. A comparison of warfarin and aspirin for the prevention of recurrent ischemic stroke. *N Engl J Med* 2001;345:1444–1451.
77. Major Ongoing Stroke Trials. *Stroke* 2001;32:1449–1457.
78. The International Cooperative Study of Extracranial/Intracranial Arterial Anastomosis (EC/IC Bypass Study): methodology and entry characteristics. The EC/IC Bypass Study Group. *Stroke* 1985;16: 397–406.
79. Gumerlock MK, Coull BM, Howieson J, et al. Late stenosis of a superficial temporal-middle cerebral artery bypass: angiographic and histological findings. *Neurosurgery* 1985;16:650–657.
80. Gumerlock MK, Ono H, Neuwelt EA. Can a patent extracranial-intracranial bypass provoke the conversion of an intracranial arterial stenosis to a symptomatic occlusion? *Neurosurgery* 1983;12: 391–400.
81. Hopkins LN, Budny JL. Complications of intracranial bypass for vertebrobasilar insufficiency. *J Neurosurg* 1989;70:207–211.
82. Hopkins LN, Budny JL, Castellani D. Extracranial-intracranial arterial bypass and basilar artery ligation in the treatment of giant basilar artery aneurysms. *Neurosurgery* 1983;13:189–194.
83. Matsushima Y, Aoyagi M, Fukai N, et al. Angiographic demonstration of cerebral revascularization after encephalo-duro-arterio-synangiosis (EDAS) performed on pediatric moyamoya patients. *Bull Tokyo Med Dent Univ* 1982;29:7–17.
84. Mori T, Fukuoka M, Kazita K, et al. Follow-up study after intracranial percutaneous transluminal cerebral balloon angioplasty. *AJNR Am J Neuroradiol* 1998;19:1525–1533.

85. Mori T, Mori K, Fukuoka M, et al. Percutaneous transluminal cerebral angioplasty: serial angiographic follow-up after successful dilatation. *Neuroradiology* 1997;39:111–116.
86. Nahser HC, Henkes H, Weber W, et al. Intracranial vertebrobasilar stenosis: angioplasty and follow-up. *AJNR Am J Neuroradiol* 2000;21:1293–1301.
87. Eckard DA, Zarnow DM, McPherson CM, et al. Intracranial internal carotid artery angioplasty: technique with clinical and radiographic results and follow-up. *AJR Am J Roentgenol* 1999;172: 703–707.
88. Song JK, Eskridge JM. Intracranial angioplasty and thrombolysis. *Neurosurg Clin N Am* 2000;11: 49–65, viii.
89. Alazzaz A, Thornton J, Aletich VA, et al. Intracranial percutaneous transluminal angioplasty for arteriosclerotic stenosis. *Arch Neurol* 2000;57:1625–1630.
90. McKenzie JD, Wallace RC, Dean BL, et al. Preliminary results of intracranial angioplasty for vascular stenosis caused by atherosclerosis and vasculitis. *AJNR Am J Neuroradiol* 1996;17:263–268.
91. Takis C, Kwan ES, Pessin MS, et al. Intracranial angioplasty: experience and complications. *AJNR Am J Neuroradiol* 1997;18:1661–1668.
92. Eskridge JM, Newell DW, Winn HR. Endovascular treatment of vasospasm. *Neurosurg Clin N Am* 1994;5:437–447.
93. Marks MP, Marcellus M, Norbash AM, et al. Outcome of angioplasty for atherosclerotic intracranial stenosis. *Stroke* 1999;30:1065–1069.
94. Roubin GS, Yadav S, Iyer SS, et al. Carotid stent-supported angioplasty: a neurovascular intervention to prevent stroke. *Am J Cardiol* 1996;78:8–12.
95. Theron J. [Protected carotid angioplasty and carotid stents]. *J Mal Vasc* 1996;21(Suppl A):113–122.
96. Theron J. Cerebral protection during carotid angioplasty. *J Endovasc Surg* 1996;3:484–486.
97. Yadav JS, Roubin GS, Iyer S, et al. Elective stenting of the extracranial carotid arteries. *Circulation* 1997;95:376–381.
98. Yadav JS, Roubin GS, King P, et al. Angioplasty and stenting for restenosis after carotid endarterectomy. Initial experience. *Stroke* 1996;27:2075–2079.
99. Rasmussen PA, Perl J, Barr JD, et al. Stent-assisted angioplasty of intracranial vertebrobasilar atherosclerosis: an initial experience. *J Neurosurg* 2000;92:771–778.
100. Al-Mubarak N, Gomez CR, Vitek JJ, et al. Stenting of symptomatic stenosis of the intracranial internal carotid artery. *AJNR Am J Neuroradiol* 1998;19:1949–1951.
101. Phatouros CC, Higashida RT, Malek AM, et al. Endovascular stenting of an acutely thrombosed basilar artery: technical case report and review of the literature. *Neurosurgery* 1999;44:667–673.
102. Gomez CR, Misra VK, Campbell MS, et al. Elective stenting of symptomatic middle cerebral artery stenosis. *AJNR Am J Neuroradiol* 2000;21:971–973.
103. Gomez CR, Misra VK, Liu MW, et al. Elective stenting of symptomatic basilar artery stenosis. *Stroke* 2000;31:95–99.
104. Mori T, Kazita K, Chokyu K, et al. Short-term arteriographic and clinical outcome after cerebral angioplasty and stenting for intracranial vertebrobasilar and carotid atherosclerotic occlusive disease. *AJNR Am J Neuroradiol* 2000;21:249–254.
105. Horowitz MB, Pride GL, Graybeal DF, et al. Percutaneous transluminal angioplasty and stenting of midbasilar stenoses: three technical case reports and literature review. *Neurosurgery* 1999;45:925–930.
106. Mori T, Kazita K, Mori K. Cerebral angioplasty and stenting for intracranial vertebral atherosclerotic stenosis. *AJNR Am J Neuroradiol* 1999;20:787–789.
107. Connors JJ 3rd. Intracranial angioplasty. In: Connors JJ 3rd, Wojak JC, eds. *Interventional neuroradiology*. Philadelphia: W.B. Saunders, 1999.
108. Berger PB. Clopidogrel after coronary stenting. *Curr Interv Cardiol Rep* 1999;:263–269.
109. Berger PB, Bell MR, Rihal CS, et al. Clopidogrel versus ticlopidine after intracoronary stent placement. *J Am Coll Cardiol* 1999;34:1891–1894.
110. Waksman R, Ajani AE, White RL, et al. Prolonged antiplatelet therapy to prevent late thrombosis after intracoronary gamma-radiation in patients with in-stent restenosis: Washington Radiation for In-Stent Restenosis Trial plus 6 months of clopidogrel (WRIST PLUS). *Circulation* 2001;103: 2332–2335.
111. Petruk KC, West M, Mohr G, et al. Nimodipine treatment in poor-grade aneurysm patients. Results of a multicenter double-blind placebo-controlled trial. *J Neurosurg* 1988;68:505–517.
112. Joshi S, Meyers P, Wang M, et al. Intraarterial verapamil decreases vascular resistance in conductance arteries of human subjects. 2002 (letter).
113. Feng L, Fitzsimmons BF, Young WL, et al. Intraarterially administered verapamil as adjunct therapy for cerebral vasospasm: safety and 2-year experience. *AJNR Am J Neuroradiol* 2002;23:1284–1290.

114. Herrick IA, Gelb AW. Occlusive cerebrovascular disease: anesthetic considerations. In: Cottrell JE, Smith DS, eds. *Anesthesia and neurosurgery.* St. Louis: Mosby, 1999.

115. Gasche Y, Copin JC, Sugawara T, et al. Matrix metalloproteinase inhibition prevents oxidative stress-associated blood-brain barrier disruption after transient focal cerebral ischemia. *J Cereb Blood Flow Metab* 2001;21:1393–1400.

116. Montaner J, Alvarez-Sabin J, Molina CA, et al. Matrix metalloproteinase expression is related to hemorrhagic transformation after cardioembolic stroke. *Stroke* 2001;32:2762–2767.

117. Sumii T, Lo EH. Involvement of matrix metalloproteinase in thrombolysis-associated hemorrhagic transformation after embolic focal ischemia in rats. *Stroke* 2002;33:831–836.

118. Del Zoppo GJ, Hallenbeck JM. Advances in the vascular pathophysiology of ischemic stroke. *Thromb Res* 2000;98:73–81.

119. Del Zoppo GJ, Higashida RT, Furlan AJ, et al. PROACT: a phase II randomized trial of recombinant pro-urokinase by direct arterial delivery in acute middle cerebral artery stroke. PROACT Investigators. Prolyse in Acute Cerebral Thromboembolism. *Stroke* 1998;29:4–11.

120. Kase CS, Furlan AJ, Wechsler LR, et al. Cerebral hemorrhage after intra-arterial thrombolysis for ischemic stroke: the PROACT II trial. *Neurology* 2001;57:1603–1610.

121. The National Institute of Neurological Disorders rt-PA Stroke Study Group. Generalized efficacy of t-PA for acute stroke. Subgroup analysis of the NINDS t-PA Stroke Trial. *Stroke* 1997;28:2119–2125.

122. Wardlaw JM. Overview of Cochrane thrombolysis meta-analysis. *Neurology* 2001;57Suppl 2):69–76.

123. Topol EJ, Califf RM, Weisman HF, et al. Randomised trial of coronary intervention with antibody against platelet IIb/IIIa integrin for reduction of clinical restenosis: results at six months. The EPIC Investigators. *Lancet* 1994;343:881–886.

124. Meyers PM, Higashida RT, Phatouros CC, et al. Cerebral hyperperfusion syndrome after percutaneous transluminal stenting of the craniocervical arteries. *Neurosurgery* 2000;47:335–343.

125. Gossetti B, Martinelli O, Guerricchio R, et al. Transcranial Doppler in 178 patients before, during, and after carotid endarterectomy. *J Neuroimaging* 1997;7:213–216.

126. Jorgensen LG, Schroeder TV. Defective cerebrovascular autoregulation after carotid endarterectomy. *Eur J Vasc Surg* 1993;7:370–379.

127. Penn AA, Schomer DF, Steinberg GK. Imaging studies of cerebral hyperperfusion after carotid endarterectomy. Case report. *J Neurosurg* 1995;83:133–137.

128. Baker CJ, Mayer SA, Prestigiacomo CJ, et al. Diagnosis and monitoring of cerebral hyperperfusion after carotid endarterectomy with single photon emission computed tomography: case report. *Neurosurgery* 1998;43:157–160.

129. Kidwell CS, Saver JL, Mattiello J, et al. Diffusion-perfusion MRI characterization of post-recanalization hyperperfusion in humans. *Neurology* 2001;57:2015–2021.

130. Mori T, Fukuoka M, Kazita K, et al. Follow-up study after percutaneous transluminal cerebral angioplasty. *Eur Radiol* 1998;8:403–408.

131. Mani RL, Eisenberg RL. Complications of catheter cerebral arteriography: analysis of 5,000 procedures. II. Relation of complication rates to clinical and arteriographic diagnoses. *AJR Am J Roentgenol* 1978;131:867–869.

132. Mani RL, Eisenberg RL. Complications of catheter cerebral arteriography: analysis of 5,000 procedures. III. Assessment of arteries injected, contrast medium used, duration of procedure, and age of patient. *AJR Am J Roentgenol* 1978;131:871–874.

133. Mani RL, Eisenberg RL, McDonald EJ, et al. Complications of catheter cerebral arteriography: analysis of 5,000 procedures. I. Criteria and incidence. *AJR Am J Roentgenol* 1978; 131:861–865.

134. Derdeyn CP, Videen TO, Yundt KD, et al. Variability of cerebral blood volume and oxygen extraction: stages of cerebral haemodynamic impairment revisited. *Brain* 2002;125(Pt 3):595–607.

135. Baron JC, Bousser MG, Rey A, et al. Reversal of focal "misery-perfusion syndrome" by extra-intracranial arterial bypass in hemodynamic cerebral ischemia. A case study with 15O positron emission tomography. *Stroke* 1981;12:454–459.

136. Yamauchi H, Fukuyama H, Nagahama Y, et al. Significance of increased oxygen extraction fraction in five-year prognosis of major cerebral arterial occlusive diseases. *J Nucl Med* 1999;40:1992–1998.

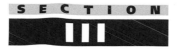

FUTURE DIRECTIONS

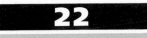

CURRENT STATUS OF CLINICAL TRIALS AND IMPLICATION OF ANTI-EMBOLI PROTECTION

BRAJESH K. LAL
ROBERT W. HOBSON II

Stroke is the third most common cause of death and the leading cause of disability in the United States. Management of identifiable risk factors and careful selection of patients for operative intervention constitute the current approach toward reducing the morbidity and mortality associated with stroke. Carotid endarterectomy (CEA), performed with a low periprocedural complication rate, is the only form of mechanical cerebral revascularization for which definitive evidence of clinical effectiveness has been reported. Recently, retrospective case reports and case series have demonstrated the feasibility of carotid artery stenting (CAS) as a possible alternative to CEA. In the tradition of the two previous National Institutes of Health (NIH)-sponsored trials, the North American Symptomatic Endarterectomy Trial (NASCET) and Asymptomatic Carotid Atherosclerosis Study (ACAS), the NIH has sponsored a clinical trial (Carotid Revascularization Endarterectomy Versus Stent Trial, or CREST) that is currently underway to determine the efficacy and risks of CAS compared to CEA. Recently published nonrandomized single-center and multiinstitutional studies have reported 30-day stroke and death rates from CAS ranging from 2.8% to 12%. *In vivo* experience confirms that perioperative neurological events correlate with atheroembolization. *Ex vivo* experiments demonstrate that CAS is associated with atheroembolization. Therefore, a concern exists regarding the generation of atheroembolic particles during guide wire, balloon, and stent manipulation of atherosclerotic plaques within the carotid artery. This has resulted in increased interest in the concomitant use of Anti-Embolization devices during CAS that have a demonstrated capacity to capture atheroembolic debris. The CREST trial incorporates the use of one such Anti-Embolic protection device, the AccuNet.

EPIDEMIOLOGY

Stroke is the third most common cause of death in North America, and approximately 500,000 new strokes are reported annually in the United States (1). Seventy-five percent of these strokes occur in the distribution of the carotid arteries. Stroke is also the leading cause of disability among elderly Americans. Although there has been a 50% reduction in mortality over the last two decades, 21% of survivors will still have a second stroke, and 7% a third stroke (2). Forty percent will require special nursing home care, whereas 10% will require institutionalization. Among strokes of a thromboembolic cause, carotid occlusive disease is the most common. The 30-day and 5-year mortality rates for stroke that occurs in the carotid distribution are 17% and 40%, respectively, although as many as 150,000 stroke-related fatalities are documented annually (2). The American Heart Association esti-mated that the cost of stroke in the United States approximated 18 billion dollars in 1993 (1).

PATHOPHYSIOLOGY

The unique hemodynamics at the carotid bifurcation predispose this area to atherosclerosis. Along the inner wall of the carotid bulb, blood flow remains laminar, with high velocity and high shear stress. Conversely, along the outer wall, there are areas of flow separation, stasis, turbulent flow, and a complex oscillating shear stress pattern that predispose to athero-sclerotic plaque deposition (3). Although neurological events have been attributed to progres-sive stenosis and decreased blood flow from enlarging atherosclerotic plaques, such events are usually secondary to atheroemboli from the carotid lesion. Loss of the fibrous cap with exposure of atherosclerotic debris to the flow lumen appears to be responsible for these embolic complications (4). Additional factors such as adequacy of collateralization, plaque ulceration, hypotension, or low cardiac output also play a contributory role. The histologic composition and architecture of the plaque has recently come under increasing scrutiny as a possible indicator of "plaque instability."

In a series of experiments using explanted carotid plaques, Ohki et al. (5) demonstrated that subjecting them to CAS resulted in the generation of several atheroembolic particles. In another experiment, Ohki et al. (6) subjected similar plaques to CAS in the presence of an Anti-Embolic filter protection device. All devices captured atherosclerotic debris with variable efficacy. In addition, transcranial Doppler studies have confirmed the generation of multiple emboli in the middle cerebral artery during carotid stenting (7). Preliminary experience with the use of Anti-Embolization devices during CAS has shown encouraging results in terms of safety and efficacy (8–10). Moreover, embolic particles have been re-covered from several cases in which protection devices have been used (8–10). Therefore, use of these devices *in vivo* could prevent distal embolization of atherosclerotic debris during balloon dilation and stent deployment, and prevent neurological complications.

RATIONALE FOR CAROTID ENDARTERECTOMY

The first randomized controlled trial comparing pharmacologic to surgical treatment of carotid occlusive disease appeared in 1970 (11). Although the study demonstrated that the patients undergoing CEA had a lower incidence of stroke and death during long-term follow-up, this benefit was offset by a high perioperative stroke rate. With improved surgical technique and selection of patients for operation, a significant decrease in the complication rate of this procedure has been reported (12). The controversy over proper management of carotid stenosis prompted several randomized controlled multiinstitutional trials during the past two decades (13). They have provided statistically reliable results that form the basis of current management recommendations.

Symptomatic Carotid Stenosis

Several centers in North America and internationally participated in NASCET, which stud-ied patients with recent hemispheric and retinal TIAs or nondisabling strokes and ipsilateral high-grade stenosis (70% to 99%) of the internal carotid artery (ICA) (14). In the NASCET data, life-table estimates of the cumulative risk of stroke at 2 years were 26% in the medical group versus 9% in the surgical group [absolute risk reduction ($\pm$ SE), 17 $\pm$ 3.5%; $p<0.001$]. The corresponding estimates for major or fatal ipsilateral stroke were 13.1% versus 2.5% [absolute risk reduction ($\pm$ SE), 10.6 $\pm$ 2.6%; $p<0.001$] and for any stroke or death were 32% versus 16% [absolute risk reduction ($\pm$ SE), 16.5 $\pm$ 4.2%; $p<0.001$]. The European Carotid Surgery Trial (ECST) published a confirmatory report demonstrating significant benefit for CEA and optimal medical therapy versus best medical care alone (15). Finally, the Veterans Affairs (VA) Symptomatic trial also confirmed benefit for CEA in a small number of patients; the trial was closed after initial announcement of the NASCET data (16). Recently, the NASCET trialists have reported benefit from CEA in patients with 50% to 69% stenosis (17). The 5-year rate of ipsilateral stroke was 15.7% among patients treated surgically and 22.2% in those treated medically. However, the benefit was not significant for women. The results of these clinical trials have determined the indications for CEA in symptomatic patients.

Asymptomatic Carotid Stenosis

The VA Cooperative Study Group enrolled men with asymptomatic carotid stenosis with diameter reduction of more than or equal to 50% (18). Although the combined rate of transient neurological events and stroke was reduced after CEA, the ACAS investigators were the first to report reduction in stroke alone after CEA (12). In patients with more than or equal to 60% diameter reducing stenosis, the projected 5-year ipsilateral stroke rates for surgically treated patients was 5.1%, whereas it was 11.0% for the medically treated group [aggregate risk reduction, 53%; 95% confidence interval (CI), 22-72%]. These trials have established the beneficial role of CEA in reducing the risk of neurological sequelae in patients with asymptomatic carotid stenosis.

Recommendations for Carotid Endarterectomy

Therefore, a series of randomized clinical trials over the past two decades have determined that CEA, performed with a low periprocedural complication rate, is an optimal form of mechanical cerebral revascularization for extracranial carotid occlusive disease. These trials have reshaped the way carotid stenosis is treated across the world and resulted in a dramatic increase in the number of CEAs performed (19).

CAROTID ARTERY STENTING

Carotid artery stenting is a relatively new endovascular procedure that has been used increasingly in recent years. Its popularity is due, at least in part, to the perceived advantages of a less invasive treatment for extracranial carotid occlusive disease. Several anecdotal reports, case series, and single institutional trials or registries have reported support for this approach.

Carotid Angioplasty Alone

The first reports of a multicenter prospective protocol-based study of CAS, the North American Percutaneous Transluminal Angioplasty Register, were published in 1993 (20,21). Initial results were reported on 165 angioplasty procedures in 147 symptomatic patients with a mean stenosis of 84% (range 70% to 99%) (20). The mean residual stenosis after angioplasty was 37% ($p < 0.01$). This corresponded to an immediate success rate of 83% (95% CI, 76% to 88%). Death from all causes occurred in 3%, and stroke occurred in an additional 6% of procedures. The 30-day combined rate of death and stroke from all causes was 9% (95% CI, 5% to 15%). Data concerning the rate of restenosis in 44 lesions with angiographic follow-up at a mean of 260 days were published in another report (21). The definition of restenosis was more than 70% stenosis on angiographic evaluation. Of the 37 lesions that were successfully treated with angioplasty, restenosis occurred in 8 (22%; 95% CI, 10% to 38%). Of those that developed restenosis, five of eight patients (63%) were symptomatic at the time of follow-up. Cox proportional hazards modeling demonstrated that symptoms and the degree of stenosis before angioplasty were independent predictors of angiographic restenosis in follow-up. These data suggested that restenosis would be a significant problem after carotid angioplasty (CA) alone and stimulated clinicians to perform stenting after angioplasty as a routine practice.

Selective Carotid Artery Stenting

In 1996, Diethrich et al. (22) reported the results of CAS in 110 symptomatic patients with more than or equal to 70% stenoses from a single institution. There was one technical failure (0.9%) with conversion to CEA. Two deaths (1.8%) occurred (one from stroke and one from a cardiac event). Seven strokes (2 major, 1.8%, and 5 minor, 4.5%) and five transient neurologic events (4.5%) occurred. On the basis of this early experience, the authors concluded that the incidence of periprocedural neurologic complications was excessive. In an accompanying editorial, Diethrich (23) suggested that CAS be restricted to cases of carotid restenosis after prior CEA, instances in which the internal carotid stenosis was anatomically higher than readily treated by CEA, and in radiation-induced stenosis.

Self-expanding Stents

A larger prospective protocol-based study of CAS in 204 patients was reported by Mathur et al. (24). Seventy-five percent of the patients had significant coronary artery disease, and 70% of the patients had medical comorbidities that would have made them ineligible for the NASCET study. Of the 238 arteries that were treated (204 patients), 145 (61%) were in symptomatic patients [60 strokes; 85 transient ischemic attacks (TIAs)] and 93 were in asymptomatic patients. Nine percent had an occluded contralateral carotid artery, 15% had restenosis after previous CEA, and 18% had complex ulcerated lesions. Technical success was achieved in 99% of cases. In two patients, the carotid artery could not be accessed by the transfemoral approach. In one patient, the procedure was aborted after initial angiography was complicated by an air embolism. Of the 204 patients, there was one death (0.5%) and two major strokes (0.98%; NIH stroke scale more than 4, with residual disability more than 30 days). One stroke was due to stent thrombosis, and the other was due to a cardiogenic embolus. Minor strokes (NIH stroke scale less than 3, with resolution within 30 days) were observed in 15 patients (7.4%). During follow-up, one additional minor ischemic stroke has occurred in these 204 patients. Three patients have experienced TIAs, with no evidence of stent restenosis. Four patients died during follow-up (one each from congestive heart failure, pneumonia, intracranial hemorrhage, and renal failure). Repeat carotid imaging (angiography or ultrasound scanning) was performed in 75% of patients at 6 months of follow-up. Restenosis (more than 70% diameter reduction) has been documented in five of the 104 patients (5%) who were restudied. Stent deformation occurred in 14% of the balloon-expandable stents that were deployed. As a result of these data, a self-expandable stent has been recommended for use by the CREST investigators.

Carotid Artery Stenting for North American Symptomatic Endarterectomy Trial and Asymptomatic Carotid Atherosclerosis Study Eligible Patients

Recently, Roubin et al. updated their previous reports (25). This study followed 528 consecutive patients (604 hemispheres/arteries) undergoing carotid stenting. There was a 0.6% (n = 3) fatal stroke rate and 1% (n = 5) nonstroke death rate at 30 days. The major stroke rate was 1% (n = 6), and the minor stroke rate was 4.8% (n = 29). The overall 30-day stroke and death rate was 7.4% (n = 43). The best predictor of 30-day stroke and death was age 80 or more years. The authors concluded by stating that CAS can be performed with an acceptable 30-day complication rate and that CAS may be comparable to CEA. They emphasized the need for a NIH-supported, randomized trial comparing the two treatment modalities. In a recent update on 40 NASCET-eligible patients, Gomez et al. (26) reported one transient neurologic event (2.5%) and no deaths, major stroke, or myocardial infarctions. These investigators suggested a comparability of complications between CAS and CEA.

Randomized Controlled Trials of Carotid Artery Stenting Versus Carotid Endarterectomy

Currently, one randomized clinical trial to compare the efficacy of CAS and CEA is ongoing in Europe, the Carotid and Vertebral Artery Transluminal Angioplasty Study (CAVATAS) (27). Investigators are comparing surgical intervention and angioplasty for treatment of carotid and vertebral occlusive lesions. Results for 504 patients from phase I of the multicenter trial were published in 2001 (28). A total of 251 patients were randomized to CA, whereas 253 were randomized to CEA. In the CA group, salvage stenting was used in 26% of patients. An independent neurologist followed up patients. The rates of major outcome events within 30 days of treatment did not differ significantly between CA and CEA groups (6.4% versus 5.9% for disabling stroke or death; 10.0% versus 9.9% for any stroke lasting more than 7 days, or death). At 1 year after treatment, severe (70% to 99%) ipsilateral carotid stenosis was more usual after endovascular treatment [25 (14%) versus 7 (4%), $p < 0.001$]. However, no substantial difference in the rate of ipsilateral stroke was noted at 3 years follow-up ($p = 0.9$). Phase II of the trial will be initiated later this year and will use angioplasty-stenting in all symptomatic carotid cases. These are currently the only data available from a randomized controlled comparison of CEA versus CA; however, their influence may be blunted by the somewhat higher than expected complication rate in the CEA group and the use of angioplasty alone in the CA group.

Alberts et al. (29) described the methods of another randomized clinical trial that compared carotid stenting versus endarterectomy in symptomatic patients (stenosis, 50% to 99%) that was sponsored by the Schneider Corporation (now Boston Scientific Vascular, Natick, MA, manufacturers of the Wallstent endoprosthesis) (29). The stated aim of the trial was to determine whether carotid stenting is equivalent to CEA in the prevention of any ipsilateral stroke, periprocedural death (within 30 days), or vascular death within 1 year of treatment. However, this trial has been discontinued because of procedural and recruitment difficulties. The other attempt at a randomized trial was plagued by an excessively high complication rate in the CAS group, which resulted in its discontinuance (30).

CURRENT STATUS OF CAROTID ARTERY STENTING

These reports collectively demonstrate the technical feasibility of performing endovascular revascularization for treatment of occlusive cerebrovascular disease in selected patients; however, no definitive comparative clinical study of CAS and CEA has been published. Although CAS has been proposed as an alternative to CEA, the safety and clinical effectiveness of CAS has not been established. Currently available reports point towards the possibility of clinical equivalence; however, they do not fulfill the rigorous criteria of level-1 evidence. The two published randomized trials were not sufficiently powered to resolve the questions of comparative efficacy, durability, safety, or cost-efficacy of CAS versus CEA.

Based on our experience with CAS, and on a review of results from retrospective analyses and two prospective clinical trials, we believe that a state of "clinical equipoise" exists between CEA and CAS. Freedman has noted that: "Clinicians have preferences for a given intervention based on their specialties and prior training. However, once various specialists are treating the same entity with different procedures and achieving 'acceptable' clinical results, a state of equipoise may be present. If so, it then becomes ethical for a clinician to participate in a Randomized Clinical Trial recognizing the uncertainty of the new procedure's effectiveness"(40).

A recently published Science Advisory from the American Heart Association concluded that "...with few exceptions, use of carotid stenting should be limited to well-designed, well-controlled randomized studies with careful dispassionate oversight" (41). The safety and efficacy of any new therapy must be clearly established in a controlled and adequately monitored clinical trial under Institutional Review Board (IRB) and Food and Drug Administration (FDA) guidelines. On the basis of the conclusions of a multidisciplinary panel at the Montefiore Vascular Symposium, only specific subgroups of patients should currently be considered for CAS (31).

Although there is no direct *in vivo* evidence that Anti-Embolic devices reduce the incidence of neurological complications, *ex vivo* evidence suggests that these devices capture atheroembolic debris and prevent their distal embolization. Based on these considerations, the Multidisciplinary Consensus Committee convened in New York recommended that CAS be performed with Anti-Embolic protection, once these devices become available (31).

CAROTID REVASCULARIZATION ENDARTERECTOMY VERSUS STENT TRIAL: A RANDOMIZED CLINICAL TRIAL CONTRASTING CAROTID ARTERY STENTING WITH CAROTID ENDARTERECTOMY

The NIH has recently approved funding for the CREST investigators from the National Institute of Neurological Disorders and Stroke for a trial to compare the efficacy of CEA and CAS in symptomatic patients with high grade more than or equal to 70% stenosis.

Aims

The primary outcome events for this clinical trial include: (a) any stroke, myocardial infarction, or death during the 30-day perioperative or periprocedural period, or (b) ipsilateral stroke after 30 days. Endpoints will be reviewed by an Adjudication Committee, blinded to the assigned treatment. Stroke will be determined by a positive TIA/stroke questionnaire that is confirmed by an evaluation of a neurologist. Myocardial infarction will be determined by electrocardiography and enzyme abnormalities. Secondary goals include: (a) describing differential efficacy of the two treatments in men and women, (b) contrasting perioperative (30-day) morbidity and post procedural (after 30 days) mortality rates for the CEA and CAS procedures, (c) estimating and contrasting restenosis rates for the two procedures, (d) identifying subgroups of participants at differential risk for the two procedures, and (e) evaluating differences in health-related quality of life issues and cost effectiveness.

Participation and Credentialing

Recognizing that CAS is a relatively new procedure, each participating center is required to complete a credentialing phase to reassure clinicians that the safety of these procedures has been reviewed and established before the randomized phase of the trial proceeds. This requires the performance of up to 20 interventional procedures at each participating center to the satisfaction of CREST's Interventional Management Committee. Once completed, randomization of patients between the two treatments then proceeds. At the present time, 26 centers have enrolled in the study, 23 are in their credentialing phase, and three are in the randomization phase.

Design

Patients will be evaluated at baseline, at 24 hours before the procedure, at 30 days, at 6 months, and thereafter at 6-month intervals. Baseline procedures will include a brief medical history and physical examination, a risk factor evaluation, the performance of neurologic status questionnaires, a neurologic examination, an electrocardiogram, and a baseline carotid duplex scan. The 30-day follow-up will include evaluation of the neurologic status through questionnaires, an electrocardiogram, and a follow-up carotid duplex scan. All 6-month follow-up visits will include a brief physical examination, the completion of the neurologic questionnaire, a risk factor evaluation, and a carotid duplex scan.

All patients with a positive neurologic status questionnaire will be evaluated by a neurologist. The sample size for the study is approximately 2,500 symptomatic patients, which will be sufficient to detect a relative difference of 25% to 30% between treatment groups. Lesser differences would be considered sufficiently small to declare the treatments equivalent. A differential efficacy assessment of CEA and CAS that is based on gender is a secondary goal for CREST. In patients with high-grade asymptomatic stenosis that were reported by ACAS, CEA offered a 66% reduction in events over a 5-year period for men, but only a 17% reduction for women (12). In NASCET, male patients demonstrated greater benefit after CEA than women for 50% to 69% stenosis (12,14). Although the causes for these examples of differential efficacy between genders are not well understood, the effect may be attributed to a higher complication rate for CEA in women, possibly caused by their reported smaller arterial sizes and a greater surgical morbidity. Unfortunately, neither ACAS nor NASCET suspected the possibility of a differential gender effect and were therefore not appropriately powered to investigate it. However, given the results of these two randomized clinical trials, a requirement for *a priori* plans to evaluate the possibility of a differential gender effect has become an important component of CREST. Centers are being selected with a goal as high as 50% for women in the randomized sample of patients and a minimum of 40%.

Methods

Centers are being allowed reasonable latitude in the technical aspects of performing CEA in the manner that participating surgeons prefer. The use of general or local anesthesia,

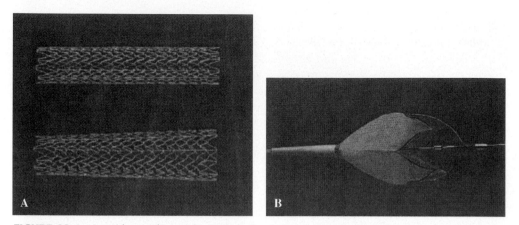

FIGURE 22-1. Carotid stent (AccuLink, Guidant Co., Indianapolis, IN) and Anti-Embolic device (AccuNet, Guidant Co.) being used by the Carotid Revascularization Endarterectomy Versus Stent Trial (CREST) investigators for performing CAS. **A:** AccuLink stents are made of self-expanding nitinol and are available in two configurations: straight (*above*) and tapered (*below*), each in several diameters and lengths. **B:** The AccuNet Anti-Embolic device is made of polyurethane and is available in several diameters. (See also the color section following page 164 of this text.)

mandatory or selective shunting, and direct or eversion endarterectomy are accepted standard approaches to CEA. Because CAS is a relatively new procedure, the protocol described above is adhered to in all centers. All procedures are being performed using self-expanding nitinol stents under the protection of an Anti-Embolic filter device (Fig. 22-1).

CONCLUSIONS

Current clinical practice dictates that CAS be considered in limited subsets of patients only. The conducting of clinical trials (CREST and others) will provide level-1 and level-2 evidence from which a firm clinical recommendation can be established. Until these data are available during the next several years, the performance of CAS should be limited to randomized clinical trials and defined unique subsets of high-risk patients. CEA continues to be recommended for the treatment of most patients with symptomatic and asymptomatic extracranial carotid occlusive disease.

REFERENCES

1. American Heart Association. *2001 heart and stroke statistical update.* Dallas : American Heart Association, 2001.
2. Chambers BR, Norris JW, Shurvell BL, et al. Prognosis of acute stroke. *Neurology* 1987;37:221–225.
3. Zarins CK, Giddens DP, Bharadvaj BK, et al. Carotid bifurcation atherosclerosis. Quantitative correlation of plaque localization with flow velocity profiles and wall shear stress. *Circ Res* 1983;53:502–514.
4. Falk E. Why do plaques rupture? *Circulation* 1992;86:III30–III42.
5. Ohki T, Marin ML, Lyon RT, et al. Ex vivo human carotid artery bifurcation stenting: correlation of lesion characteristics with embolic potential. *J Vasc Surg* 1998;27:463–471.
6. Ohki T, Roubin GS, Veith FJ, et al. Efficacy of a filter device in the prevention of embolic events during carotid angioplasty and stenting: an ex vivo analysis. *J Vasc Surg* 1999;30:1034–1044.
7. Benichou H, Bergeron P. Carotid angioplasty and stenting: will periprocedural transcranial Doppler monitoring be important? *J Endovasc Surg* 1996;3:217–223.

8. Adami CA, Scuro A, Spinamano L, et al. Use of the Parodi anti-embolism system in carotid stenting: Italian trial results. *J Endovasc Ther* 2002;9:147–154.
9. Cremonesi A, Castriota F. Efficacy of a nitinol filter device in the prevention of embolic events during carotid interventions. *J Endovasc Ther* 2002;9:155–159.
10. Macdonald S, Venables GS, Cleveland TJ, et al. Protected carotid stenting: safety and efficacy of the MedNova NeuroShield filter. *J Vasc Surg* 2002;35:966-972.
11. Fields WS, Maslenikov V, Meyer JS, et al. Joint study of extracranial arterial occlusion. V. Progress report of prognosis following surgery or nonsurgical treatment for transient cerebral ischemic attacks and cervical carotid artery lesions. *JAMA* 1970;211:1993–2003.
12. Executive Committee for the Asymptomatic Carotid Atherosclerosis Study. Endarterectomy for asymptomatic carotid artery stenosis. *JAMA* 1995;273:1421–1428.
13. Barnett HJ, Plum F, Walton JN. Carotid endarterectomy—an expression of concern. *Stroke* 1984; 15:941–943.
14. Beneficial effect of carotid endarterectomy in symptomatic patients with high-grade carotid stenosis. North American Symptomatic Carotid Endarterectomy Trial Collaborators. *N Engl J Med* 1991;325: 445–453.
15. Randomised trial of endarterectomy for recently symptomatic carotid stenosis: final results of the MRC European Carotid Surgery Trial (ECST). *Lancet* 1998;351:1379–1387.
16. Mayberg MR, Wilson SE, Yatsu F, et al. Carotid endarterectomy and prevention of cerebral ischemia in symptomatic carotid stenosis. Veterans Affairs Cooperative Studies Program 309 Trialist Group. *JAMA* 1991;266:3289–3294.
17. Barnett HJ, Taylor DW, Eliasziw M, et al. Benefit of carotid endarterectomy in patients with symptomatic moderate or severe stenosis. *N Engl J Med* 1998;339:1415–1425.
18. Hobson RW, Weiss DG, Fields WS, et al. Efficacy of carotid endarterectomy for asymptomatic carotid stenosis. The Veterans Affairs Cooperative Study Group. *N Engl J Med* 1993;328:221–227.
19. Cronenwett JL, Birkmeyer JD. Carotid artery disease. In: *The Dartmouth atlas of vascular health care*. Chicago: AHA Press, 2000.
20. The NACPTAR Investigators. Update of the immediate angiographic results and in-hospital central nervous system complications of cerebral percutaneous transluminal angioplasty. *Circulation* 1995;92: 383.
21. The NACPTAR Investigators. Restenosis following cerebral percutaneous transluminal angioplasty. *Stroke* 1995;26:186.
22. Diethrich EB, Ndiaye M, Reid DB. Stenting in the carotid artery: initial experience in 110 patients. *J Endovasc Surg* 1996;3:42–62.
23. Diethrich EB. Indications for carotid artery stenting: a preview of the potential derived from early clinical experience. *J Endovasc Surg* 1996;3:132–139.
24. Mathur A, Roubin GS, Iyer SS, et al. Predictors of stroke complicating carotid artery stenting. *Circulation* 1998;97:1239–1245.
25. Roubin GS, New G, Iyer SS, et al. Immediate and late clinical outcomes of carotid artery stenting in patients with symptomatic and asymptomatic carotid artery stenosis: a 5-year prospective analysis. *Circulation* 2001;103:532–537.
26. Gomez C, Roubin G, Vitek J. Safety of carotid artery stenting in NASCET comparable patients. *Neurology* 1998;50:76A.
27. Brown MM. Carotid angioplasty and stenting: are they therapeutic alternatives? *Cerebrovasc Dis* 2001; 11(Suppl 1):112–118.
28. Endovascular versus surgical treatment in patients with carotid stenosis in the Carotid and Vertebral Artery Transluminal Angioplasty Study (CAVATAS): a randomised trial. *Lancet* 2001;357:1729–1737.
29. Alberts MJ, McCann R, Smith TP. Carotid atherosclerosis. *J Neurovasc Dis* 1997;11:228–234.
30. Naylor AR, Bolia A, Abbott RJ, et al. Randomized study of carotid angioplasty and stenting versus carotid endarterectomy: a stopped trial. *J Vasc Surg* 1998;28:326–334.
31. Veith FJ, Amor M, Ohki T, et al. Current status of carotid bifurcation angioplasty and stenting based on a consensus of opinion leaders. *J Vasc Surg* 2001;33:S111–S116.
32. Hobson RW, Goldstein JE, Jamil Z, et al. Carotid restenosis: operative and endovascular management. *J Vasc Surg* 1999;29:228–235.
33. Chakhtoura EY, Hobson RW, Goldstein J, et al. In-stent restenosis after carotid angioplasty-stenting: incidence and management. *J Vasc Surg* 2001;33:220–225.
34. Lattimer CR, Burnand KG. Recurrent carotid stenosis after carotid endarterectomy. *Br J Surg* 1997; 84:1206–1219.

35. Healy DA, Zierler RE, Nicholls SC, et al. Long-term follow-up and clinical outcome of carotid restenosis. *J Vasc Surg* 1989;10:662–668.
36. Treiman GS, Jenkins JM, Edwards WH Sr, et al. The evolving surgical management of recurrent carotid stenosis. *J Vasc Surg* 1992;16:354–362.
37. Yadav JS, Roubin GS, King P, Iyer S, Vitek J. Angioplasty and stenting for restenosis after carotid endarterectomy. Initial experience. *Stroke* 1996;27:2075–2079.
38. New G, Roubin GS, Iyer SS, et al. Safety, efficacy, and durability of carotid artery stenting for restenosis following carotid endarterectomy: a multicenter study. *J Endovasc Ther* 2000;7:345–352.
39. Hobson RW, Lal BK, Chakhtoura EY, et al. Carotid artery closure for endarterectomy does not influence results of angioplasty-stenting for restenosis. *J Vasc Surg* 2002;35:435–438.
40. Freedman B. Equipoise and the ethics of clinical research. *N Engl J Med* 1987;317:141–145.
41. Bettmann MA, Katzen BT, Whisnant J, et al. Carotid stenting and angioplasty: a statement for healthcare professionals from the Councils on Cardiovascular Radiology, Stroke, Cardio-Thoracic and Vascular Surgery, Epidemiology and Prevention, and Clinical Cardiology, American Heart Association. *Stroke* 1998;29:336–338.

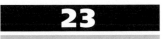

23

STATISTICAL AND EXPERIMENTAL DESIGN ISSUES IN THE EVALUATION OF CAROTID ARTERY STENTING

GEORGE HOWARD
BRENT J. SHELTON
VIRGINIA J. HOWARD

Carotid artery stenting (CAS) was developed in the 1980s and has been a rapidly expanding medical treatment for the treatment of advanced carotid atherosclerosis. Because carotid endarterectomy (CEA) has had many years to evolve, it is a well-perfected and generally accepted approach for the management of carotid atherosclerosis. Nevertheless, endarterectomy is a treatment with substantial morbidity and mortality, with perioperative stroke and death rates generally in the 3% to 6% range (1–4). Because of this considerable perioperative morbidity and mortality associated with endarterectomy, CAS has the possibility of not only being equivalent in risk to endarterectomy, but potentially superior. Being a new treatment, however, carotid stenting also has the possibility of being inferior to endarterectomy.

Numerous studies have been conducted to investigate the safety and efficacy of CAS. These studies have used different study designs, varying statements of the study hypotheses, and have varied substantially in statistical analysis approaches. The differences in the study design and approaches have led to differences in statistical methods and the interpretation of the study findings. In this chapter, we review alternative study designs and their associated statistical challenges and interpretations.

ISSUES IN THE ESTIMATION OF "RARE" EVENT RATES

For statistical purposes, and regardless of study design, perhaps the greatest challenge to the analysis of carotid stenting (and endarterectomy) is introduced by the great clinical success achieved by the operators placing the stents (and surgeons conducting endarterectomy), and the need to make very precise statements of the performance of the procedures. The most common endpoint in studies evaluating the success of CAS is the periprocedural stroke and death rate. Unfortunately for statistical evaluation, the event rate is very low (hopefully in the 2% to 4% range), and for stenting to be acceptable, event rates below very low thresholds (perhaps below 5%, and certainly below 8% to 10%) must be shown.

The most common approach to describe the anticipated magnitude of the variation between estimates of a parameter is to provide 95% confidence intervals for the parameter. For example, the estimated stroke and death rate could be estimated to be 3% with 95% confidence intervals from 1% to 5%. A slightly incorrect interpretation of these confidence limits is that there is a 95% chance that the true parameter is within the range defined by the confidence interval. The correct interpretation is that if we repeated the experiment a large number of times, and calculated confidence intervals in this manner, then 95% of the time these limits would include the true parameter. In the example, the 3% is a guess (or estimate) of the true and unknown parameter (the event rate), but (again, only slightly incorrectly) there is a 95% chance that the true parameter is between 1% and 5%. From this example, the *guess* of the true event rate is a low 3% rate, but we would be confident that the true parameter is not higher than 5%.

Suppose that a study is designed to establish the performance of endovascular treatment ("stenting") in asymptomatic patients. In this case, one could *a priori* hypothesize that the anticipated event rate would be 3% (arbitrarily chosen, but representative), and that one would not support stenting if the event rate were 5% or higher. This 2% difference between the expected rate (3%) and the upper boundary of acceptability (5%) is a very narrow range over which to define the success or failure of stenting. In this case, an estimate of a 3% event rate, with 95% confidence intervals from 1% to 5%, provides some assurance that stenting can be performed safely, and as such, the study is of considerable value. However, an alternative study with the same 3% event rate but with 95% confidence intervals from 0% to 10% is of little value. This is because the range is so wide it includes values that would be "acceptable" as well as values that would be considered "unacceptable." As such, the estimated event rate from a study is meaningless without reflecting on the *reliability* of the estimate as described by the 95% confidence intervals (or as described by some other statistical approach).

As described above, the anticipated event rate following CEA is low (say 3%), and for stenting to be considered successful, it must be established that it can be performed with an event rate below a rate only slightly higher than for endarterectomy, perhaps in the range of 5% to 8%. In this environment, substantial caution should be expressed in the interpretation of studies that report event rates but fail to report confidence limits (or some other measure of reliability of the estimates), as these studies have only marginal value. The literature, particularly abstract presentations at national meetings, is rich with relatively small studies that do provide some information but should be interpreted with substantial caution (5–10).

That the reliability of reported estimates is critical is demonstrated in Fig. 23-1, which

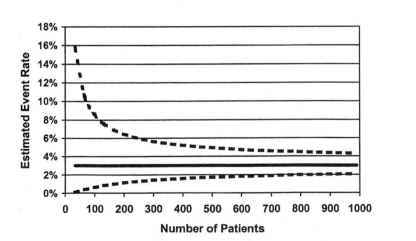

FIGURE 23-1. Estimated 95% confidence intervals (dashed lines) shown about an estimated 3% event rate (solid line) as a function of the study sample size.

shows the upper and lower bound of 95% confidence intervals at about an estimated event rate of 3% as a function of the sample size. Although the 3% event rate was arbitrarily chosen to display the width of the confidence intervals, this figure demonstrates that a large sample size is required to make definitive statements. For example, in studies with as many as 200 subjects, if the estimated event rate is 3% then the 95% confidence intervals are from 1.5% to 6.5%, a range that may be considered sufficiently wide to influence the interpretation of the study. That is, if the true event rate were 1.5%, then stenting would be accepted as successful, but if the true event rate were 6.5%, it would be rejected as too high risk. In this case, we cannot be confident which of these situations is true. As the sample size increases beyond 500 patients in the series, then in the case where the estimated event rate is 3%, the upper 95% confidence interval is finally below 5%. However, substantially increasing the sample size to 1,000 patients (very rare in stenting series), the 95% confidence interval at about an estimated 3% event rate is still only 2.0% to 4.3%. As such, the very low event rate and the need to state estimated event rates with substantial precision requires very large series, and although smaller series do provide important information, they should be interpreted with substantial caution.

EXPERIMENTAL DESIGN AND INTERPRETATION OF OUTCOMES

In general, two types of studies have been employed to assess the performance of CAS: (a) registries, and (b) randomized clinical trials. Both approaches offer important, but different, information regarding the safety and efficacy of CAS. A registry is a series of patients, all treated by CAS, whereas the randomized clinical trial takes groups of patients and randomly assigns them to stenting versus alternative treatments.

For both the registry and randomized approach, well-designed studies should have clearly defined eligibility and outcome criteria. Importantly, however, the criteria for inclusion in the clinical study and the definitions of endpoints can differ substantially between series, and substantial caution should be taken in making comparisons between series. For example, in a prospective report of the 5-year experience from a single group of stent operators, the perioperative stroke and death rate in 287 asymptomatic patients was 6.3% (11), which on the surface is somewhat above the "event" rate from asymptomatic endarterectomy studies such as 2.3% rate quoted in the Asymptomatic Carotid Atherosclerosis Study (ACAS) (1). On the surface, this difference gives rise to concerns that stenting may not be as safe as the better-established endarterectomy. However, high-risk asymptomatic patients are included in the stent study, whereas they were excluded from ACAS, resulting in studies with virtually no or little overlap in patient populations. As such, the standard to compare these results is, at best, confounded.

Importantly, somewhat subtle differences in the patient populations between series can underlie observed differences in event rates, and as such, substantial caution should be expressed in comparing event rates from series of patients receiving stents in registry studies to historic results among patients receiving endarterectomy. This gives rise to the great shortcoming of registries—that absent clear clinical success (for example, a large series with the upper confidence interval of the event rate below 1% or 2%) or clear clinical failure (for example, a large series with a lower confidence limit above 8% to 10%), it is very difficult to interpret the results of a registry of stent patients. Unfortunately, the majority of registries should be expected to have event rates that fall into the "middle ground" between success and failure, making the selection of criteria to define success problematic. The lack of a control population similar to the stent patients in every way but the delivery of stent (the great shortcoming of registries) is exactly the great strength of the randomized clinical trial approach, where randomization is very likely to ensure that the only difference between the stent and endarterectomy series is the procedure itself.

There are also several strengths of a registry approach, however. Perhaps the greatest is that all patients in the study receive a stent, providing the largest possible sample size of patients treated with stents, and thereby providing the most precise assessment (i.e., smallest 95% confidence intervals on event rates) of stent performance. In addition, randomization is not possible in selected populations, for example, those with a high bifurcation that places them at high risk for endarterectomy but not for placement of a stent. Finally, because the randomization process does not have to be discussed during the informed consent process, recruitment to a registry may be easier than recruitment to a randomized trial.

A topic that is closely related to trial design is the potential impact of government versus industry sponsorship of studies. Clearly, there are many well-designed and executed trials with industry, as well as governmental, sponsorship. However, there is also a literature that has documented that industry-sponsored research may potentially provide an assessment of the differences in treatments that is biased in favor of the industry-supported treatment, a bias that is not as pronounced in government-supported studies (12–14). For example, Djulbegovic et al. (13) evaluated trials contrasting alternative treatments for multiple myeloma. The impact of the source of the sponsorship nearly reached statistical significance ($p = 0.06$), with the 35 studies supported by industry having a higher quality score than the 95 government-sponsored studies (quality score of 2.9 ± 1.3 versus 2.4 ± 0.8; $p = 0.06$). However, there was a highly significant ($p = 0.004$) difference in the likelihood of finding that the "new" treatment was superior with 74% of the industry-sponsored studies showing benefit for the new therapy, whereas only 47% of those sponsored by government showed a benefit for the new therapy, suggesting a bias in the reporting of the results (13). Although the report suggested that industry-sponsored studies were more likely to indicate the superiority of the "new" treatment because of study design features that favored the new treatment, it did not fully investigate whether the industry studies were more likely to favor the "new" treatment because they had a sufficient sample size to provide adequate power to detect a difference that truly existed (i.e., were higher quality studies because they had a sufficient sample size to "see" differences).

Conversely, very subtle choices in trial design could be instituted that would tend to benefit the "new" treatment. In the case of CAS, the eligibility criteria could be set to admit a larger proportion of patients, such as endarterectomy redos, who are at high risk for surgical intervention but not for endovascular intervention. In addition, the definition of endpoints could be selected to include myocardial infarctions in addition to stroke and death endpoints, with myocardial infarctions included because they are potentially more likely to occur in the endarterectomy-treated group than among those with stents. There are numerous other approaches that can be unconsciously used to offer a slight benefit to the stent treatment group, and it is very unlikely that the scientific report would describe the decision-making process in sufficient detail to allow the objective detection of these subtle actions. Importantly, this concern is not raising an issue regarding the unethical decision making by the investigators or industry sponsors, but rather the cumulative effect of small subtle decisions that benefit one treatment group.

DIFFERENCE VERSUS EQUIVALENCY RANDOMIZED TRIALS

Within the conduct of a randomized trial, there are two frequently employed formats for the study hypothesis that are intended to answer different, but closely related, questions.

Suppose that the comparison between the treatment groups will be made on the basis of the proportion of study participants having reached an endpoint in the endarterectomy group (p_{CEA}) and in the stent group (p_{CAS}). The "traditional" statement hypothesis test is to assume the null hypothesis of no difference between the treatment groups (H_0: p_{CEA} = p_{CAS}), as compared to the alternative hypothesis that the two treatment groups are not equal (H_A: $p_{CEA} \neq p_{CAS}$). The one-to-one relationship between hypothesis testing and 95% confidence intervals permits a visual representation of the three possible outcomes of a "traditional" hypothesis test (see Fig. 23-2A). The difference between the two treatments groups can be estimated by the difference in the proportions of patients with events (i.e., $p_{CAS} - p_{CEA}$); note that testing if this difference is equal to zero is equivalent to testing if the event rates in the two groups are equal. This difference can be estimated with two-sided 95% confidence intervals as shown in Fig. 23-2A, with three possible outcomes. First, if the lower boundary of the 95% confidence interval does not include zero (top panel), the associated statistical test will reject the null hypothesis that the two groups are equal, and the study will conclude that the new treatment (stenting) is superior at the α = 0.05 level. If the 95% confidence intervals include zero (middle panel), the associated statistical test will be unable to reject the null hypothesis of no difference between the two groups. Finally, if the upper boundary of the 95% confidence interval does not include zero (lower panel), the associated statistical test will conclude that the null hypothesis should be rejected, and the study will conclude that the old treatment (endarterectomy) is superior.

The advantage of the "traditional" approach to the formation of the hypothesis test is if the null hypothesis is rejected, the investigators can definitively declare that there is evidence that the two treatments differ in event rates. The great shortcoming of the "traditional" approach is that if the null hypothesis is not rejected, all that can be concluded is "there is no evidence in these data that the two treatment groups have a different event rate." That is, in this case, the null hypothesis is *not* accepted, and it is inappropriate to state that "there is no difference between the groups"; rather, it is appropriate to state only that there is not evidence of a difference. This distinction, which to some investigators appears to be a relatively small difference in interpretation, is in fact substantially different in the appropriate interpretation of results. Frequently, investigators confuse this condition and very inappropriately conclude that when there is not evidence to reject the null hypothesis, then it has been proven that the event rates in the two groups are equal. This is quite wrong; all that has been proven is that there is not sufficient evidence to show which treatment is superior.

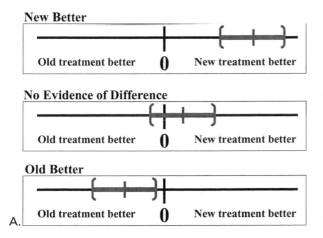

FIGURE 23-2. A: possible outcomes from a "traditional" hypothesis approach. Outcomes are shown on a scale centered at zero (0). Differences to the left of the scale indicate the old treatment is superior, whereas differences to right indicate the new treatment is superior. Shown on the scale is a hypothetical estimated difference between treatment groups (*shown by the gray vertical bar*) and hypothetical 95% two-sided confidence intervals (*shown by gray parentheses and horizontal bar*).

(Continues)

However, showing that the event rates in the two groups are equal in risk is sometimes the entire reason for performing a study. Specifically in the case of CAS, it could be argued that the endovascular approach is less invasive and costly than endarterectomy, and as such, if it can be shown that the endovascular approach is at least as good as endarterectomy, then this could be considered sufficient evidence for a recommendation for the use of the endovascular technique. Blackwelder (15) led the charge to address this challenge by proposing "equivalency" designs, a design which, in his words, is intended to "prove the null hypothesis" that two treatments are equal. The fundamental concept of an equivalency study is motivated by the observation that although you can accept the alternative hypothesis, you can only fail to reject the null hypothesis. In light of this observation, Blackwelder proposed to state the null hypothesis in terms of a difference or "effect" between the two groups, specifically that the old treatment (endarterectomy in this case) is better than the new treatment (endovascular techniques in this case), and the alternative hypothesis such that the two treatments are equal ("no effect") or that the new treatment is better. By specifying the null hypothesis in this format, in the case where the null hypothesis is rejected (and the alternative hypothesis accepted), then the researcher will be actively concluding that the two groups are equal (or the new treatment is better).

Mathematically, the null hypothesis of an equivalency study is (H_0: $p_{CEA} + \delta < p_{CAS}$), where δ is a small increment or "pad" to determine the neighborhood about zero (or no difference) that is to be considered as "not different." For example, if δ is 0.02 (2%), then this would be equivalent to assuming that if the event rate between the treatments (CEA versus CAS) did not differ by more than 2%, then they would be considered "equivalent." The alternative hypothesis in the equivalence design is (H_A: $p_{CEA} + \delta \geq p_{CAS}$). Importantly, if the null hypothesis that the old treatment is better (i.e., that endarterectomy has an event rate that is at least δ less than endovascular therapy) is rejected, then it can be definitively stated that the endovascular therapy is "as good or better" than endarterectomy. Note that although most traditional hypothesis testing is performed in the "two-sided" format (i.e., testing if either treatment is superior), most equivalency testing is performed in a "one-sided" format (i.e., testing the "unidirectional" hypothesis of whether the new treatment is as good or better than the old treatment).

The interpretation of equivalency testing can also be described by the analogous 95% confidence intervals. Figure 23-2B shows the spectrum of possible differences between the

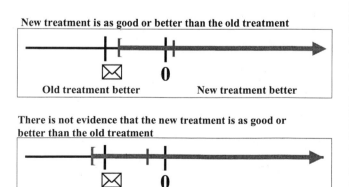

FIGURE 23-2. B: Possible outcomes from an "equivalence" hypothesis approach. Outcomes are shown on a scale centered at zero (0). Also shown on the scale is the difference permitted to where the two treatments can still be declared as equivalent (δ). Differences to the left of the scale indicate that the old treatment is superior, whereas differences to right indicate that the new treatment is superior. Shown on the scale is a hypothetical estimated difference between treatment groups (*shown by the gray vertical bar*) and hypothetical 95% one-sided confidence intervals (*shown by gray left bracket and horizontal bar*).

proportions of events in the two treatments, with δ slightly below zero (in the direction of the old treatment being superior) and showing the region where the two treatments are considered as having "equal" incidence of events. The one-sided 95% confidence interval (corresponding to the one-sided hypothesis) reflects the hypothesis that focuses on the difference in the proportion of patients with events. As shown by this figure, there are only two possible outcomes of equivalency testing: (a) shown in the top panel, if the lower limit of the 95% confidence interval does not include δ, then the hypothesis test will conclude that there is evidence that the new treatment (endovascular treatment) is "as good or better" than the old treatment (endarterectomy), or (b) as shown in the bottom panel, if the lower limit of the 95% confidence interval includes δ, then the hypothesis test will conclude that there is not evidence in these data that the new treatment is as good or better than the old treatment. Like the traditional hypothesis, the null hypothesis (corresponding to the second of the outcomes) is not accepted, it is just not rejected, and as such, failure to reject the equivalency analysis null hypothesis should not be interpreted as evidence that the new treatment is inferior—only that there is not evidence that it is equal or superior to the new treatment.

There is the scientific equivalent of an "urban legend" that equivalency studies require a smaller sample size than the traditional difference approach. Although there is a minor potential reduction in sample size associated with the one-sided hypothesis normally employed in an equivalency analysis (as compared to the two-sided hypothesis frequently used in traditional hypotheses), the design parameters of the experiments can imply that the sample size for an equivalency study can be larger, smaller, or similar to that of the traditional approach. Specifically, the sample size of a traditional difference hypothesis is largely determined by the difference in the proportion of events between the treatments required to be "clinically significant." For example, a much larger sample size is required to detect a 3% difference in treatment effects than a 5% difference in treatment effects. Likewise, the sample size of an equivalency study is largely determined by the magnitude of δ, where the sample size required will be substantially larger if a difference smaller than 3% is required to consider treatments "the same," as compared to the sample size if differences as large as 5% can be considered "the same." As such, the sample size for one approach can be greater or less than the other depending on the magnitude of the related parameters that define what a "clinically significant" difference is and what magnitude of difference is so small such that it can be considered "the same."

Obviously, if there were a clearly better way to formulate hypotheses in statistical testing, then there would not be two alternative analysis designs frequently employed in the assessment of endovascular therapy. The advantages of the traditional test are: (a) when the null hypothesis is rejected, there is the ability to definitively state that one of the treatments is superior to the other, and (b) there is the opportunity to show that the new treatment is superior to the old, *or* that the old treatment is superior to the new. The impact of the latter point is that in the case of the comparison of carotid stenting and endarterectomy, should endarterectomy actually be the superior treatment, then the traditional difference approach would allow a definitive statement that this is the case, as compared to the much weaker conclusion of "there is not evidence in these data that endovascular treatment is as good or better than endarterectomy" that would result from the equivalence approach. Conversely, the advantage of the equivalence approach is that in the case where there is no difference between the treatments, the equivalence approach permits a definitive statement, as compared to the much weaker conclusion of "there is not evidence in these data that the treatments differ." In addition to this substantial strength, the equivalence approach has the notable shortcoming of having to "defend" the choice of δ. That is, if the null hypothesis is rejected and the alternative hypothesis accepted, the statement that "there is evidence that the new treatment is as good or better" can be made, but it must come with the proviso that 'as good' is defined as "not more than X% (δ) worse."

ALTERNATIVE APPROACHES FOR STATISTICAL TESTING

There have been two commonly used approaches to the testing of differences between treatment groups in the assessment of endovascular techniques: (a) estimation of event rate, and (b) "survival" or time-to-event analysis. In studies with very short follow-up, such as those examining in-hospital or 30-day events [for example, MacDonald et al. (16)], it is relatively unlikely that the outcome of study participants will be unknown or that participants will be withdrawn from the study for reasons unrelated to the study outcome (e.g., cancer or accidental deaths). In this case, reporting the proportion of patients with events is a reasonable approach to analysis. However, with an increasing length of follow-up, a larger number of patients will be lost to follow-up or withdrawn from the study for other medical causes (e.g., cancer or accidental deaths). Because participants have a variable length of follow-up, they have varying opportunities to have events, and there must be an accounting of the differences in the "exposure time" of the patients (17). Analyses that account for these varying opportunities experienced by patients are referred to as "survival" or "time-to-event" analyses, and the most frequent approaches are Kaplan-Meier curves and proportional hazards analysis. Although it is not inappropriate to use these time-to-event techniques for data that do not contain censored observations, the converse is not true. Studies where patients are followed for a variable length of time, but the results report proportion of patients with events, calculated by dividing the number of patients with events by the number of patients studied, should be interpreted with substantial skepticism because the proportion of patients with events will be systematically underestimated.

INTERIM ANALYSIS

Both for the safety of patients in the research studies and to ensure that results are promptly made available to the clinical community, it is important to monitor a study and stop at the earliest point that the conclusion regarding the study outcome can be made from the data. However, without appropriate statistical adjustments, even in the absence of a true difference between treatment groups, multiple tests for treatment differences will increase the likelihood of concluding that a difference exists (i.e., will increase α above 0.05). In simple terms, the more times you look for a difference, the more likely you are to find it (even if it does not truly exist).

Statistical methods have been developed to protect from falsely reporting a difference between treatment groups when one does not exist and still perform serial examinations of potential differences between treatment groups. Conceptually, these approaches allocate or "spend" the alpha of 0.05 across the multiple tests in a manner that the likelihood of declaring a significant difference between groups across the array of multiple tests remains at the 0.05 level. Commonly used stopping rules include O'Brien and Fleming (18) or Lan and DeMets (19) boundaries that "spend" little of the alpha early and keep the final test of significance at the end of the study near 0.05, Pocock boundaries that "spend" the significance evenly over all interim analyses (20), and Peto et.al. (21), which spends moderately at early examinations with an intermediate final test of significance. The choice between these alternative approaches is difficult, and somewhat arbitrary, and should be subject to external peer review and approval prior to study initiation.

Perhaps the most important aspect of awareness of these alternative approaches for "spending the alpha" is to be acutely aware of trials that could have terminated early without the *a priori* planning involved in one of the approaches described above. Regardless of whether the company or an independent Data and Safety Monitoring Board was responsible for an unplanned termination of a study, if a study is stopped without proper planning for the opportunity to stop the study prior to its planned termination, the likelihood of declaring a significant difference between treatments can be substantially unduly increased (that is, the significance can be substantially overstated). Unplanned assessments of efficacy and unplanned terminations of trials is a potential approach to inappropriately declaring differences between treatments.

CONCLUSIONS

There are not substantial unique statistical issues in approach and methods to assess the efficacy of endovascular therapies. However, several aspects of assessing the efficacy of CAS are particularly statistically challenging. First (and perhaps foremost) is that the general goal of carotid stent studies is to estimate a proportion of patients with "events" in the case where we anticipate that that proportion is quite small. Estimating such a small percentage with reasonable reliability implies that studies must have a substantial sample size. As a corollary of this observation, small studies assessing the efficacy of endovascular therapies lack reliability and should be interpreted with caution. Second, the confidence that can be drawn from a study is substantially affected by the study design. Although registries are logistically easier to conduct and do provide information, the results should be interpreted with substantial caution, as differences between populations raise concerns regarding the "reference" rate of events used to compare the observed event rate in the registry. Third, there are several approaches to the formulation of the hypothesis to be employed in a randomized trial assessment of efficacy, with the two most common approaches being the traditional difference formulation and the equivalence formulation. Both of these approaches have strengths and weaknesses, and the interpretation of results of a study must be carefully interpreted within the context of the approach taken to formulate the hypothesis. Finally, great caution should be taken to plan both the appropriate analysis and to plan for appropriate interim assessments of differences between treatment groups.

REFERENCES

1. Executive Committee for the Asymptomatic Carotid Atherosclerosis Study. Endarterectomy for asymptomatic carotid artery stenosis. *JAMA* 1995;273:1421–1428.
2. Barnett HJM, Taylor DW, Eliasziw M, et al. Benefit of carotid endarterectomy in patients with symptomatic moderate or severe stenosis. *N Engl J Med* 1998;339:1415–1425.
3. Rothwell PM, Slattery J, Warlow CP. A systematic review of the risks of stroke and death due to endarterectomy for symptomatic carotid stenosis. *Stroke* 1996;27:260–265.
4. Rothwell PM, Slattery J, Warlow CP. A systematic comparison of the risks of stroke and death due to carotid endarterectomy for asymptomatic and asymptomatic stenosis. *Stroke* 1996;27:266–269.
5. Sinclair L, Kenney C, Button A, et al. Complication rates after internal carotid stenting in high-risk symptomatic patients. *Stroke* 2002;33:345.
6. Malisch TW, North EA, Alberts MJ, el al. When is carotid stenting really necessary? Results of a conservative algorithm. *Stroke* 2002;33:348.

7. Becker U, Gahn G, Hallmeyer-Elgner S, et al. Clinical risk and silent ischemic lesions after unprotected percutaneous transluminal stent angioplasty of the internal carotid artery. *Stroke* 2002;33:413.
8. Ireland JK, Chaloupka JC, Weigele JB, et al. Potential utility of carotid stent assisted percutaneous transluminal angioplasty in the treatment of symptomatic carotid occlusive disease in patients with high neurological risk. *Stroke* 2003;34:308.
9. Gomez CR, Misra VK, Campbell MS, et al. Elective stenting of intracranial stenosis is a safe and durable procedure. *Stroke* 2003;34:307.
10. Qureshi AI, Boulos AS, Kim SH, et al. Carotid angioplasty and stent placement using the Filterwire[EX] for distal protection: an international multicenter study. *Stroke* 2003;34:307.
11. Roubin GS, New G, Iyer SS, et al. Immediate and late clinical outcomes of carotid artery stenting in patients with symptomatic and asymptomatic carotid artery stenosis: a 5-year prospective analysis. *Circulation* 2001;103:532–537.
12. Davidson RA. Sources of funding and outcome of clinical trials. *J Gen Intern Med* 1986;1:155–158.
13. Djulbegovic B, Lacevic M, Cantor A, et al. The uncertainty principle and industry-sponsored research. *Lancet* 2000;356:635–638.
14. Kjaergard LL, Als-Nielsen B. Association between competing interests and authors' conclusions: epidemiological study of randomized clinical trials published in BMJ. *Br Med J* 2002;325:249.
15. Blackwelder WC "Proving the null hypothesis" in clinical trials. *Control Clin Trials* 1982;3:345–353.
16. MacDonald S, Venables GS, Cleveland TJ, et al. Protected carotid stenting: safety and efficacy of the MedNova NeuroShield filter. *J Vasc Surg* 2002;35:966–972.
17. Hobson RW 2nd. Update on the Carotid Revascularization Endarterectomy versus Stenting Trial (CREST) protocol. *J Amer Coll Surg* 2002;194:S9–S14.
18. O'Brien PC, Fleming TR. A multiple testing procedure for clinical trials. *Biometrics* 1979;35:549–556.
19. Lan KKG, DeMets DL. Discrete sequential boundaries for clinical trials. *Biometrika* 1983;70:659–663.
20. Pocock SJ Group sequential methods in the design and analysis of clinical trials. *Biometrika* 1977;64:191–199.
21. Peto R, Pike MC, Armitage P, et al. Design and analysis of randomized clinical trials requiring prolonged observation of each patient. *Br J Cancer* 1976;34:586–612.

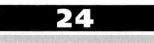

CLINICAL INVESTIGATIONS AND PROTOCOLS

CHRISTINA M. BRENNAN
PALLAVI KUMAR
GARY S. ROUBIN

Carotid artery stenting (CAS) is considered a minimally invasive technique for treating carotid artery disease, particularly in those patients at high risk from surgery. In patients with significant disease, where the degree of stenosis is greater than 70% to 80% for asymptomatic patients and greater than 50% for symptomatic patients, CAS is a viable alternative to carotid endarterectomy (CEA). Symptomatic patients are defined as those patients who have experienced a minor or major stroke, transient ischemic attack (TIA), or amaurosis fugax ipsilateral to the diseased carotid artery. To date, the Food and Drug Administration (FDA) has not approved stents or an Anti-Embolization device for use in CAS, and the procedure therefore remains under intense investigation. As such, CAS with the use of Anti-Embolization protection (i.e., filter and balloon occlusion devices) is typically carried out under Investigational Device Exemption (IDE) protocols approved by the FDA.

Carotid stenting may offer certain advantages to CEA in patients who are at increased risk for the surgical procedure. Specifically, those benefits include:

- Less invasive approach to treatment
- No anesthesia requirement
- Continuous neurological monitoring intraprocedurally as compared with CEA (performed under general anesthesia)
- Avoiding cervical dissection complications associated with CEA (such as cranial nerve injury, cervical wound hematoma)
- The ability to access anatomically or surgically inaccessible lesions
- Shorter hospital stay (typically 24 hours postprocedure)
- Minimization of embolization of particulate matter through the use of neuroprotective devices

SCREENING

I. Initial Screening

Patients are routinely admitted on an ambulatory basis for diagnostic brachiocephalic angiography and possible CAS. Initial screening of all patients is performed in order to determine their eligibility for the related clinical protocol. High surgical risk eligibility/inclusion criteria include the following categories: anatomical conditions, comorbid conditions (Class I), and comorbid conditions (Class II). Each category comprises specific criteria, and is defined below:

A. Anatomical High-risk Conditions—One Criterion Qualifies
- Surgically inaccessible lesions above C-2 or below the level of the clavicle
- Spinal immobility of the neck due to cervical arthritis or other cervical disorders
- Previous head/neck radiation therapy or surgery that included the area of stenosis or ipsilateral radical neck dissection for the treatment of cancer
- Restenosis after a previous or unsuccessful attempt of CEA
- Presence of a tracheostoma
- Presence of laryngeal palsy

B. Comorbid Conditions (Class I)—One Criterion Qualifies
- Congestive heart failure (Class III/IV)
- Unstable angina
- Requirement for staged and scheduled coronary artery bypass graft (CABG) or valve replacement procedures more than 30 days following the stent procedure
- Chronic obstructive pulmonary disease (COPD) with a forced expiratory volume (FEV) 1 less than 30%
- Left ventricular ejection fraction (LVEF) less than 30%
- Age 80 years or more (in recent IDE trials, this has been the single entry criterion)

C. Comorbid Conditions (Class II)—Two Criteria Qualify
- Age 75 years or more
- Recent myocardial infarction more than 72 hours and less than 30 days
- Two or more major diseased coronary arteries that require revascularization

D. General Inclusion Criteria—All Required for Eligibility
- Age 18 years or more
- Patients may be asymptomatic or symptomatic (minor or major stroke, TIA, or amaurosis fugax ipsilateral to the diseased carotid artery within 6 months prior to treatment)
- The target lesion is in the common carotid artery, internal carotid artery, or carotid bifurcation
- Patients taking warfarin may be included if the dosage is decreased to result in an international normalized ratio (INR) of 1.5 or less
- Patient is willing to comply with follow-up requirements as per study guidelines
- Patient has signed the informed consent
- Life expectancy of at least a year from the date of enrollment or procedure

E. General Exclusion Criteria—Patients Are Typically Excluded if Any of the Following Apply
- Total occlusion of the target carotid artery treatment site
- Myocardial infarction within 72 hours prior to the index procedure
- Stroke within 7 days prior to the procedure
- NIH Stroke Scale score more than or equal to 15 within 7 days prior to the procedure
- Patient has excessive peripheral vascular disease that precludes safe sheath insertion
- Patient has allergy or contraindication to aspirin (ASA), ticlopidine, clopidogrel, heparin, bivalirudin, nickel, titanium, or a sensitivity to contrast media that cannot be adequately premedicated
- Patient has a platelet count of less than 50,000 cells/mm^3 or a white blood cell count (WBC) of less than 3,000 cells/mm^3

- Patient is unwilling or unable to comply with procedural and postprocedural requirements
- Dementia or confusion that precludes thorough understanding of risks and benefits associated with angiography and intervention

II. Secondary Screening

A second screening phase is integrated during the CAS procedure. At the time of the prestenting angiography, patients will be assessed for angiographic and anatomical eligibility. Only patients meeting the angiographic inclusion criteria and in whom no exclusion criteria are present are typically treated using stenting.

- Vessels with less than 50% stenosis are generally not treated, as the disease may be treated medically
- Lesions showing a marked degree of tortuosity or calcification are also not appropriate for intervention, as catheter maneuvering and device delivery are hindered by these conditions

INFORMED CONSENT

Once eligibility has been determined, the background, benefits, and risks of the proposed procedures and any related research protocols are discussed in detail with the patient. The patient (or the patient's legal representative) must sign the hospital's Institutional Review Board (IRB) approved informed consent prior to participation in the procedure. Informed consent is mandatory and must be obtained from all patients prior to their participation in the study. Informed consent must be in accordance with 21CFR, Part 50, and the Declaration of Helsinki. A typical informed consent includes the following subsections:

A. Full name/title of the research protocol
B. Name of principal investigator conducting the trial
C. Purpose: This section describes the purpose of the study, specifically to determine the safety and effectiveness of a new experimental device in an experimental procedure called carotid stent-supported angioplasty. This section also discloses total enrollment for the trial.
D. Procedure: This section describes the requirements to be met by the patient in order to participate in the study. Included here are the preprocedural workup, the actual stenting procedure, and postprocedural requirements and follow-up for the course of the study.
E. Risks: A full outline of the risks associated with the study procedure is detailed to include procedure-related risks as well as stent-related risks. General risks are stratified into common, less common, and rare occurrences of complications. Less common risks include but are not limited to the need for repeat procedure or stroke. Rare risks include myocardial infarction or death.
   - Procedure-related risks
     Common: discomfort and hypotension
     Less common: bleeding, infection, and hematoma at groin access site
     Rare: dissection of arteries, nerve damage at the site of catheter insertion
   - Stent-related risks
     Less common: bleeding or dislodgement of plaque, resulting in transient ischemic

symptoms, such as difficulties with speech, visual disturbances, upper/lower extremity weakness. Dilatation of treatment balloons may result in bradycardia, possibly requiring temporary pacing and/or medication.

Rare: stroke, coma, or death. There is also the possibility that the narrowing or blockage of the treated artery may restenose.

- Protection device-related risks
  Common: hypotension
  Less common: embolization
  Rare: dissection, perforation, rupture of the carotid artery, abrupt vessel closure, injury to the carotid artery requiring emergency vascular surgery, seizures, difficulty, or inability to open, close, or remove the protective device.
- Contrast/drug-related risks
  Rare: contrast or procedure-related medication allergies. Occasionally, contrast or medications may be toxic and cause tissue or organ damage. Such damage could result in minor injury, or in rare cases, death.

F. Benefits: This section discusses the possible benefits of CAS. As there is no FDA approval for either the stents or protection devices, procedural success cannot be predicted with certainty. The use of local anesthesia to the groin access site, as opposed to the use of general anesthesia for surgical carotid intervention, is another benefit outlined here.

G. Alternatives: Alternative therapies for the treatment of carotid artery disease include CEA and medical therapy.

H. Confidentiality: If patients consent to participate in research protocols, all personal information will be maintained confidentially and will not be released without permission with the following exceptions. The patients' personal information may be shared to the extent necessary, with the IRB, the treating physician, other healthcare providers, the FDA, or as required by law. If this study is a multicenter trial, the patients' information may also be shared for the purposes of data analysis. On all study-related forms, patients will be identified only by initials and assigned patient numbers. Patients' medical records will be maintained at the hospital and will be subject to state and federal laws and regulations concerning the confidentiality and privacy of medical records.

I. Voluntary participation and withdrawal: This section discloses the voluntary nature of research protocols, and the right of the patient to withdraw from the study at any time. Refusal to participate or withdrawal from the study will not result in any loss of benefits to which patients are otherwise entitled.

J. Costs and payment: Patients are not paid to participate in these studies. Many of the diagnostic exams are considered routine and will be billed to patients' insurance providers.

K. Questions/contact information: This section discloses the contact information of the principal investigator(s) and/or a member of the IRB, to whom any procedure-related inquiries may be directed.

L. Statement of consent: The patient (or the patient's legal representative) must fully comprehend and sign the entire informed consent in order to participate in any research trials.

HEALTH INSURANCE PORTABILITY AND ACCOUNTABILITY ACT OF 1996 REGULATIONS

On April 14, 2003, the standards of privacy for individuals' health information in the United States took effect. The entities covered under the Health Insurance Portability and

Accountability Act of 1996 (HIPAA), which include health plans, health care clearinghouses, and health care providers, are now subject to the protectional provisions set forth by the Department of Health and Human Services. These provisions place limits on the use of personal medical information and require written consent by the individual to allow use of health information for purposes other than health care. As carotid stenting is performed primarily under research protocols, and patient information is routinely submitted to various third parties for non-health care-related purposes, obtaining consent under the guidelines of the HIPAA regulations is essential.

PREPROCEDURE

The following baseline testing must be performed for all patients prior to the index procedure (Table 24-1).

A. Informed consent: Consent must be obtained from the patient or the patient's legal representative
B. Baseline head computed tomography (CT)/magnetic resonance imaging (MRI): A CT scan or MRI scan should be performed within 30 days prior to the procedure
C. Baseline carotid duplex ultrasound scan: A carotid duplex scan should be performed within 30 days prior to the procedure
D. History/physical: Here, the data are documented that the patient meets screening criteria and does not have any exclusion criteria
E. Baseline neurological assessment: A neurological assessment administered by a neurologist or neurosurgeon who is certified in the administration of the National Institute of Health Stroke Scale (NIHSS) should be performed within 7 days prior to the procedure
F. Laboratory tests
  ■ A complete blood count (CBC) with differential for patients who are taking ticlopidine, platelet count, hemoglobin, hematocrit, and electrolytes should be performed within 7 days prior to procedure.

TABLE 24-1. PREPROCEDURE TESTING

	Preprocedure		
	Within 30 Days	Within 7 Days	Within 24 Hours
Informed consent	✓		
History/physical exam		✓	
Neurological assessment		✓	
Ultrasound	✓		
CT/MRI	✓		
Laboratory tests			
CBC/differential[a]		✓	
Electrolytes		✓	
CK			✓
CK-MB			✓
PT, PTT, INR			✓
Pregnancy test			✓
EKG			✓

[a] CBC with differential required for patients on ticlopidine.
CT, computed tomography; MRI, magnetic resonance imaging; CBC, complete blood count; CK, creatine kinase, CK-MB, creatine-kinase, MB fraction; PT, prothrombin; PTT, partial thromboplastin time; INR, international normalized ratio; EKG, electrocardiogram.

- Creatine kinase (CK), creatine kinase-MB fraction (CK-MB), prothrombin (PT), partial thromboplastin time (PTT), and INR levels should be collected within 24 hours of the index procedure.
- A pregnancy test is required for female patients of child-bearing potential

A. Electrocardiogram: A 12 lead electrocardiogram (EKG) should be obtained within 24 hours of the index procedure.

PREPROCEDURE MEDICATIONS

- Aspirin: acetylsalicylic acid (ASA; 325 mg twice daily) should be given for at least 72 hours prior to the procedure. If ASA is administered on the day of the procedure, an enteric, noncoated formulation is required (Table 24-2).
- Clopidogrel (Plavix): The patient should have a total dose of 450 mg of clopidogrel prior to the stenting procedure. If the patient is already on a 5-day course of clopidogrel, a loading dose is not required. If clopidogrel is contraindicated, the patient should receive ticlopidine (total dose of 1,000 mg) instead. If the patient is already on ticlopidine therapy (more than 2 days), a loading dose is not required.

PERIPROCEDURAL MEDICATIONS

- The use of medications with potential sedative effects (Fentanyl, Versed, Valium) should be avoided prior to and during the procedure. These medications can impact the ability to assess peri-procedural and post-procedural changes in neurological status.

TABLE 24-2. CONCOMITANT MEDICATIONS

Medication	Preprocedure	Procedure	Postprocedure (30 Days)	Postprocedure (More Than 30 Days)
Aspirin	325 mg bid, starting 3 days prior to procedure if possible	650 mg	325 mg qd	325 mg qd indefinitely
Clopidogrel	75 mg (starting 5 days prior to procedure)	75 mg[a]	75 mg[b]	
Ticlopidine	250 mg bid	250 mg bid[c]	250 mg[d]	
Heparin		PRN, to maintain ACT at greater than 250 sec		
Bivalirudin		PRN, to maintain ACT at greater than 250 sec		

[a] Loading dose of 450 mg required if 5-day course of clopidogrel was not administered.
[b] Patients with previous radiation to the neck should be maintained on clopidogrel 75 mg qd for 6–12 months.
[c] Loading dose of 1,000 mg required if 5-day course of ticlopidine was not administered.
[d] Patients with previous radiation to the neck should be maintained on ticlopidine 250 mg qd for 6–12 months.
bid, twice daily; qd, every day; PRN, as necessary; ACT, activated clotting time.

TABLE 24-3. POSTPROCEDURE TESTING

	Postprocedure
	Time Frame
Physical exam	Physical exam must be performed within 24 hrs following the procedure
Neurological assessment	Postprocedure neurological assessment should be performed by a neurologist or neurosurgeon within 24 hrs following the intervention, or earlier in the case of a change in the patient's clinical status
Ultrasound	Carotid duplex ultrasound within 24 hrs following the procedure
CT/MRI	CT/MRI required if there is a change in patient's neurological status
CBC/differential[a]	CBC within 24 hrs following the procedure
Electrolytes	Electrolytes within 24 hrs following the procedure
CK, CK-MB	CK, CK-MB to be performed at 8–12 hrs, 12–16 hrs, and 16–24 hrs (or hospital discharge) following the procedure. CK-MB is required only if the CK value is two times the upper limits of normal as defined by hospital laboratory
EKG	Conduct a 12-lead EKG at any time following the procedure

[a] CBC with differential required for patients on ticlopidine.
CT, computed tomography, MRI, magnetic resonance imaging; CBC, complete blood count; CK, creatine kinase; CK-MB, creatine kinase-MB fraction; EKG, electrocardiogram.

■ Heparin or Bivalirudin: should be given intravenously after insertion of sheath. The dosing should be sufficient to maintain the activated clotting time (ACT) at greater than 250 seconds.

POSTPROCEDURE MEDICATIONS

All patients should receive 325 mg ASA indefinitely as well as either clopidogrel (75 mg every day) or ticlopidine (for those patients intolerant to clopidogrel) for a minimum of 4 weeks following the procedure. Coumadin should be managed to ensure an INR of less than 1.7 prior to procedure and may be reinstituted postprocedure.

FOLLOW-UP ASSESSMENTS

Follow-up visits should be conducted at 1 month, 6 months, 12 months, and yearly thereafter at the physician's discretion. The primary concerns during the follow-up period include close monitoring of stent positioning, restenosis, and neurological changes (Table 24-3). Meticulous records should be maintained throughout the follow-up period, as well as during the baseline hospital course. Follow-ups include a clinical evaluation, neurological assessment, a carotid duplex ultrasound, review of antiplatelet therapy, and EKG. In addition, an assessment of any adverse events occurring from last to current contact points should be recorded at each follow-up visit. The table below is a summary of the recommended follow-up assessments (Table 24-4).

NEUROLOGICAL ASSESSMENT

Neurological assessment should be administered by a neurologist or neurosurgeon, other than the treating interventionalist. This physician should be certified in the administration

TABLE 24-4. FOLLOW-UP TESTING

	Follow-up			
	1 mo	6 mo	12 mo	Annually
Physical exam	✓	✓	✓	✓
Neurological assessment	✓	✓	✓	✓
Ultrasound	✓	✓	✓	✓
CT/MRI				
EKG				✓

CT, computed tomography; MRI, magnetic resonance imaging; EKG, electrocardiogram.

of the NIHSS. The assessment typically includes the NIHSS, the Modified Barthel Scale (MBI), the Modified Rankin Scale (MRS), and the Glasgow Outcome Scale (GOS). Neurological assessments should be performed preprocedure, periprocedure, and postprocedure.

The preprocedure or baseline neurological assessment should be performed within 7 days prior to the intervention, preferably within 24 hours of the procedure. Similarly, the postprocedure neurological assessment should be performed by a neurologist or neurosurgeon within 24 hours following the intervention, or earlier in the case of a change in the patient's clinical status. It is recommended that the same neurologist or neurosurgeon perform both preprocedure and postprocedure assessments in order to ensure clinical consistency in patient evaluation.

A neurologist, neurosurgeon, or surrogate must be present in order to monitor the neurological status of the patient periprocedurally. The treating interventionalist may serve as the surrogate, concurrently performing the procedural neurological evaluation throughout the interventional procedure. Nurses and technicians can also serve as surrogates if a neurologist or neurosurgeon has trained them in administering the required examinations. A recommended method used for periprocedural neurological assessment involves placing a rubber squeeze toy with an audible squeaker in the patient's hand contralateral to the target lesion. The patient will be asked to squeeze the toy at specific times corresponding to completion of various steps of the procedure. Those time points are typically during deployment of the embolic protection device, prestent balloon dilatation, stent deployment, poststent balloon dilatation, and following removal of the embolic protection device.

Figure 24-1 (see below) represents a sample NIHSS. The neurologist or neurosurgeon should administer the Stroke Scale items in the order in which they are listed. The following are instructions provided by the NIH regarding scoring of patients across all categories.

NATIONAL INSTITUTES OF HEALTH STROKE SCALE

1a–Level of Consciousness (LOC): The investigator must choose a response, even if a full evaluation is prevented by such obstacles as an endotracheal tube, language barrier, or orotracheal trauma/bandages. A three is scored only if the patient makes no movement (other than reflexive posturing) in response to noxious stimulation.

1b–LOC questions: The patient is asked the month and his/her age. The answer must be correct; there is no partial credit for being close. Aphasic and stuporous patients who do not comprehend the questions will score two. Patients unable to speak because of endotracheal intubation, orotracheal trauma, sever dysarthria from any cause, language barrier, or any other problem not secondary to aphasia are given a score of one. It is important that

Patient Name:_____

NIH Stroke Scale

Date of evaluation

☐☐ ☐☐ ☐☐
m m   d d   y y

Scale Definitions

Level of consciousness
(LOC)

☐

0= Alert, keenly responsive: 1= Drowsy; arousable by minor stimulation to obey, answer, or respond: 2= Stuporous; requires repeated stimulation to attend, or is obtunded and requires strong or painful stimulation to make movements (not stereotype). 3= Coma, responds only with reflex motor or autonomic effects or totally unresponsive, flaccid araflexic

LOC questions

☐

0= Answers both questions correctly. 1= Answers one question correctly. 2= Answers neither question correctly. 9= Untestable

LOC commands

☐

0= Performs both tasks correctly, 1= Performs one task correctly. 2= Performs neither task correctly

Best Gaze

☐

0= Normal; 1= Partial gaze palsy. 2= Forced deviation, or total gazed paresis is not overcome by the oculocephatic maneuver

Visual

☐

0= No visual loss: 1= Partial hemianopia: 2=Complete hemianopia: 3=Bilateral hemianopia (blind including cortical blindness): 9= Untestable

Facial Palsy

☐

0= Normal facial movement; 1= Minor paresis (flattened nasolabial fold, asymmetry on smiling); 2= Partial paresis (total or near total paralysis of lower face); 3= Complete paresis (absence of facial movement in upper and lower face)

L arm motor

☐

R arm motor

☐

Scoring for Arms and Legs: 0= No drift: 1= Drift: 2= Some effort against gravity: 3= No effort against gravity, limb falls; 4= No movement: 9= Untestable

L leg motor

☐

Amputation, joint fusion

Explanation_____(L) arm: (R) arm___   (L) leg_____ (R) leg_____

R leg motor

☐

Limb ataxia

☐

0= Absent; 1= Present unilaterally in either arm or leg; 2= Present unilaterally in arm and leg or bilaterally; 3= Untestable

Sensory

☐

0= Normal, no sensory loss; 1= Partial loss; patient feels pinprick is less sharp or is dull on the affected side; or there is a loss of superficial pain with pinprick but patient is aware he/she being touched; 2= Dense loss. Patient is not aware of being touched

Best language

☐

0= No aphasia; normal, 1= Mild to moderate aphasia; 2= Severe aphasia; 3= Mute

Dysarthria

☐

0= Normal articulation; 1= Mild to moderate dysarthria; 2= Near unintelligible or worse; 9= Untestable

Extinction and inattention

☐

0= No neglect (no flexion after 5 seconds); 1= Partial neglect; 2= Complete neglect

R distal motor function

☐

0= Normal; 1= At least some extension after 5 seconds, but not fully extended. Any movement in the fingers which is not a response to a command is not scored; 2= No voluntary extension after 5 seconds. Movement of the fingers at another time is not scored

L distal motor function

☐

Total

☐

Other neurological factors **not** affecting NIH Scores: _____

_____

_____   _____
Evaluator's Name   Evaluator's Signature   Date

FIGURE 24-1. Sample National Institutes of Health Stroke Scale (NIHSS) (adapted from www.nih.gov).

only the initial answer be graded and that the examiner not "help" the patient with verbal or nonverbal cues.

1c–LOC commands: The patient is asked to open and close the eyes and then to grip and release the nonparetic hand. Substitute another one-step command if the hands cannot be used. Credit is given if an unequivocal attempt is made but not completed because of weakness. If the patient does not respond to command, the task should be demonstrated to them (pantomime) and the result scored (i.e., follows none, one, or two commands). Patients with trauma, amputation, or other physical impediments should be given suitable one-step commands. Only the first attempt is scored.

2–Best gaze: Only horizontal eye movements will be tested. Voluntary or reflexive (oculocephalic) eye movements will be scored but caloric testing is not done. If the patient has a conjugate deviation of the eyes that can be overcome by voluntary or reflexive activity, the score will be one. If a patient has an isolated peripheral nerve paresis [cranial nerve (CN) III, IV, or VI], score a one. Gaze is testable in all aphasic patients. Patients with ocular trauma, bandages, preexisting blindness, or other disorder of visual acuity or fields should be tested with reflexive movements and a choice made by the investigator. Establishing eye contact and then moving about the patient from side to side will occasionally clarify the presence of a partial gaze palsy.

3–Visual: Visual fields (upper and lower quadrants) are tested by confrontation, using finger counting, or visual threat as appropriate. Patient must be encouraged, but if patient looks at the side of the moving fingers appropriately, this can be scored as normal. If there is unilateral blindness or enucleation, visual fields in the remaining eye are scored. Score one only if a clear-cut asymmetry, including quadrantanopia, is found. If the patient is blind from any cause, score three. Double simultaneous stimulation is performed at this point. If there is extinction, the patient receives a one, and the results are used to answer question 11.

4–Facial palsy: Ask or use pantomime to encourage the patient to show teeth or raise eyebrows and close eyes. Score symmetry of grimace in response to noxious stimuli in the poorly responsive or noncomprehending patient. If facial trauma/bandages, orotracheal tube, tape, or other physical barrier obscures the face, these should be removed to the extent possible.

5 and 6–Motor arm and leg: The limb is placed in the appropriate position: extend the arms (palms down) 90 degrees (if sitting) or 45 degrees (if supine) and the leg 30 degrees (always tested supine). Drift is scored if the arm falls before 10 seconds or the leg before 5 seconds. The aphasic patient is encouraged using urgency in the voice and pantomime but not noxious stimulation. Each limb is tested in turn, beginning with the nonparetic arm. Only in the case of amputation or joint fusion at the shoulder or hip may the score be "nine" and the examiner must clearly write the explanation for scoring as a "nine."

7–Limb ataxia: This item is aimed at finding evidence of a unilateral cerebellar lesion. Test with eyes open. In case of visual defect, insure testing is done in intact visual field. The finger-nose-finger and heel-shin tests are performed on both sides, and ataxia is scored only if present out of proportion to weakness. Ataxia is absent in the patient who cannot understand or is paralyzed. Only in the case of amputation or joint fusion may the item be scored "nine," and the examiner must clearly write the explanation for not scoring. In case of blindness, test by touching nose from extended arm position.

8–Sensory: Sensation or grimace to pin prick when tested or withdrawal from noxious stimulus in the obtunded or aphasic patient. Only sensory loss attributed to stroke is scored as abnormal and the examiner should test as many body areas [arms (not hands), legs, trunk, face] as needed to accurately check for hemisensory loss. A score of two, "severe or total," should be given only when a severe or total loss of sensation can be clearly demonstrated. Stuporous and aphasic patients will therefore probably score one or zero. The patient with brain stem stroke who has bilateral loss of sensation is scored two. If the patient does not respond and is quadriplegic score two. Patients in coma (item 1a = three) are arbitrarily given a two on this item.

9–Best language: A great deal of information about comprehension will be obtained during the preceding sections of the examination. The patient is asked to describe what is happening in the attached picture, to name the items on the attached naming sheet, and to read from the attached list of sentences. Comprehension is judged from responses here as well as to all of the commands in the preceding general neurological exam. If visual loss interferes with the tests, ask the patient to identify objects placed in the hand, repeat, and produce speech. The intubated patient should be asked to write. The patient in a coma (question 1a = three) will arbitrarily score three on this item. The examiner must choose a score in the patient with stupor or limited cooperation, but a score of three should be used only if the patient is mute and follows no one-step commands.

10–Dysarthria: If patient is thought to be normal, an adequate sample of speech must be obtained by asking the patient to read or repeat words from the attached list. If the patient has severe aphasia, the clarity of articulation of spontaneous speech can be rated. Only if the patient is intubated or has other physical barrier to producing speech may the item be scored "nine," and the examiner must clearly write an explanation for not scoring. Do not tell the patient why he/she is being tested.

11–Extinction and inattention (formerly Neglect): Sufficient information to identify neglect may be obtained during the prior testing. If the patient has a severe visual loss preventing visual double simultaneous stimulation, and the cutaneous stimuli are normal, the score is normal. If the patient has aphasia but does appear to attend to both sides, the score is normal. The presence of visual spatial neglect or anosognosia may also be taken as evidence of abnormality. Because the abnormality is scored only if present, the item is never untestable.

*Additional item, not a part of the NIH Stroke Scale score:

A–Distal motor function: The patient's hand is held up at the forearm by the examiner, and the patient is asked to extend his/her fingers as much as possible. If the patient can't or doesn't extend the fingers, the examiner places the fingers in full extension and observes for any flexion movement for 5 seconds. The patient's first attempts only are graded. Repetition of the instructions or of the testing is prohibited.

MODIFIED RANKIN SCALE

The Modified Rankin Scale is typically used as an outcome measure for recovering stroke patients (Fig. 24-2). The scoring of this scale is based on 6 levels of ability, ranging from "no symptoms" to "severe disability." Often, if a patient is unable to provide accurate answers (i.e., overestimates ability to perform certain tasks and activities), it is recommended that a caregiver or family member be interviewed independently.

GLASGOW OUTCOME SCALE

The GOS (Fig. 24-2) is primarily used as an indicator of outcomes following a stroke or other brain injury and should therefore be taken into consideration as one component of a complete neurological exam that includes the other stroke scales (Fig. 24-3). However, it

Modified Rankin Scale

Date of evaluation

☐☐ ☐☐ ☐☐
m m   d d   y y

Grade (0–6)

☐

Grade	Description
0	No symptoms at all.
1	No significant disability despite symptoms: able to carry out all usual duties and activities.
2	Slight disability; unable to carry out all previous activities but able to look after own affairs without assistance.
3	Moderate disability; requiring some help, but able to walk without assistance.
4	Moderate to severe disability; unable to walk without assistance, and unable to attend to own bodily needs without assistance.
5	Severe disability; bedridden, incontinent, and requiring constant nursing care.
6	Death.

Glasgow Outcome Scale

Date of evaluation

☐☐ ☐☐ ☐☐
m m   d d   y y

Grade (1–5)

☐

Grade	Description
1	Death
2	Persistent vegetative state
3	Severe disability (conscious, but disabled)
4	Moderate disability (disabled but independent)
5	Good recovery

Evaluator's Name

Evaluator's Signature   Date

FIGURE 24-2. Sample Modified Rankin Scale and Glasgow Outcome Scale (adapted from www.nih.gov).

can be useful in ascertaining physical independence in patients without neurological deficits. In patients that have not suffered any type or neurological insult, the GOS score is generally observed to be 5.

ULTRASOUND EXAMINATION

A carotid duplex ultrasound study should be performed within 30 days prior to the procedure to ascertain carotid artery disease and to determine eligibility for CAS. A carotid duplex

Modified Barthel Scale

Date of evaluation ☐☐ ☐☐ ☐☐
                    m m d d y y

Bowel control	☐	0= Incontinent (or needs to be given enema); 5= Occasional accidents (<1/week) or needs help with enema or suppository; 10= Continent; no accidents. Able to use enema or suppository, if needed.
Bladder control	☐	0= Incontinent, or catheterized and unable to manage; 5= Occasional accident (<1/day) or needs help with external device; 10= Continent; no accidents. Able to care for collecting device if used.
Grooming	☐	0= Needs help in grooming 5= Independent; can wash face, comb hair, brush teeth, shave (can manage plug if electric razor).
Toilet use	☐	0= Dependent; 5= Needs help for balance, handling, or toilet paper; 10= Independent; can get on and off, handle clothes, wipe, empty and clean bedpan.
Feeding	☐	0= Dependent; 5= Needs help; e.g., for cutting food; 10= Independent; able to put on assistive device. Eats in reasonable time.
Bathing	☐	0= Dependent; 5= Independent; able to use bath tub, shower, or take complete sponge bath without supervision.
Walking	☐	0= Dependent; 5= Unable to walk, but independent with wheelchair for 50 yards; 10= Can walk with help for 50 yards; 15= Independent for 50 yards. May use assistive devices, except for rolling walker.
Dressing	☐	0= Dependent; 5= Needs help but does at least half of task within reasonable time; 10= Independent; can tie shoes, fasten fasteners, undress.
Stairs	☐	0= Unable; 5= Needs help or supervision; 10= Independent up and down. May use assistive devices.
Chair/bed transfers	☐	0= Dependent; 5= Able to sit but needs maximum assistance to transfer; 10= Minimum assistance or supervision; 15= Independent. Can lock a wheelchair, lift footrests, get out.

TOTAL ☐

_____   _____   _____
Evaluator's Name   Evaluator's Signature   Date

FIGURE 24-3. Sample Modified Barthel Scale (adapted from www.nih.gov).

study should be performed in order to determine the vessel patency at postprocedure, 1 month, 6 months, 12 months, and yearly intervals. The purpose of this exam is to identify significant stenosis and/or occlusions in the bilateral, common, internal, and external carotid arteries, as well as to identify abnormal flow directions in the vertebral arteries. It is recommended that this ultrasound scan be performed by a vascular laboratory that is certified by the Intersocietal Commission for Accreditation of Vascular Laboratories (ICAVL).

The ultrasonic scanner should be equipped with a 4 to 7.7-MHz ultrasound transducer that is capable of two-dimensional B-mode imaging, pulse Doppler waveform analysis, and measurement of the angle between the ultrasound beam and the vessel access. In order to ensure optimal imaging, Doppler exam angles should use Doppler ultrasound beams at 60 degrees to the vessel access with angle cursor parallel to the vessel wall. The patient is normally supine on the examination table, with the head slightly extended to provide better access to the neck. A bilateral exam is recommended for all scans. The exam can be completed in 30 minutes.

Abbreviations used in ultrasound label imaging: CCA, common carotid artery; ICA, internal carotid artery; ECA, external carotid artery; P, proximal; M, mid; D, distal; PSV, peak systolic velocity; EDV, end diastolic velocity.

Recorded images should include the CCA, ICA, and ECA with pictures that show the location of the disease and/or carotid stent.

ICA must be visualized. CCA has characteristic diastolic reversal. A "thump" may be heard at the stump. The distal ICA velocity should be measured a minimum of 1 cm distal to the stent (postprocedurally).

Another means of determining severity of carotid artery stenosis (Table 24-5) is the commonly used ICA/CCA ratio. ICA/CCA ratios greater than or equal to 4.0 indicate 70% or greater degree of stenosis. Ratios less than 4.0 indicate stenosis less than 70%

$$\frac{\text{ICA}}{\text{CCA}} \text{ Ratio} = \frac{\text{Maximum PSV of DCCA, PICA, or MICA}}{\text{Maximum PSV of DCCA or MCCA}}$$

TABLE 24-5. CLASSIFICATION OF CAROTID ARTERY STENOSIS

Percent Stenosis	PSV	EDV
Normal	20–130 cm/sec	NA
Less than 50%	120–180 cm/sec	NA
50% to 79%	180–250 cm/sec	< 140 cm/sec
80% to 99%	>300 cm/sec	>140 cm/sec
Occluded (100%)	No flow	No flow

PSV, peak systolic velocity; EDV, end diastolic velocity; NA, not applicable.

INDEX

Note: Page numbers in *italics* indicate figures; "t" following a page number indicates a table.